PATHOGENESIS AND MECHANISMS OF
LIVER CELL NECROSIS

PATHOGENESIS AND MECHANISMS OF LIVER CELL NECROSIS

Edited by

D. KEPPLER

Biochemisches Institut, University of Freiburg im Breisgau

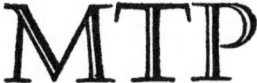

Published by
MTP Press Ltd.
St. Leonard's House,
Lancaster.

ISBN-13: 978-94-011-6620-1   e-ISBN-13: 978-94-011-6618-8
DOI: 10.1007/978-94-011-6618-8

First published 1975

Made and printed in Great Britain by
The Garden City Press Limited
Letchworth, Hertfordshire SG6 1JS

Contents

List of contributors

B. Agostini, Max-Planck-Institut für Medizinische Forschung, Abteilung Physiologie, D 69 Heidelberg, FRG

K. Aterman, Department of Pathology, Dalhousie University, Halifax, N.S. Canada, and the Julius Maximilian University of Würzburg, FRG

A. Bernelli-Zazzera, Instituto di Patologia Generale, 20133 Milano, Italy

A. Bingen, Laboratoire de Virologie de l'Université Louis Pasteur et Groupe de Recherches I.N.S.E.R.M. sur la Pathogénie des Infections Virales, 67000 Strasbourg, France

P. Czygan, Medizinische Universitätsklinik (Ludolf-Krehl-Klinik), D 69 Heidelberg, FRG

K. Decker, Biochemisches Institut der Medizinischen Fakultät, Universität Freiburg im Breisgau, D 78 Freiburg, FRG

M. U. Dianzani, Institute of General Pathology of the University of Turin, 10125 Turin, Italy

M. Elharrar, Laboratoire de Virologie de l'Université Louis Pasteur et Groupe de Recherches I.N.S.E.R.M. sur la Pathogénie des Infections Virales, 67000 Strasbourg, France

E. Farber, Fels Research Institute and Departments of Pathology and Biochemistry, Temple University School of Medicine, Philadelphia, Pennsylvania 19140, USA

H. Faulstich, Max-Planck-Institut für Medizinische Forschung, Abteilung Chemie, D 69 Heidelberg, FRG

U. Fauser, Medizinische Universitätsklinik, D 69 Heidelberg, FRG

L. Fiume, Istituto di Patologia Generale, 40126 Bologna, Italy

M. Frimmer, Institut für Pharmakologie und Toxikologie im Fachbereich Veterinärmedizin der Justus Liebig-Universität Giessen, 63 Giessen, FRG

J. L. Gendrault, Laboratoire de Virologie de l'Université Louis Pasteur et Groupe de Recherches I.N.S.E.R.M. sur la Pathogénie des Infections Virales, 67000 Strasbourg, France

J. R. Gillette, Laboratory of Chemical Pharmacology, National Heart and Lung Institute, Bethesda, Maryland 20014, USA

V. M. Govindan, Max-Planck-Institut für Medizinische Forschung, Abteilung Chemie, D 69 Heidelberg, FRG

E. Gravela, Institute of General Pathology of the University of Turin, 10125 Turin, Italy

H. Greim, Institut für Toxikologie der Universität Tübingen, D 74 Tübingen, FRG

Ch. Herfarth, Chirurgische Klinik der Universität Ulm, D 79 Ulm, FRG

W. Hoffmann, Pathologisches Institut der Universität, D 69 Heidelberg, FRG

D. Keppler, Biochemisches Institut der Medizinischen Fakultät, Universität Freiburg im Breisgau, D 78 Freiburg, FRG

A. Kirn, Laboratoire de Virologie de l'Université Louis Pasteur et Groupe de Recherches I.N.S.E.R.M. sur la Pathogénie des Infections Virales, 67000 Strasbourg, France

A. E. M. McLean, Department of Experimental Pathology, University College Hospital Medical School, London WC1, England

J. Möhr, Abteilung Medizinische Informatik, Dept. Biometrie u. Medizinische Informatik der Medizinischen Hochschule Hannover, D 3 Hannover, FRG

P. Otto, *Gastroenterologische Abteilung, Medizinische Hochschule Hannover, D 3 Hannover-Kleefeld, FRG

H. Popper, Mount Sinai School of Medicine of the City University of New York, New York NY 10029, USA

U. N. Riede, Pathologisches Institut der Universität Freiburg im Breisgau, D 78 Freiburg, FRG

W. Sandritter, Pathologisches Institut der Universität Freiburg im Breisgau, D 78 Freiburg, FRG

D. Sasse, Anatomisches Institut (III) der Universität Freiburg im Breisgau, D 78 Freiburg, FRG

A. Schafer, Max-Planck-Institut für Medizinische Forschung, Abteilung Chemie, D 69 Heidelberg, FRG

E. Schmidt, Gastroenterologische Abteilung, Medizinische Hochschule Hannover, D 3 Hannover-Kleefeld, FRG

F. W. Schmidt, Gastroenterologische Abteilung, Medizinische Hochschule Hannover, D 3 Hannover-Kleefeld, FRG

L. Schwarz, Institut für Toxikologie der Universität Tübingen, D 74 Tübingen, FRG

T. F. Slater, Biochemistry Department, Brunel University, Uxbridge, Middlesex, England

J. L. Van Lancker, Department of Pathology, UCLA Centre for Health Sciences, Los Angeles, Calif. 90024, USA

I. Vido, Gastroenterologische Abteilung, Medizinische Hochschule Hannover, D 3 Hannover-Kleefeld, FRG

Th. Wieland, Max-Planck-Institut für Medizinische Forschung, Abteilung Chemie, D 69 Heidelberg, FRG

K. Wrogemann, Department of Biochemistry, University of Manitoba, Winnipeg, Ma., Canada

G. Yüce, Department of Pathology, Dalhousie University, Halifax, N.S., Canada

Preface

The pathogenesis of cell death and necrosis in the liver is a central topic of research in liver disease. A molecular understanding of events and sequences leading to cellular death provides the basis for preventive and therapeutic efforts. This volume originates from a "Workshop on Experimental Liver Injury" held on November 9 and 10, 1974, in Freiburg, Germany. Recent progress in the elucidation of the mode of action includes agents inducing liver cell necrosis by a primary disturbance of nucleotide and nucleic acid metabolism as well as hepatotoxins characterized by a primary attack on cellular membranes. I hope that this book will contribute to an increasing understanding of disease mechanisms.

Freiburg im Breisgau   Dietrich Keppler
June 1975

Acknowledgments

The generous support from Dr. H. Falk, Freiburg, has been a prerequisite for the organisation and publication of the meeting on "Pathogenesis and Mechanisms of Liver Cell Necrosis". I wish to express my sincere thanks for this sponsorship. I am indebted to those who acted as chairmen during the meeting:
Professors H. Remmer (Tübingen), M. Frimmer (Giessen), W. Gerok (Freiburg), H. Popper (New York), H. Schimassek (Heidelberg), and K. Decker (Freiburg).
Finally, I want to express my gratitude to my wife Karin for her help and support.

CHAPTER 1

Morphology of liver cell necrosis

W. Sandritter and U. N. Riede*

Cell death frequently accompanies pathologic processes and is a constant factor in the life cycle of an individual[1]. For this reason a pathologist claims to be familiar with and understand necrosis. To our surprise we have realised that very little is known about the biochemistry of dying cells and the morphology of dying and necrotic cells[2-7].

Liver parenchymal cells which are put in a fixation solution such as formalin or glutaraldehyde immediately after death of the animal are subject to acute chemical death. Such cells are not considered necrotic since an acute cell death occurs without structural alterations. *Necrosis* is *qua definitione* an intravital cell or tissue death, which is associated with definite characteristics, i.e. death leads to secondary changes in the cell structures—'necrophanerosis'. Therefore, from the morphological point of view necrosis refers to local tissue or cell death, an intravital necrosis of cells with associated morphological characteristics. The term 'necrobiosis' is used in connection with physiological cell death or also if death of the cell occurs slowly. 'Autolysis' refers to postmortem cell changes, which take place in a similar way to intravital necrosis. *Coagulation necrosis* can be distinguished from colliquative necrosis, according to the macroscopical appearance. The term coagulation necrosis was introduced by Weigert in 1880, to describe the transformation of cells into a mass similar to coagulated fibrin, i.e. yellow, dry and solid[8]. *Colliquative necrosis* leads to liquefaction of the tissue. Caseation in tuberculosis is a special form of necrosis which occupies a bridging position between coagulation and colliquation.

The first cellular changes on the way to cell death are a so-called degenerative (in contrast to the functional) swelling of nucleus and cytoplasm. According to general opinion the failure of the sodium pump due to ATP-deficiency causes an influx of sodium and calcium, whilst

* Recipient of the DFG grant Ri 271/1

potassium is shifted into the extracellular fluids. This change in permeability can also be observed under the light microscope by staining the cell with vital dyes, e.g. eosin[2]. The dissolution of the cell connection is a further sign of membrane damage[7,9]. Cloudy swelling[10], hydropic changes or also fatty changes can appear as a sign of necrobiosis. The intensified staining affinity for eosin, due to denatured cytoplasmic proteins with release of basic groups, is one of the most certain signs of necrosis[2]. In the next step of necrosis the cytoplasmic structures and the cell margins which are visible under a light microscope disappear.

NUCLEAR CHANGES ASSOCIATED WITH NECROSIS

It is remarkable that the activity of succinic dehydrogenase remains unchanged for up to eight hours even though the mitochondria are seriously damaged[11-13]. The first change in the cell nucleus seems to be an aggregation of chromatin of the nuclear membrane[4]. This process is said to be reversible and is called *Kernwandhyperchromatose*[4]. This is one of the most sensitive indicators of cell injury[4,7] and appears even before the loss of the matrix granules of the mitochondria. Thirty minutes later the interchromatin granula aggregate. After two hours a maximum chromatin aggregation is observed, corresponding to the granular-hyperchromatic nucleus of Altmann[13]. A focal dilatation of the nuclear envelope follows[4]. Two hours later the chromatin condenses and finally appears more compact and homogeneous.

This process results in *nuclear pyknosis*[2,6]. After 8–12 hours the chromatin appears more and more blurred and during a period of up to 24 hours an almost complete loss of chromatin takes place. *Karyolysis* is often described[6,12] and is considered to be a consequence of release of the cellular (lysosomal) DNA-ase and cathepsin[3]. In other cells, after undergoing pyknosis, the nucleus and envelope may rupture (karyorrhexis)[6,12,14].

Analysing these nuclear changes with the aid of histochemistry, the reduction of membrane permeability and dissociation of the nucleoprotein lead to nuclear staining with nile blue sulphate, acridine orange and other vital stains. The increased Fast-green stainability of histones is due to the increased release of basic charge groups[15]. At the same time the HCl-lability during the Feulgen hydrolysis increases[15], while the Feulgen-DNA-values drop[17]. The hyperchromasia[18] of pyknotic cell nuclei can be explained by the condensation of the chromatin. Furthermore, it is possible to demonstrate (Figure 1.1) that pyknotic cell nuclei bind more eosin as a consequence of the release of basic groups of the histone[15].

The most serious interference with structure and function of the nucleolus is brought about by complete blockade of the transcription[19].

On the molecular level this is the common final pathway of many lethal cell injuries, e.g. after ischaemia[3-5], phalloidin intoxication[20,21]

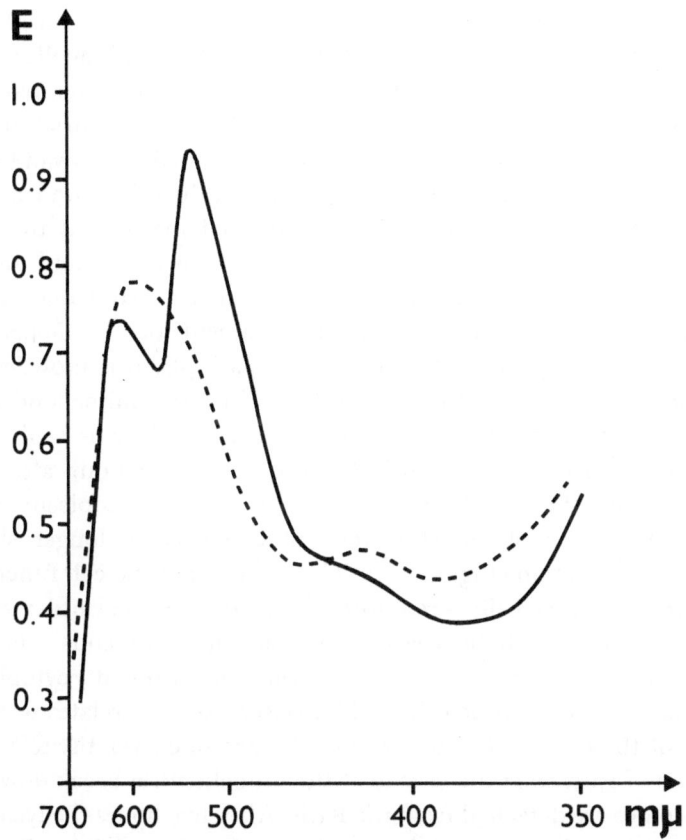

FIGURE 1.1   Spectrum of absorption of liver cell nuclei after haematoxiline-eosin staining. The necrotic (heavy line) and the normal (dotted line) liver cell nuclei show a peak at 615 mμ. This peak results from the absorption of the haematoxiline staining. The normal liver cell nuclei show a second peak at 530 μm as a result of the increased affinity to the eosin stain

and administration of antibiotics[22]. In such cases the nucleolus becomes smaller and all nucleolar components which are part of the nucleolar structure including the nucleolar-associated chromatin are separated completely. This process is called *nucleolar segregation*[13]. At the end of necrosis the various nucleolar structural components disappear.

CYTOPLASMIC CHANGES ASSOCIATED WITH NECROSIS

Having considered the nuclear changes of necrosis, let us now turn to the ultrastructural cytoplasmic changes (Table 1.1) and consider the timetable of an ischaemic necrosis[3,5,23,24]. The target organelles of the ischaemic necrosis are the mitochondria. Fifteen minutes after loss of the oxygen supply a decrease in the number of the mitochondrial grana is observed[23]. At the same time the already mentioned 'Kernwandhyperchromatose' appears. After 30 min of ischaemia the mitochondria begin to swell with partial loss of the mitochondrial matrix. At this stage blebs and disruptions of the cell membrane[9] are also found and the SER loses its typical configuration and vesiculates. After one hour of ischaemia the typical topographic arrangement of the hepatocytic mitochondria disappears[24]. Normally the ergastoplasm is crowded in a cytoplasmic region close to the nucleus, while the mitochondria are accumulated in a cytoplasmic zone close to the nucleus as well as in a middle and peripheral cell zone (Figure 1.2). One hour after total ischaemia only the membrane structure of the ergastoplasm is still found in the same place, while the mitochondria no longer show a regional accumulation (Figure 1.2). This means that the cell function— and therefore the cell life—requires a three-dimensional order system of the different metabolic spaces. This arrangement ends when the irreversibility threshold is reached with subsequent cytoplasmic homogenisation of necrotic cells[24]. This observation correlates well with changes of the electrical impedance of the necrotic liver tissue[25]. After two hours of ischaemia the cristae of the mitochondria break down and the ribosomes are detached from the RER. After five hours the lysosomal membranes are disrupted and hydrolases are released into the cytoplasm and into the extracellular space. Only after 10 hours of ischaemia are chromatolysis and disaggregation of the nucleoli observed. At this time the cell only contains cytoplasmic membrane debris[3].

Table 1.1 TIMETABLE OF THE NUCLEAR AND CYTOPLASMIC CHANGES DURING ISCHAEMIC LIVER CELL NECROSIS

Lysosomes	Nucleus	Peroxisomes	Mitochondria	Cell membrane	Endopl. reticulum	Time
	'Kernwandhyper-chromatosis'		Ischaemia Mitochondrial contraction			15 min
	Chromatin condensation		Partial loss of grana mitochondrialia			
Cytoplasmic sequestration increase in number			High amplitude swelling	Cell swelling (hydrops)		
			Matricolysis	Formation of blebs, agonal cell movement	SER vesiculation	30 min
Swelling	Aggregation of interchrom. granules	Matricolysis reduction of peroxisomal number	Loss of mitochondrial topography; total loss of grana	Membrane interruptions loss of cell contacts	Fragmentation, dilatation, reduction of RER membranes	1 hour
	Disaggregation of nucleolar material		Cristolysis	Loss of cell movement	Ribosomal detachment from the RER	2 hours
Membrane labilisation and rupture		Increase of uricase activity		Release of intracellular enzymes (CPK/SGOT etc.)		5 hours
Release of hydrolases	Karyolysis: chromatolysis, nucleolysis		Floccular ? ?			10 hours

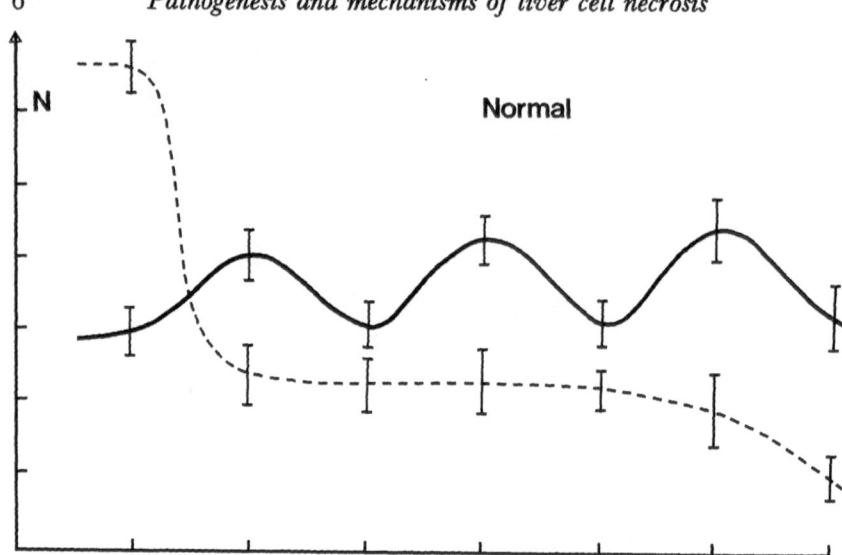

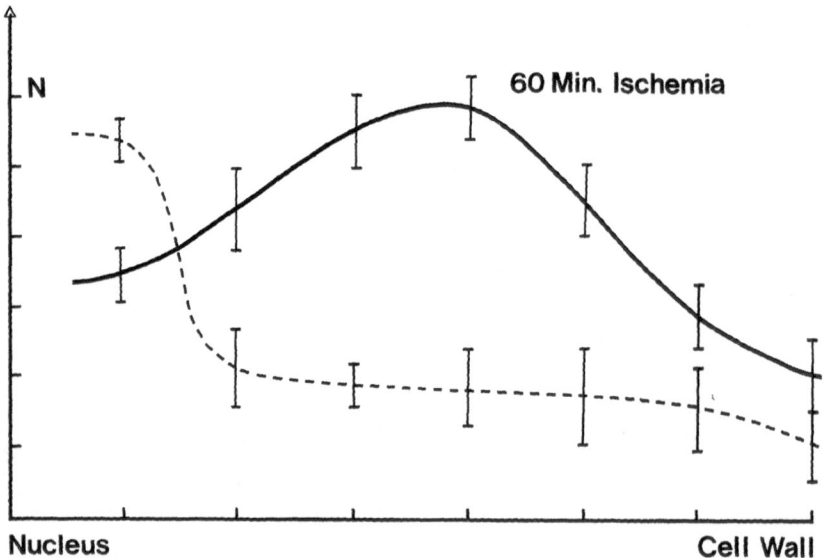

Nucleus   **Cell Wall**

FIGURE 1.2   Diagrammatic representation of the quantitative topographic distribution
of the mitochondria and the endoplasmic reticulum in the hepatocellular cytoplasm.
Normally the mitochondria (dark line) accumulate in a central (i.e. near to the nucleus),
in a middle and in a peripheral (i.e. near to the cell wall) cytoplasmic zone. The
endoplasmic reticulum (dotted line) forms a central cytoplasmic zone. In necrotic
hepatocytes after 60 min of absolute ischaemia only the membranes of the endoplasmic
reticulum are in the original area. The mitochondria seem to have a random distribution

However total liver cell necrosis occurs less frequently than *focal cytoplasmic necrosis*[26-33]. In such cases an injured and so functionless cytoplasmic region is engulfed by an ergastoplasmic cisterna[34-37]. The hydrolytic enzymes are released and break down the cisternal content (Figure 1.3). Due to the fact that such phagosomes do not include enough catabolic enzymes in comparison with the vacuolar content, for a certain time autophagocytised mitochondria can still show an intact respiratory chain[28,29]. The primary lysosomes now include additional quantities of catabolic enzymes[26]. They are moved by an intracytoplasmic transport system, the microtubules and microfibrils. Their action can be inhibited by colchicine and supported by cAMP[38,39]. Finally the lysosomal enzymes are only separated from their substrate by the lysosomal membrane. Only when the lysosomal membrane has been labilised, does a fusion of the primary lysosomes with the phagosomes as well as an exit of the catabolic enzymes into the vacuolar spaces take place[26,34].

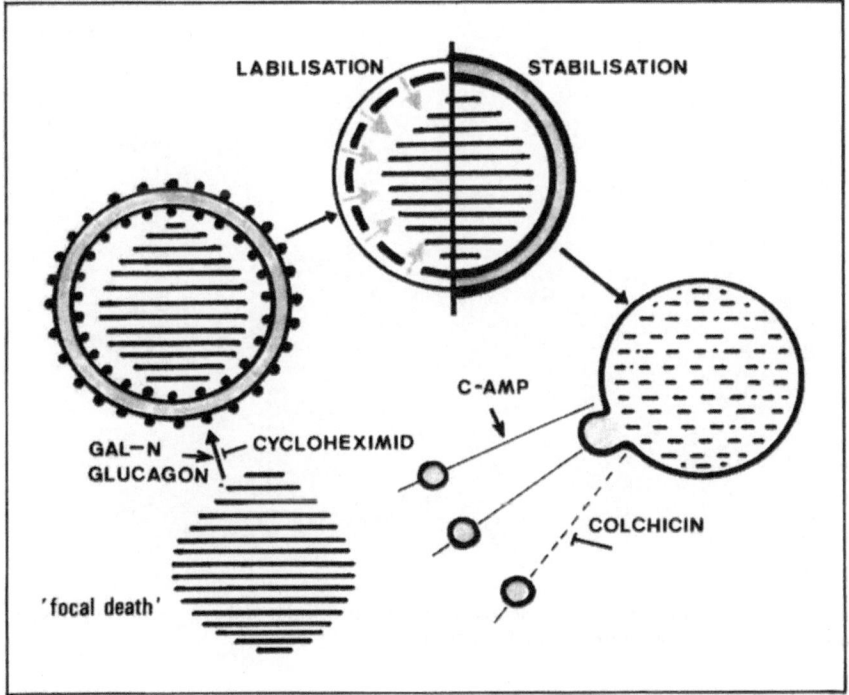

FIGURE 1.3   Diagrammatic representation of the focal cytoplasmic necrosis (autophagy)

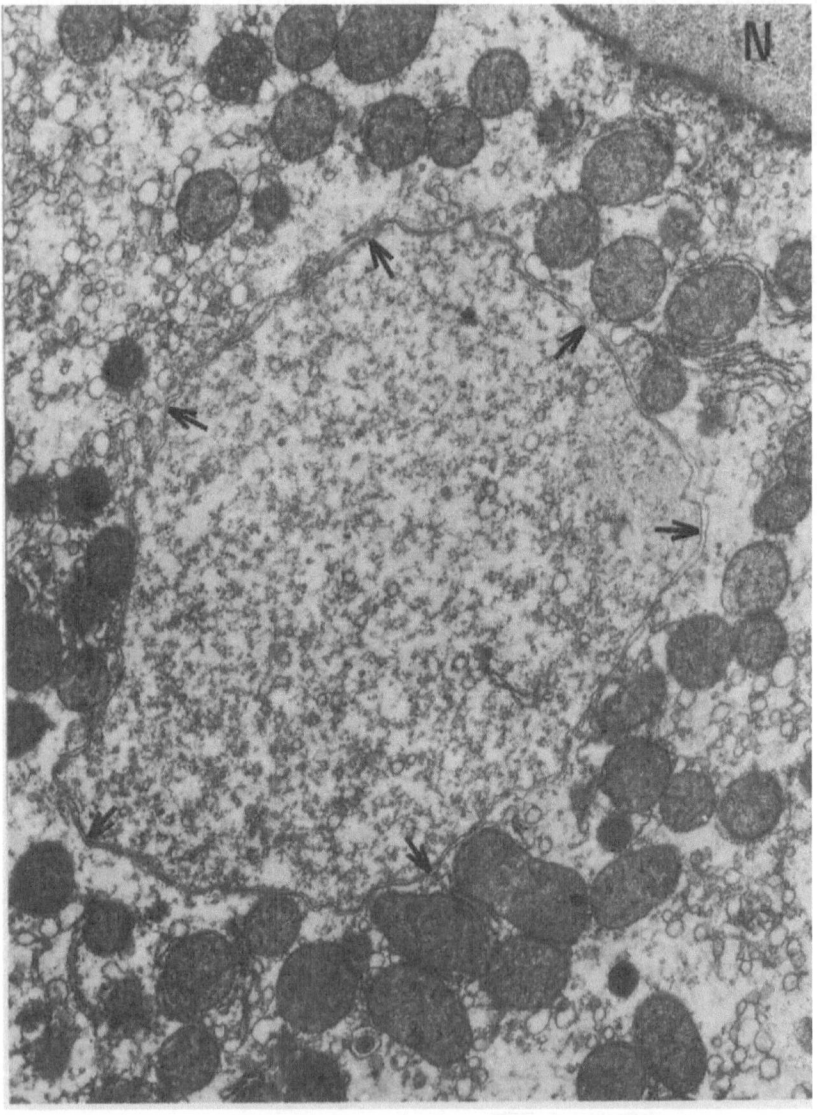

FIGURE 1.4   Giant autophagic vacuole (containing cellular debris) in rat hepatocyte one hour after absolute ischaemia ($\times$ 8000)

De Duve initially suggested that the lysosomes are 'suicide bags' of the cells[40,41]. After more than 10 years of research we know that this functional description is only correct for a few special cases[28,29]. It can hardly be presumed that all cell-damaging factors cause cell death by a direct effect on the lysosomes thus damaging the lysosomal membrane and allowing the lytic enzymes to escape into the cytoplasm. It is more likely that there are quite a number of noxious injuries which damage primary distinct cell organelles, which are afterwards sequestrated by lysosomes or lead to cell death due to their loss of function[3,7]. In this case—which is more frequent—the lysosomes can be considered as 'survival bags' for the cell[3,7]. A number of facts substantiate this belief: one hour after absolute ischaemia, giant lysosomes develop in the hepatocytes (Figure 1.4) and the volume fraction of lysosomes per hepatocyte shows a six-fold increase, compared with the controls[24]. In such cases the lysosomes probably act as 'survival bags', because the liver cell is still capable of maintaining certain partial functions for up to 10 hours in case of ischaemia[42].

This chronological process of the ischaemic liver cell necrosis is in principle valid for most of the parenchymal cells. Typical for the liver is the total organ necrosis, the acute and subacute liver dystrophy or group necrosis of the perivenous part of the liver lobule, which develops for example under oxygen deficiency. Single cell necrosis is quite often observed in viral hepatitis.

SHRINKAGE NECROSIS

A special form of single cell necrosis develops in the liver in cases with lethal cell damage after slight injurious stimulus (Figure 1.5). Deviating from the coagulation necrosis these cells shrink. Accordingly Kerr has called it shrinkage necrosis[43,44]. The first changes consist in a condensation and clumping of the cell nucleus and partly also of the cytoplasm. It is remarkable that the mitochondria remain uninjured—both structurally and probably functionally[44].

A reason for this is the fact that these cells can extrude water from the cytoplasm[43,44]. Comparing the appearance of necrobiotic cells with cells undergoing shrinkage necrosis the same process appears to be involved (Figure 1.5). The cell nucleus breaks down slowly, so that these cells appear as hyaline bodies under the light microscope. These

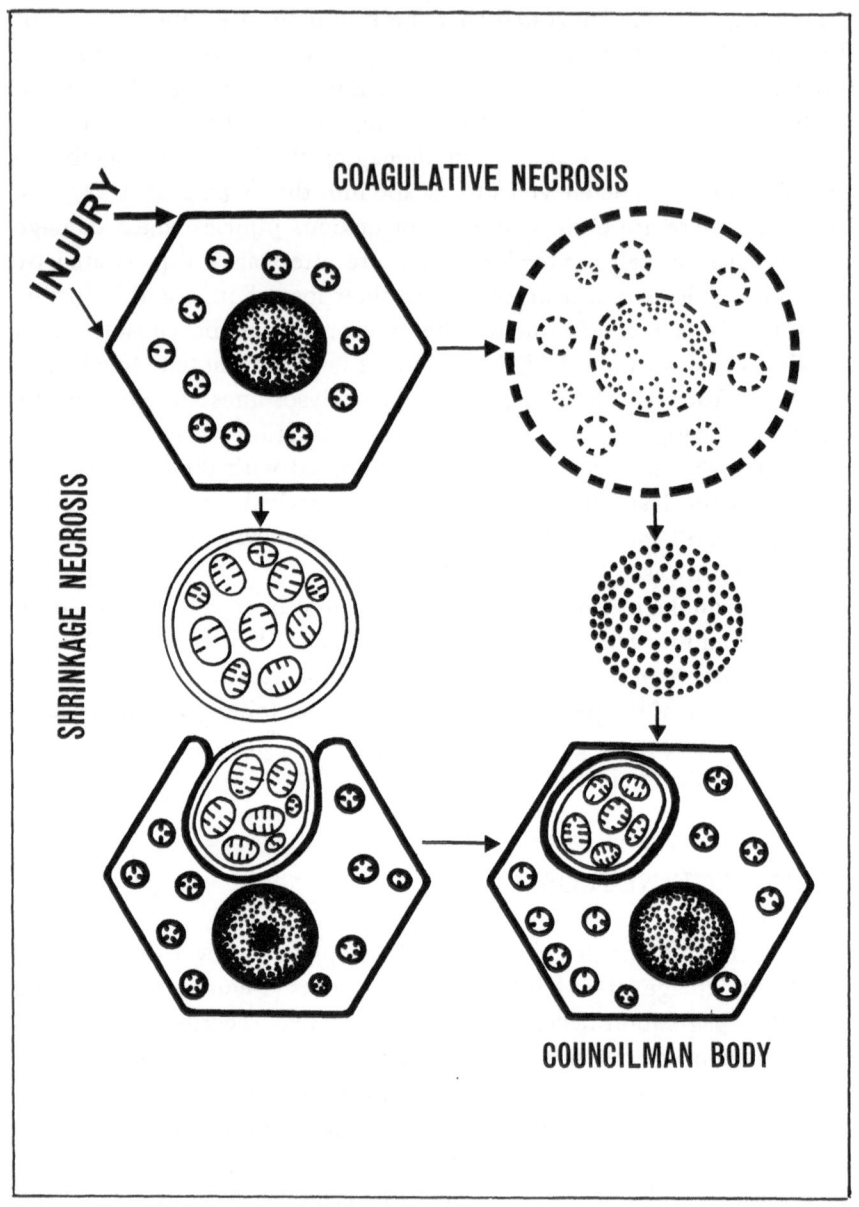

FIGURE 1.5 Diagrammatic representation of the morphogenesis of the shrinkage
necrosis and the coagulation necrosis depending on the severity of the cell injury

shrinkage-necrotic cells are later phagocytised by the surrounding hepatocytes and also by histiocytes. Under the light microscope the shrinkage-necrotic cells appear as round, denucleated and eosinophilic inclusions and are called 'Councilman bodies' (Figure 1.5). In the interior of the phagolysosomes the intracellular digestion of these Councilman bodies begins and gradually their cytoplasm appears similar to a normal coagulation necrosis[43]. The phagocytised Councilman bodies are decomposed to a homogeneous amorphous vacuolar content and finally only residual bodies are left. Light microscopically they are defined as peribiliary bodies and can be discharged into the bile capillaries (Figure 1.5) via the process of *cell defaecation*[43,44].

In single cell or also larger necrosis in the liver, the phagocytosis of the cells and regeneration probably play the most important part[6]. A formation of connective tissue can also take place and cause a cirrhosis. In other organs the usual way is the granulocytic demarcation followed by resorption. Softening, as is the case in the brain and pancreas, leaves a cavity. In tuberculosis calcification is often found.

The electron microscopist has a static view vaguely reminiscent of a Victorian family photograph, with the components frozen into formal rigidity. But we have already seen in time lapse microcinematography that the cytoplasmic and nuclear content show characteristics of living dynamism[45,46]. Shortly before cell death the cell exhibits dramatic convulsive movements and extends numerous pseudopodia. The cell then assumes a globular shape and swells. The mitochondria stop moving through the cytoplasm[48] and the cell is disrupted and dies.

The described *agonal pattern of cellular movement* is similar in many respects to that in the initial phase of mitosis[45]. Thus death and regeneration look alike.

REFERENCES

1. Starre, I. G. and Otten, L. (1974). Embryogenesis of calliphora erythrocephalea Meigen. Cell death in the central nervous system during late embryogenesis. *Cell. Tiss. Res.*, **151**, 219–228
2. Majno, G., La Guattata, M. and Thompson, T. E. (1960). Cellular death and necrosis: Chemical, physical and morphological changes in rat liver. *Virchows Arch. Pathol. Anat.*, **333**, 421–465
3. Trump, B. F., Goldblatt, P. J. and Stowell, R. E. (1965). Studies of necrosis *in vitro* of mouse hepatic parenchymal cells. Ultrastructural, and cytochemical alterations of cytosomes, cytosegresomes, multivesicular

bodies and microbodies and their relation of the lysosome concept. *Lab. Invest.*, **14**, 1946–1968

4. Trump, B. F., Goldblatt, P. J. and Stowell, R. E. (1965). Studies of mouse liver necrosis *in vitro*. Ultrastructural and cytochemical alterations in hepatic parenchymal cell nuclei. *Lab. Invest.*, **14**, 1969–1999

5. Trump, B. F., Goldblatt, P. J. and Stowell, R. E. (1965). Studies of necrosis *in vitro* of mouse hepatic parenchymal cells. Ultrastructural alterations in endoplasmic reticulum, Golgi apparatus, plasma membrane and lipid droplets. *Lab. Invest.*, **14**, 2000–2028

6. Robbins, S. L. (1974). *Pathologic Basis of Disease* (Philadelphia, London, Toronto: W. S. Saunders Co.)

7. Scarpelli, D. G. and Trump, B. F. (1974). *Cell Injury* (Kalamazoo, Michigan: Upjohn Company)

8. Weigert, C. (1880). Über die pathologischen Gerinnungsvorgänge. *Virchows Arch. Pathol. Anat.*, **79**, 87–103

9. David-Ferreira, J. F. and David-Ferreira, K. L. (1973). Gap junction-ribosome association after autolysis. *J. Cell Biol.*, **58**, 226–230

10. Zollinger, H. U. (1948). Trübe Schwellung und Mitochondrien. *Schweiz. Z. Pathol.*, **11**, 617–634

11. Goldblatt, P. J., Trump, B. F. and Stowell, R. (1965). Studies on necrosis of mouse liver *in vitro*. Alterations in some histochemically demonstrable enzymes. *Amer. J. Pathol.*, **47**, 183–207

12. Latta, H., Osvaldo, L., Jackson, J. D. and Cook, M. L. (1965). Changes in renal cortical tubules during autolysis. *Lab. Invest.*, **14**, 635–657

13. Altmann, H. W. and Müller, H. A. (1974). Grundlagen der Karyologie. In: *Angewandte Zytologie und ihre Grundlagen*, 2–31 (G. Seifert, editor) (Stuttgart: Gustav Fischer Verlag)

14. Altmann, H. W. and Bannasch, P. (1966). Die intravitale Karyorrhexis der exokrinen Pankreaszellan im elektronenmikroskopischen. *Bild. Z. Zellforsch.*, **71**, 53–68

15. Noeske, K. and Ebner, H. (1965). Zum Problem der Hyperchromasie. *Verh. Dtsch. Ges. Pathol.*, **49**, 327–330

16. Krygier-Stojalowska, A. (1974). Personal communication

17. Leuchtenberger, C. (1950). A cytochemical study of pycnotic nuclear degeneration. *Chromosoma*, **3**, 449–473

18. Klebs, M. (1889). *Die Allgemeine Pathologie*, **Vol. 2** (Jena: Fischer-Verlag)

19. Simard, R. and Bernhard, W. (1966). Le phenomen de la segregation nucleolaire. *Int. J. Cancer*, **1**, 463–482

20. Marinozzi, V. and Fiume, L. (1971). Effects of α-amanitin on mouse and rat liver cell nuclei. *Exp. Cell Res.*, **67**, 311–345

21. Fiume, L., Marinozzi, V. and Nardi, F. (1969). The effects of amanitin poisoning on mouse kidneys. *Brit. J. Exp. Pathol.*, **50**, 270–298

22. Perry, R. P. (1963). Selective effects of actinomycin D on the intracellular distribution of RNA synthesis in tissue culture cells. *Exp. Cell Res.*, **29**, 400–427

23. Trump, B. F., Goldblatt, P. J. and Stowell, R. E. (1965). Studies on necrosis of mouse liver *in vitro*. Ultrastructural alterations in the mitochondria of hepatic parenchymal cells. *Lab. Invest.*, **14**, 343–371
24. Sandritter, W., Riede, U. N. (1974). Unpublished data
25. Pliquett, F., Krug, H., Cossel, L. and Förster, W. (1974). Comparative passive electrical light and electron microscopical investigations on the model of autolysis of the liver tissue. *Acta Histochem*, **49**, 106–122
26. Novikoff, A. B. (1964). GERL, its form and function in neurons of rat spinal ganglia. *Biol. Bull.*, **127**, 358–365
27. Riede, U. N., Seebass, C. and Rohr, H. P. (1971). Ultrastrukturell-morphometrische Untersuchungen an der Leberparenchymzelle der Ratte nach Hemmung der Proteinsynthese durch Cycloheximid. *Virchows Arch. Abt. B. Zellpath.*, **9**, 16–27
28. Arstila, A. U., Shelburne, J. D. and B. F. Trump (1972). Studies on cellular autophagocytosis. A histochemical study on sequential alterations of mitochondria in the glucagon induced autophagic vacuoles of rat liver. *Lab. Invest.*, **27**, 317–323
29. Shelburne, J. D., Arstila, A. U. and Trump, B. F. (1973). Studies on cellular autophagocytosis. *Amer. J. Pathol.*, **72**, 521–540
30. Rohr, H. P., Brunner, H. R., Rasser, Y. M., Von Matt, C. A. and Riede, U. N. (1973). Einfluß des Hungers auf die quantitative Cytoarchitektur der Rattenleberzelle. I. Absoluter Hunger und Wiederauffütterung. *Beitr. Pathol.*, **149**, 347–362
31. Riede, U. N., Hodel, J., Von Matt, C. A., Rasser, Y. and Rohr, H. P. (1973). Einfluß des Hungers auf die quantitative Cytoarchitektur der Rattenleberzelle. II. Chronischpartieller Hunger. *Beitr. Pathol.*, **150**, 246–260
32. Riede, U. N., Rasser, Y. M. and Rohr, H. P. (1974). Influence of lead-overload on the quantitative cytoarchitecture of juvenile rat hepatocytes. *Beitr. Pathol.*, **152**, 383–394
33. Riede, U. N., Kreutzer, W., Robausch, T., Kiefer, G. and Sandritter, W. (1974). Influence of partial exsiccosis on the quantitative cytoarchitecture of rat hepatocytes. *Beitr. Pathol.*, **153**, 379–394
34. Arstila, A. U. and Trump, B. F. (1969). Autophagocytosis: origin of membranes and hydrolytic enzymes. *Virchows Arch. Abt. B. Zellpath.*, **2**, 85–90
35. Helminen, H. J. and Ericsson, J. L. E. (1972). Ultrastructural studies on prostatic involution in the rat. Evidence for focal irreversible damage to epithelium and heterophagic digestion in macrophages. *J. Ultrastruct. Res.*, **39**, 443–455
36. Lockshin, R. A. and Beaulaton, J. (1974). Programmed cell death. *J. Ultrastruct. Res.*, **46**, 43–62
37. Nevalainen, T. J. and Janigan, D. T. (1974). Degeneration of mouse pancreatic acinar cells during fasting. *Virchows Arch. Abt. B. Zellpath.*, **15**, 107–118
39. Seiden, D. (1973). Effects of colchicine on myofilament arrangement

and the lysosomal system in skeletal muscle. *Z. Zellforsch.*, **144**, 467–473

40. De Duve, Ch. (1963). The lysosome. *Sci. Amer.*, **208**, 64–78
41. De Duve, Ch. and Wattiaux, R. (1966). Functions of lysosomes. *Ann. Rev. Physiol.*, **28**, 435–492
42. Nunley, W. C., Schuit, K. E., Dickie, M. W. and Kinlaw, J. B. (1972). Delayed, *in vitro* hepatic post mortem autolysis. *Virchows Arch. Abt. B. Zellpath.*, **11**, 289–302
43. Kerr, J. F. R. (1971). Shrinkage necrosis: a distinct mode of cellular death. *J. Pathol.*, **105**, 13–20
44. Kerr, J. F. R. (1974). Some lysosome functions in liver cells reacting to sublethal injury. In: *Lysosomes in Biology and Pathology*, 364–394 (J. T. Dingle, editor) (Amsterdam, London: North-Holland Publ. Co.)
45. Sandritter, W. (1965). Unpublished data
46. Chayen, J. and Bitensky, L. (1973). Cell injury. In: *Cell Biology in Medicine*, 595–680 (E. E. Bittar, editor) (New York, London, Sydney, Toronto: John Wiley & Sons)

CHAPTER 2

Morphologic features of hepatocellular necrosis in human disease

H. POPPER

Necrosis of the hepatocytes, as a rule associated with disappearance of cells or their breakdown products, is usually accompanied by an inflammatory reaction composed of macrophages, lymphocytes and occasionally, neutrophilic and eosinophilic granulocytes; particularly with single cell necrosis this is histologically more conspicuous than the loss of the hepatocytes[1]. In the following discussion the topographic localisation and size of the necrosis is correlated with its functional significance and various aetiologic examples of necrosis are discussed with some emphasis on the features of cholestatic necrosis to provide a basis for the subsequent discussion on the mechanism of necrosis induced by hepatotoxic bile acids by Greim *et al.* (Chapter 18).

DISTRIBUTION OF NECROSIS

Necrosis may involve single or very small groups of cells and is usually initiated by injury to the cell membrane. If the formation of blebs is followed by their rupture, the cell content is expelled into the surrounding fluid and the cell outline is no more visible; therefore this *focal necrosis* is better recognised by the accumulation of inflammatory cells replacing the necrotic hepatocytes. It is not always easy to separate this cytolytic form of necrosis from an accumulation of inflammatory cells in sinusoids and tissue spaces without necrosis. In other instances the injury of the cell membrane leads to loss of the cell water with persistence of the necrotic cells containing pyknotic or no nuclei. These acidophilic bodies are expelled into the tissue space where they become victims of phagocytosis by macrophages.

Focal necrosis associated with accumulation of neutrophilic granulocytes while the rest of the hepatocytes appear normal, may occur as a
result of injury to the liver due to an operation[2]. Under these circumstances even large numbers of such focal necroses spread throughout the
parenchyma are not accompanied by a significant loss of liver function.
This indicates that the integrity of the surrounding parenchyma com-
pensates for the loss of the hepatocytes. By contrast, in any form of
hepatitis in which focal necrosis is associated with alterations of the
surrounding viable hepatocytes, a more or less severe deficiency of
hepatic function can be demonstrated. This deficit is thus the result of a
hardly recognisable injury (as seen under a light microscope) to the
viable and surviving hepatocytes. The damage of their organelles is
readily recognised by electron microscopy. Since animal experiments
have indicated that removal of a considerable amount of the liver need
not be associated with a conspicuous functional deficit, the loss of
hepatocytes alters liver function significantly in extensive necrosis only.

These considerations also hold true for *zonal necrosis* which may be
either centrolobular, and far less frequently in the intermediate zone, or
around the portal tracts. As a rule the lost hepatocytes are replaced by
regeneration with the exception of sustained exposure to the offending
agent, persisting local inflammation, nutritional deficiency, anaemia, or
old age.

Necrosis connecting bridge-like central and portal canals, designated
as subacute hepatic necrosis[3], is significant from the point of view of
prognosis as well as of evolution. If found in biopsy specimens, for
instance in viral hepatitis, the possibility of progression to massive
necrosis has to be entertained. Even more important is the fact that this
bridging necrosis may, after collapse of the necrotic area, result in a
persisting bridging septum which disturbs hepatic circulation by
permitting bypass of blood from the portal tracts to the central zone,
escaping exposure to hepatocytes. Sustained inflammation in the area
of this bridging septum in viral hepatitis may lead to a chronic active
hepatitis potentially proceeding to cirrhosis. In alcoholic liver injury
such a connection of the originally centrolobular injury in form of
central hyaline necrosis and sclerosis with the portal tracts results in a pull
between both areas as the first step in the transition from alcoholic
hepatitis to cirrhosis[4]. Thus, alcoholic and viral hepatitis-induced liver
injury cause similar architectural deformities despite great differences in
cytologic features. This is one of the reasons why the end stage of

cirrhosis need not reflect the aetiology, particularly if the initiating hepatitis has disappeared. The question why the bridging necrosis develops in a given area of the parenchyma and not in others is related to the concept of the structural unit of the liver. Some investigators wish to replace the widely used concept of the lobule with its centre around the efferent veins by the acinar concept well-developed by Rappaport[5]. These acini are conceived to exist with the portal structures as their centre and the efferent veins on their periphery. This concept postulates that the oxygen tension decreases towards the periphery of the acini and since the acinar borders extend throughout the lobule, the bridging necrosis developing in the areas of lowest oxygen tension, traverses the lobular parenchyma. Recently Oomen[6] has offered a different—a columnar—concept based on the presence within the lobular or acinar parenchyma of terminal afferent and efferent vessels demonstrated by injection preparations[7]. This concept is particularly useful in understanding the selection of the planes of bridging necrosis.

Massive necrosis designates both in viral but also in alcoholic liver injury[4] the loss of all liver cells in one contiguous lobule with resulting massive collapse or submassive collapse if irregular islands of parenchyma persist. Massive necrosis may involve only a small portion of the lobule and then it may give some prognostic indication as to progression[8], but it does not by itself significantly reduce hepatic function. With extensive massive collapse throughout the liver, characteristic for fulminant or acute massive necrotic hepatitis, sufficient parenchyma is destroyed to conspicuously diminish function and sometimes, especially in the fulminant form, to cause rapid demise of the patient. The prognosis in survivors as in all forms of necrosis, depends on the evolution of the inflammation, mainly reactive to the necrosis, rather than on the necrosis itself, particularly since survivors may recover perfect health after massive necrosis[9].

AETIOLOGIC CHARACTERISTICS OF HEPATIC NECROSIS

Although the responses of an organ as homogenous as the liver to injurious agents are limited, sufficient variations exist to tentatively point to an aetiologic factor. For instance, bacterial infections may be associated with focal necrosis with predominant accumulation of neutrophilic granulocytes which sometimes resembles the lesion in acute surgical injury. By contrast, in viral hepatitis the inflammatory cells in focal necrosis are mononuclear macrophages and lymphocytes. But this type of focal necrosis is not diagnostic of the disease even if associated with acidophilic bodies which are frequent in viral hepatitis. Fine structural alterations of the non-necrotic hepatocytes seen by electron microscopy[10] add some diagnostic significance. The early lesion is a shattering of the rough endoplasmic reticulum and detachment of the polysomes, with reduction of the latter in later stages. Initially this reflects the decreased secretion of proteins formed by hepatocytes such as albumin and coagulation proteins and subsequently reduced synthesis of structural hepatic proteins in addition. Some drug-induced hepatic reactions differ only slightly from viral hepatitis under the light microscope, e.g. the rare halothane-induced hepatitis. Electron microscopically though, mitochondrial injury here is characteristic[11]. This, however, does not hold true for all drug-induced hepatitides resembling viral hepatitis. For instance, the electron microscopic picture in the methyl dopa-induced reaction does not differ from that of viral hepatitis in which the endoplasmic reticulum is first altered.

These non-predictable types of hepatic drug injuries[12] are explained either by an immunologic reaction or by a peculiar, perhaps genetically or environmentally determined unusual constellation of enzymatic reactions in the hepatocytes and sometimes by both unusual immunologic and enzymatic reactions. In contrast, the predictable drug or chemical-induced injury, e.g. by carbon tetrachloride, represents a typical laboratory model of liver injury. The morphologic features are identical in the rare instances of similar human diseases, for instance as a result of poisons. A type of human intoxication which is rare but predictable is the tetracycline-induced liver injury which develops if persons with impaired renal function are given large intravenous doses of tetracycline resulting in high blood levels of the antibiotic[13]. A diffuse steatosis of the liver characterised by abundance of small fat droplets within the cytoplasm is in contrast to the common forms of extensive hepatic steatosis in that the nuclei are not dislodged from the centre of the cell and the presence of small fat droplets accentuates the cell membrane so that the hepatocytes resemble plant cells. This lesion is associated with cholestasis as well as necrosis. This cell loss accounts for the lack of hepatomegaly otherwise characteristic of fatty liver. The pathogenesis, as demonstrated in animal experiments[14], is inhibition of the formation of the apolipoprotein or of its combination with triglycerides, reducing hepatic secretion of very low density lipoproteins. The pernicious steatosis of pregnancy is morphologically the same lesion, also with a similar unfavourable clinical course. Its pathogenesis is not established. The tendency to this process might explain the greater susceptibility of pregnant women to the tetracycline steatosis if they receive large doses for pyelonephritis.

Alcoholic liver injury at least in the initial stage is characterised by degeneration and necrosis of hepatocytes in the lobular centre, associated with parenchymal accumulation of neutrophilic granulocytes. Cytoplasmic off-coloured irregular material designated as alcoholic hyalin of Mallory is a hallmark. Electron microscopically it is fine fibrillar, initially not surrounded by a membrane[15] and undergoes a characteristic evolution[16,17]. Originally it was associated with alterations of various hepatocytic organelles. It is now realised that it represents newly-formed material of unknown origin, related by some investigators to microfilaments. It does not indicate unavoidable death of the cell, particularly since cells containing hyalin may be in mitosis. The basic defect in alcoholic liver injury and possibly the one accounting for the cell necrosis is localised in the mitochondria, which show a series of changes, albeit non-specific, but apparently in greater amount than in other conditions, including breaks of their membranes. This morphological defect is supported by chemically demonstrated alterations of mitochondria[18].

Alcoholic hyalin by itself is by no means characteristic of alcoholic liver injury. It is highly indicative of it if found in centrolobular location[19] although it has also been demonstrated there in the liver injury following intestinal bypass operation for intractable obesity[20] and in rare cases of what has been called fatty-liver hepatitis in obese women. Such hyalin is also found in primary hepatic carcinoma[21] and in the lobular periphery in prolonged cholestasis and particularly in primary biliary cirrhosis[19]. Moreover, it is seen in necrotising stages of cirrhosis of any aetiology, but is frequent in Indian childhood cirrhosis and the acute stage of Wilson's disease[22], where rapid deterioration of liver function is accompanied by accumulation of very large amounts of this hyalin in hepatocytes near the septa around which new formation of fibres is conspicuous. This points to the hyalin-containing hepatocytes as a feature favouring cirrhosis formation.

Another intracellular deposit seemingly important in fibrogenesis is the PAS positive hepatocytic globule containing alpha-l-antitrypsin in genetic alpha-1-antitrypsin deficiency[23]. A demonstrated deficiency in sialyltransferase[24] may account for a defect in the normal secretion of this enzyme into the serum. That it is an inhibitor of collagenase[25] may be the hypothetical reason of the unusually dense fibrosis, mainly in the centre of the septa characteristic for this type of cirrhosis.

The fact that oxygen deficiency causes hepatic necrosis need not be further considered. Hepatic breakdown products persist for a long time and account for the eosinophilic necrosis associated with faulty nuclear staining which characterises the anoxic type of necrosis. The long persistence of the cells may be explained by suppressed phagocytic action by the oxygen deficiency and also by the usually inhibited circulation. The pathogenesis is obvious with interrupted or markedly reduced blood flow as seen after obstruction of the hepatic artery, or from disturbance of the microcirculation by fibrin thrombi, or in shock. In passive congestion brought about by cardiac failure or in diseases of the hepatic veins, the anoxia is complicated by increased intrasinusoidal pressure. Disturbance of the microcirculation with anoxic necrosis is, however, also an important element in cirrhosis when it results from the disturbance of the effective parenchymal blood flow, particularly when it is aggravated by gastrointestinal haemorrhage or shock. Eosinophilic type of necrosis is also found in some viral diseases caused by a virus other than the hepatitis virus[26]. It remains to be established whether disturbance of microcirculation or direct toxic effects cause this lesion.

HEPATIC NECROSIS FROM CHOLESTASIS

Hepatocellular necrosis develops in cholestasis more effectively in the mechanically produced obstructive type than in the metabolically induced intrahepatic forms. While evidence can be listed for a toxic effect of intracellularly retained bilirubin in brain cells and even in cultured liver cells, the main toxic agents are bile acids, the detergent function of which is well-established[27]. Morphologically[28], the initial light microscopic lesion is a loss of cytoplasm, with persistent yellow stained strands. This lesion is designated as feathery degeneration[29] and involves isolated cells in the lobular centre. Electron microscopically the hepatocytes have vesicles of various sizes containing whorl-like deposits of phospholipids. Moreover, there is evidence of mitochondrial injury reflected in curling of their cristae and biochemically, in uncoupling of the oxidative phosphorylation[30]. The main target, however, is the endoplasmic reticulum, both rough and smooth, with the smooth endoplasmic reticulum seemingly increased, also in cells without feathery degeneration[31]. The increased smooth endoplasmic reticulum is recognised under the light microscope by a ground glass appearance of the cytoplasm similar to the induction cells found after administration of drugs[32]. However, as Dr Greim will point out in Chapter 18, the increased endoplasmic reticulum is hypoactive in its enzymatic function although recent evidence suggests that phenobarbital treatment of rats with ligated bile ducts may restore at least initially the reduced microsomal enzyme activity[33]. Necrosis of the cells with feathery degeneration elicits intralobular foci of inflammation which is the result of the cholestasis and not of an independent hepatitis, from which it can be distinguished by its centrolobular localisation[28]. Intralobular inflammation is followed by portal inflammation which is found in all types of prolonged cholestasis, mechanical or metabolic, and only somewhat subdued in the steroid induced form. The portal inflammation is accompanied by proliferation and alteration of bile ductules with irregular epithelial lining. This differs from the tortuosity of pre-existing bile ducts or ductules which are usually close to the border of the portal tracts, and this strongly suggests mechanically-induced cholestasis[34]. The ductular reaction, electron microscopically characterised by conspicuous pinocytosis, has been designated as cholangiolitis and was previously considered the cause of intrahepatic cholestasis, induced by drugs for instance, when obstruction of bile ducts and liver cell injury cannot be demonstrated. By contrast, it is now assumed that the cholangiolitis is the result rather than the cause of the cholestasis. Nevertheless, the inflammation progressing to periductular fibrosis eventually produces in any type of cholestasis an intrahepatic mechanical component by compression and destruction of bile ductular channels. This peripheral cholestasis is irregularly distributed throughout the liver, but where it is present it involves uniformly all hepatocytes bordering on the portal tracts and septa. They show the same feathery degeneration as the scattered cells in centrolobular cholestasis. Progressing fibrosis may eventually lead to the biliary cirrhosis of secondary or obstructive type. The same picture is also found in late stages of primary biliary cirrhosis following septal bile duct destruction.

Under the light microscope features resembling feathery degeneration in peripheral cholestasis may also be seen in the absence of hyper-bilirubinaemia and of deposition of bile pigmented material in these or other cells. The lesion resembles also the feathery degeneration electron microscopically in that the cells contain the described vacuoles with phospholipid whorls. It is assumed but not yet proven, that this represents the effect of intracellular retention of bile acids in the absence of bilirubin and the lesion has tentatively been designated as 'cholate stasis'[35] as found, for instance, in anicteric stages of chronic active hepatitis. Under these circumstances the cells seem to favour fibrosis.

CONCLUSION

Hepatocellular necrosis can be classified morphologically by its distribution as well as by its aetiology. Except in extensive massive necrosis, the functional deficit is explained by the damage of the organelles in the surviving cells. Morphologic features more often distinguish groups of aetiologic factors than single ones, particularly because of the limited number of hepatocellular reactions to injury. Moreover, cell membrane defect is a common terminal pathway in almost all types of necrosis.

REFERENCES

1. Popper, H. (1971). The problem of hepatitis. *Amer. J. Gastroenterol.*, **55**, 335–346
2. Christoffersen, P., Poulsen, H. and Skeie, E. (1970). Focal liver cell necrosis accompanied by infiltration by granulocytes arising during operation. *Acta Hepatosplen.*, **17**, 240–245
3. Boyer, J. L. and Klatskin, G. (1970). Patterns of necrosis in acute viral hepatitis: prognostic value of bridging (subacute hepatic necrosis). *New Engl. J. Med.*, **283**, 1063–1071
4. Gerber, M. A. and Popper, H. (1972). Relation between central canals and portal tracts in alcoholic hepatitis. A contribution to the pathogenesis of cirrhosis in alcoholics. *Human Pathol.*, **3**, 163–166
5. Rappaport, A. M. and Hiraki, G. Y. (1958). Histopathologic changes in the structural and functional unit of the human liver. *Acta Anat.*, **32**, 240–255
6. Oomen, H. A. P. C. (1974). *The Liver Model in the Evaluation of Liver Biopsies* (University of Amsterdam: M.D. Thesis)
7. Takahashi, T. (1970). Lobular structures of the human liver from the

viewpoint of hepatic vascular architecture. *Tohoku J. Exp. Med.*, **101**, 119–140

8. Baggenstoss, A. H., Summerskill, W. H. J. and Ammon, H. V. (1974). The morphology of chronic hepatitis. In: *The Liver and Its Diseases*, 199–206 (F. Schaffner, S. Sherlock and C. M. Leevy, editors) (New York: Intercontinental Medical Book Corp.)

9. Karvountzis, G., Redeker, A. G. and Peters, R. L. (1974). Long term follow-up studies of patients surviving fulminant viral hepatitis. *Gastroenterology*, **67**, 870–877

10. Schaffner, F. (1970). The structural basis of altered hepatic function in viral hepatitis. *Amer. J. Med.*, **49**, 658–668

11. Klion, F. M., Schaffner, F. and Popper, H. (1969). Hepatitis after exposure to halothane. *Ann. Int. Med.*, **71**, 467–477

12. Popper, H. (1973). Drug-induced liver injury. In: *The Liver*, 182–198 (E. A. Gall and F. K. Mostofi, editors) (Baltimore: Williams and Wilkins Co.)

13. Combes, B., Whalley, P. J. and Adams, R. H. (1972). Tetracycline and the liver. In: *Progress in Liver Diseases*, **Vol. IV**, 589–596 (H. Popper and F. Schaffner, editors) (New York: Grune and Stratton)

14. Hansen, C. H., Pearson, L. H., Schenker, S. and Combes, B. (1968). Impaired secretion of triglycerides by the liver; a cause of tetracycline-induced fatty liver. *Proc. Soc. Exp. Biol. Med.*, **128**, 143–146

15. Schaffner, F. and Popper, H. (1970). Alcoholic hepatitis in the spectrum of ethanol-induced liver injury. *Scand. J. Gastroenterol.*, **Suppl. 7**, 69–78

16. Yokoo, H., Minick, O. T., Batti, F. and Kent, G. (1972). Morphologic variants of alcoholic hyalin. *Amer. J. Pathol.*, **69**, 25–40

17. Wiggers, K. D., French, S. W., French, B. A. and Carr, B. N. (1973). The ultrastructure of Mallory body filaments. *Lab. Invest.*, **29**, 652–658

18. Rubin, E. and Lieber, C. S. (1974). The effects of alcohol on the human liver. In: *The Liver and Its Diseases*, 236–244 (F. Schaffner, S. Sherlock and C. M. Leevy, editors) (New York: Intercontinental Medical Book Corp.)

19. Gerber, M. A., Orr, W., Denk, H., Schaffner, F. and Popper, H. (1973). Hepatocellular hyalin in cholestasis and cirrhosis: Its diagnostic significance. *Gastroenterology*, **64**, 89–98

20. Peters, R. L. and Reynolds, T. B. (1973). Hepatic changes simulating alcoholic liver disease post ileo-jejunal bypass. *Gastroenterology*, **65**, 564

21. Keely, A. F., Iseri, O. A. and Gottlieb, L. S. (1973). Ultrastructure of hyaline cytoplasmic inclusions in a human hepatoma: relationship to Mallory's alcoholic hyalin. *Gastroenterology*, **62**, 280–293

22. Sternlieb, I. and Scheinberg, H. (1974). Wilson's disease. In: *The Liver and Its Diseases*, 328–336 (F. Schaffner, S. Sherlock and C. M. Leevy, editors) (New York: Intercontinental Medical Book Corp.)

23. Ishak, K. G., Jenis, E. H., Marshall, M. L., Bolton, B. H. and Battistone, G. C. (1972). Cirrhosis of the liver associated with α-1-antitrypsin deficiency. *Arch. Pathol.*, **94**, 445–455

24. Kuhlenschmidt, M. S., Yunis, E. J., Iammarino, R. M., Turco, S. J., Peters, S. P. and Glew, R. H. (1974). Demonstration of sialyltransferase deficiency in the serum of a patient with α-1-antitrypsin deficiency and hepatic cirrhosis. *Lab. Invest.*, **31**, 413–419

25. Harris, E. D., Jr and Krane, S. M. (1974). Collagenases (first of three parts). *New Engl. J. Med.*, **291**, 557–563

26. Bechtelsheimer, H., Korb, G. and Gedigk, P. (1972). The morphology and pathogenesis of 'marburg virus' hepatitis. *Human Pathol.*, **3**, 255–264

27. Denk, H., Schenkman, J. B., Bacchin, P. G., Hutterer, F., Schaffner, F. and Popper, H. (1971). Mechanism of cholestasis. III. Interaction of synthetic detergents with the microsomal cytochrome P-450 dependent biotransformation system *in vitro*. A comparison between the effects of detergents, the effects of bile acids, and the findings in bile duct ligated rats. *Exp. Molec. Pathol.*, **14**, 263–276

28. Popper, H. and Schaffner, F. (1970). Pathophysiology of cholestasis. *Human Pathol.*, **1**, 1–24

29. Gall, E. A. and Dabrogorki, O. (1964). Hepatic alterations in obstructive jaundice. *Amer. J. Clin. Pathol.*, **41**, 126–139

30. Schersten, T. (1972). Metabolic differences between hepatitis and cholestasis in human liver. *Progress in Liver Diseases*, **Vol. IV**, 133–150 (H. Popper and F. Schaffner, editors) (New York: Grune and Stratton)

31. Schaffner, F., Bacchin, P. G., Hutterer, F., Scharnbeck, H. H., Sarkozi, L. L., Denk, H. and Popper, H. (1971). Mechanism of cholestasis. 4. Structural and biochemical changes in the liver and serum in rats after bile duct ligation. *Gastroenterology*, **60**, 888–897

32. Klinge, O. and Bannasch, P. (1968). Zur Vermehrung des Glatten Endoplasmatischen Reticulum in Hepatocyten Menschlicher Leberpunktate. *Verhandl Dtsch. Ges. T. Pathol.*, 568–573

33. Solymoss, B. and Zsigmond, G. (1974). Effect of microsomal enzyme inducers on the liver changes produced by common bile duct ligature. *Proc. Soc. Exp. Biol. Med.*, **147**, 430–433

34. Christoffersen, P. and Poulsen, H. (1970). Histological changes in human liver biopsies following extrahepatic biliary obstruction. *Acta Pathol. Microbiol. Scand.*, **Suppl. 212**, 150–157

35. Popper, H. (1970). Morphological and immunological studies on chronic aggressive hepatitis and primary biliary cirrhosis. In: *Immunology of the Liver*, 17–27 (M. Smith and R. Williams, editors) (London: William Heinemann Medical Books Limited)

CHAPTER 3

Hydrolases and cellular death

J. L. VAN LANCKER

INTRODUCTION

Because of the fear of one's own death, or because of the grief suffered by those who remain alive, the quick and the dead are at antipoles in the minds of man. Yet, life and death continuously interreact in the living world. In these times when food comes in cans or plastic bags with colours, shapes and sometimes tastes far removed from the original product, it is easy to forget that man kills the cows who eat the grass in the green pasture, or that the salmon swim upstream to the Kodiak shallow lakes to spawn and ultimately become the prey of bears, eagles and foxes. Animal life thrives on other forms of life.

Even the harmony of the individual living organism depends on the delicate balance between cellular proliferation and cellular death. To live we must die a little all the time.

It is likely that most cells, even those with long life spans, partially die either as a result of turnover of cellular organelles, or of discrete macromolecular destruction.

Because of this unexpected, but indissoluble marriage between life and death, the cells which have, since Virchow, become the unit of life and the target of injury can only preserve their harmony by delicately balancing anabolism and catabolism.

Such balance can be maintained in at least two ways: (1) A delicate regulation of substrate and enzyme resulting in an equilibrium which may at some time be tilted towards anabolism and at others, catabolism. (2) The maintenance of catabolic enzymes in the latent state. Only the second of these mechanisms will be discussed.

A number of mechanisms have been discovered that maintain an enzyme in a latent form, they include: the presence of allosteric effectors as is the case for the conversion of inactive to active phosphorylase; the binding of the enzyme to other macromolecules through —S—S bonds which need to be reduced for activity as is the case in some ATPases; the formation of an extended protein whose amino acid sequence must be partially amputated before it can be active as is the case with chymotrypsinogen; and the wrapping of the enzyme within an envelope impermeable to the substrate as is the case for zymogen granules and possibly lysosomes. Finally, a combination of two or more of the above mechanisms could obtain to secure latency.

To understand elementary mechanisms in cellular death, it is useful to distinguish between programmed and provoked death. The fate of the red cell best illustrates the programming of cellular death. In a well-regulated sequence of steps the genome is systematically repressed for the purpose of making one single protein, haemoglobin. The human red cell ultimately sacrifices the opportunity for reproduction and long life span for the sake of efficiency by discarding its useless nucleus. It is, however, not known whether it commits suicide or is sentenced to death by agents foreign to its intracellular environment. The fate of the epithelial cell of the skin which ultimately becomes keratinised, is not very different from that of the red cell (for review see Ref. 1).

If we know little of what causes programmed death in the red cell, we know even less of what triggers it in the foetus, where the programmed elimination of cells of various types is indispensable for development[1]. Evidence from plants where programmed death is rigidly regulated can be helpful, but even then we know little about the mechanism that triggers death.

If the harmonious deployment of cellular proliferation, cellular maturation and cellular death was never disturbed by changes in the environment, the living being could be eternal or at least live until an inherent death clock programmed to end life is put in motion.

But in this seemingly schizophrenic universe, elementary molecules of life, like nucleic acids, which probably required u.v. light to develop, were soon threatened by that very light that caused them to be born. As life further evolved, living organisms physically collided with their environment and died by trauma. They inhaled or ingested poisons and were attacked by other living organisms, often invisible ones. As a result, the rate of organismal and cellular death is greatly accelerated over what it could be without interference by the environment.

It is not known at present whether injuries accelerate a death clock, or whether they do trigger cellular death by mechanisms other than those that obtain under physiological conditions.

Now that we have reminded ourselves of the various forms of death and various types of injuries we can return to the role of hydrolases in cellular death. The question is not whether or not hydrolases play a role in cellular death. Pathologists have known for a long time that lipase causes fat necrosis and that trypsin can be responsible for necrosis of the pancreas[2,3], liver and lung[4,5]. The real question is at which point of the sequence of events that follows the onset of programmed death or the application of lethal injury, do the hydrolases act? At the very beginning triggering the sequence, at the end scavenging the remains, or sometimes in between? It is very likely that the role hydrolases play in the sequence of steps leading to cellular death depends upon the type of hydrolase.

Although in the course of the last decenni, much of the work on the role of hydrolases in cellular death was focused on acid hydrolases and although the role of that group of enzymes will be at the centre of this presentation, the existence of numerous other hydrolases cannot be ignored. In most cases their role in cellular injury is unknown, but in a few rare cases it has been shown that their role is complex in that, at the same time, they may serve to repair injuries and also cause further damage; a case at point is the parts of the mammalian enzyme involved in the sequence that leads to DNA repair.

DNA, a child of the sun, was also among its first victims—u.v. light causes among other injuries the formation of thymine dimers. Moreover, chemicals, iatrogenic or environmental, bind to the deoxypolynucleotide *in vivo*. Much of the damage to DNA is repaired by the sequential action of an endonuclease, alkaline phosphatase, and DNA polymerase[6]. But in some cases, for example, after the administration of X-radiation, the repair mechanism fails and is likely to cause double strand breaks for which no repair mechanism is yet known[7].

It is likely that a battery of catabolic enzymes are involved in DNA repair and it cannot be excluded that many enzymes still to be discovered participate in the repair of RNA, proteins and other macromolecules.

In the latter part of the 1950s de Duve and his associates in Louvain isolated a cytoplasmic organelle rich in acid hydrolases (for review see Refs. 1 and 8). The enzymes were most effective at pH 5 and exhibited latency in that full activity could only be released by blending, osmotic

shock or by the action of detergents. De Duve quite logically directly
linked the granule with cellular death by proposing what was then an
appealing, but is now an obsolete hypothesis, that of the 'suicide bag'[9].
Many followed the lead. Yet, even in face of the existing knowledge of
the time, one should have been reminded of the words of Hamlet:
'There are more things in heaven and earth, Horatio, than are dreamt
of in our philosophy'.

Indeed, already in 1938 Bradley[10] recognised that cellular death is
caused by a chain of events. A decrease in oxidising metabolism resulting
from subnormal oxygen tension in the tissues; an increase in the concentration of hydrogen ions resulting from the accumulation of acids
including lactic acid, CO_2 and other metabolites and an increase in
proteolytic activity. The mechanism of activation of proteases was not
obvious, but Willstater and Rodenwald[11] had shown that in tissues all
cathepsins do not exist in the free state, but that some remain perm-
anently bound to insoluble proteins after attempts to extract them.

Since then a number of studies on injuries that are associated with
cell death have shown that a variety of molecular alterations take place
minutes, or sometimes hours, prior to the release of acid hydrolase.

In pancreas autolysis, the release of the enzyme from zymogen
granules precedes that of the acid hydrolases from lysosomes[12]. In liver
autolysis the release of acid hydrolases occurs at a time when the levels
of ATP have fallen to zero[13]. The release of acid hydrolases starts 15
min after the onset of autolysis. After three minutes of autolysis the
levels of ATP have fallen to 5% of their normal intracellular concentration. At 10 min they are down to zero. It is also known through the
work of Judah and his associates, that severe mitochondrial alterations
take place in between five and 30 min after the onset of autolysis[14].

Vogt and Farber have presented a most elegant study of ischaemia of
the kidney which cannot be reviewed here[15]. Suffice to point out that it
was observed that most of the critical events concerning lactic acid
formation and ATP generation occur in the first minutes after the onset
of autolysis. Gottleib and Van Lancker[16] have shown that the release of
acid hydrolase does not start in kidney until 30 min after the onset of
ischaemia and reaches a peak only one hour later; again indicating that
the release of such hydrolases follows the development of other macromolecular alterations and is likely to be a consequence of the injury
rather than the primary manifestation of it. Studies on liver damage
produced by hypoxia, by Van Lancker and Lentz[17], also support the

notion that the role of lysosomal enzymes in cellular death is several steps removed from the original insult. We will return to these studies later.

X-radiation induces almost instantaneously single strand breaks, double strand breaks, cross links and base alterations. Some of the damage is repaired, some is not. With lethal doses there is interference with transcription of some enzymes. In liver, none of these effects of radiation are associated with the release of acid hydrolases[18]. In spleen of irradiated animals, interference with transcription and DNA and even the appearance of pyknosis or karyorrhexis occur up to 30 min prior to the release of acid hydrolases[19].

The administration of puromycin does not release or change the concentration of acid hydrolases and lysosomes appear hours after the block of protein synthesis[20]. The administration of carbon tetrachloride leads to an interference with protein synthesis which in turn results in triglyceride accumulation. Slater and Greenbaum have shown that these changes occur prior to the appearance of secondary lysosomes and the release of acid hydrolases[21].

One could continue to list circumstances in which the appearance of hydrolases follows other types of damage, but we will content ourselves to refer to the conclusions of Slater[22].

If, in addition to the facts just described, we take into consideration the difficulties of interpreting data on lysosomal enzyme release in inflammatory death or in physiological remodelling of tissues because of the inescapable participation of polymorphonuclears and macrophages, it seems fair to conclude that if lysosomal enzymes are likely to be ultimately involved in all forms of cellular death, they do not trigger it, but scavenge the remains long after the lesions have become irreversible[1].

CORRELATION OF MORPHOLOGICAL AND BIOCHEMICAL EVENTS

On the basis of previous work by Novikoff[23], and Ashoff and Porter[24], Swift and Hruban and his associates[25] proposed an ingenious generalisation referred to as 'focal cytoplasmic degradation'. These investigators postulated that the cell segregates pieces of cytoplasm for autodigestion by surrounding them with membranes. The cytoplasmic components are progressively digested within the confines of the membrane and dense bodies are formed as a result. The concept raised, without prejudice, meaningful questions relating to the origin of the segregating membrane, the mechanism of conversion of a double into a single membrane, the origin of the hydrolases and the mechanism of elimination of the dense bodies. Even more far reaching questions concern the factors which determine that degradation shall take place in a restricted area and the type of signal which tells the surrounding healthy cytoplasm that a portion of its being is to be digested.

The origin of the enzyme has been debated. Although we were the first to demonstrate using a biochemical approach that β-glucuronidase was synthesised in the endoplasmic reticulum[26], most of our understanding of the origin of the acid hydrolase found in the area of focal cytoplasmic degradation comes from histochemical and electron microscopic studies which cannot be reviewed critically here[27]. We will restrict our review to the biochemical approach.

We followed the labelling of β-glucuronidase with [14][C] leucine and [14][C] valine as the enzyme was synthesised in regenerating liver. The total homogenate contains at least six isozymic forms of β-glucuronidase, but only one form was found in lysosomes. The lysosomal isozyme was found in all other cell fractions except mitochondria. It was purified from each cell fraction to electrophoretic homogeneity. The enzyme associated with the lysosomes was easy to purify. The enzyme associated with microsomes or supernatant resisted solubilisation until treatment with ribonuclease. This finding suggested that the supernatant enzyme is more related to the microsomal than the lysosomal β-glucuronidase.

These findings have been confirmed in Fishman's laboratory[28]. The rapid uptake of the radioactivity in the microsomal β-glucuronidase is not followed by transfer of the radioactivity to lysosomes. In that fraction, β-glucuronidase remains cold even hours after injection of the isotope.

We then wondered what would happen to the transfer of enzymes from microsomes to lysosomes under conditions associated with focal cytoplasmic degradation of the liver; for example, after induction of severe hypoxia.

Thus, animals were partially hepatectomised, maintained under hypoxia between 22 and 24 hours and injected with the radioactive amino acid 30 min and 60 min after onset of hypoxia. Labelled β-

glucuronidase was purified from various cell fractions. The radioactivity dropped markedly in the microsomes and rose in the lysosomes. When the enzyme was purified from both microsomes and lysosomes no changes in specific radioactivity in other cell fractions were observed either. Everything thus happened as if the lysosomal enzymes, which in the intact liver could not be transferred from endoplasmic reticulum to the lysosomes, were after hypoxia dumped into foci of cytoplasmic degradation.

In 1964 we proposed[26] a new mechanism for the introduction of acid hydrolase into foci of cytoplasmic degradation; namely, a direct transfer from endoplasmic reticulum. Our arguments were:

1. the lack of convincing evidence for the existence of primary lysosomes except in inflammatory cells;
2. the presence of large amounts of some latent hydrolase in the endoplasmic reticulum;
3. the sudden transfer of enzyme from endoplasmic reticulum to areas of focal cytoplasmic degradation, under conditions when most anabolic events are inhibited.

Although we do not imply that such a mechanism prevails under all circumstances, it is likely to obtain when cells die in part or as a whole. The concept has the advantage of simplicity and if correct, it would suggest that the hydrolases associated with the endoplasmic reticulum may have physiologic functions that remain to be discovered. Recently this hypothesis has received support from electron microscopic studies in tetrahymina[29]. The implication is that acid hydrolases are not set apart to execute cells but play important physiological roles and that such roles may directly involve the enzyme associated with the endoplasmic reticulum.

Of course, such a physiological role was not overlooked by de Duve[8] and it is now clear that the lysosomes, a child of the test tube which became a constellation of particles when seen by the electron microscopist, participates in multiple physiological functions. But as Kipling used to say, 'This is another story' and it has been told by others better than it could be done here.

Can we in any way guess as to why some areas of cytoplasm become segregated? Let's assume that there is no qualitative, but only quantitative differences between the mechanism of formation of focal cytoplasmic degradation in cells that survive the process and cells that die. Is

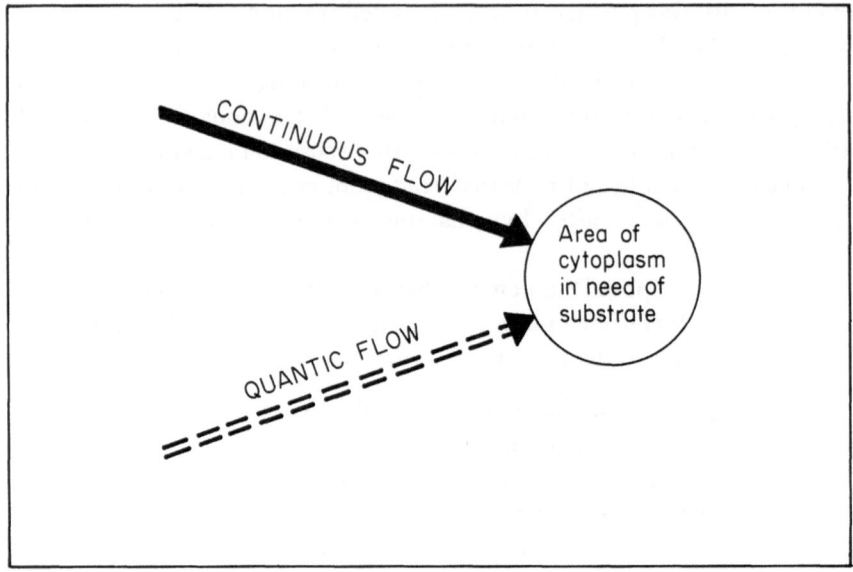

FIGURE 3.1 (see text)

it also not fair to assume that the concentration throughout the cytoplasm of macromolecular or other components that are needed in the
cytoplasm for maintenance of the integrity of the membranes, replacement of structural protein or other essential events is not uniform and
that the supply of such components in an area in need may not be continuous, but quantic (Figure 3.1). Therefore, while some areas may be
freshly supplied by the needed substrate, others may be close to depletion. These are threshold zones. Other parts may be somewhere in
between abundance and famine. Often, because of a programmed
event or because of an injury, the supply of substrates to the threshold
zones will be reduced, switching the equilibrium from anabolism to
catabolism. Such areas are then segregated from the still healthy
cytoplasm by membranes from which hydrolases are released (Figure
3.2).

CONCLUSION

Whenever a cell dies, in part or as a whole, areas of cytoplasm are
segregated for autolysis and at some point of their development the

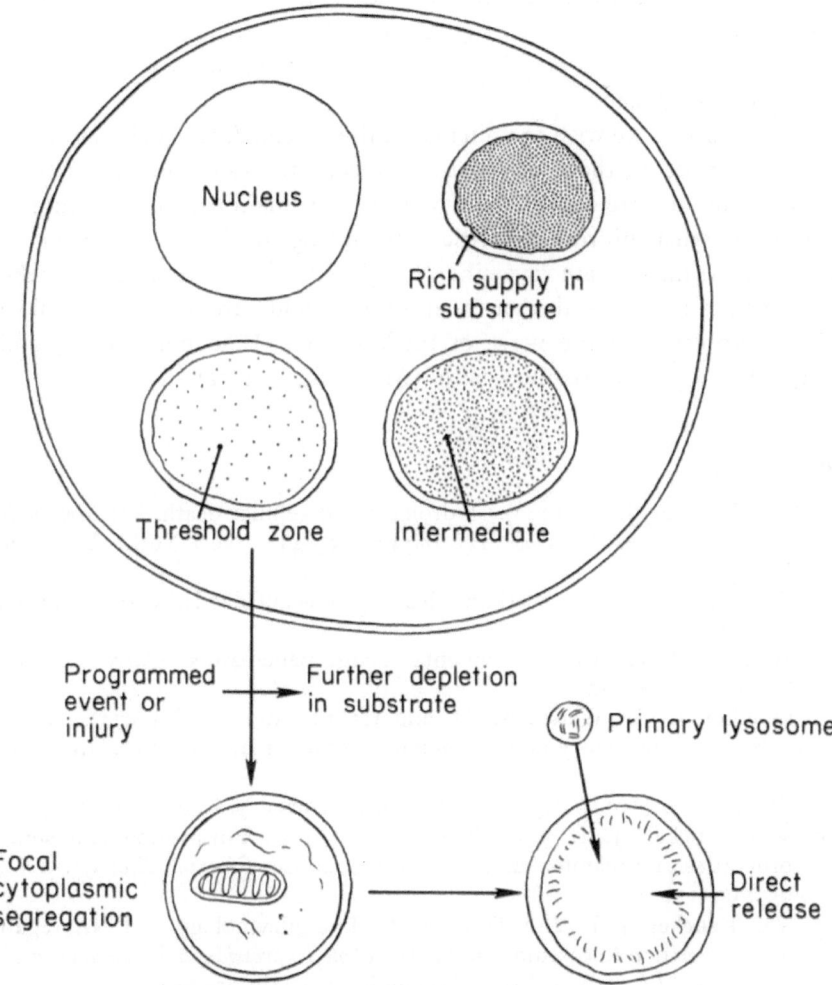

FIGURE 3.2   Focal cytoplasmic segregation and the release of hydrolases

segregated areas contain hydrolases which may have been introduced either by fusion with primary lysosomes or by direct release of the enzyme from the endoplasmic reticulum into the autolytic vacuole. Certainly when hydrolases appear, the equilibrium in the segregated area is switched from anabolic to catabolic pathways and the trend towards autodigestion becomes irreversible.

Other macromolecular alterations almost always precede autodigestion and therefore it would seem that either they trigger the event or are located in the sequence of events that follow the application of the injury somewhere between the primary alteration and the scavenging of the dying cytoplasm.

In any case, if we wish to understand the mechanism of cellular death, we must focus on those events that precede the development of focal cytoplasmic degradation. Identify the first manifestation of injury, determine what injuries are critical in causing death and the extent to which those injuries are reversible. Only such an approach can help the physician to reach his ultimate goal, prevent and cure disease. A goal so nicely expressed in the verse of Shakespeare, 'Find her disease, and purge it to a sound pristine health' (Macbeth, V-3-52).

REFERENCES

1. Van Lancker, J. L. (1970). Hydrolases and cellular death. In: *Metabolic Conjugation and Metabolic Hydrolysis*, 355–418 (New York: Academic Press)
2. Polya, E. (1908). Die Werkung des Trypsins auf das Lebende Pankreas. *Pflügers Arch.*, **121**, 483
3. Wanke, M. (1970). Experimental acute pancreatitis. *Current Topics Pathol.*, **52**, 64–142
4. Guenter, C. A., Welch, M. H. and Hammarsten, J. F. (1971). Alpha$_1$ antitrypsin deficiency and pulmonary emphysema. *Ann. Rev. Med.*, **22**, 283–292
5. Sharp, H. L. (1971). Alpha-1-antitrypsin deficiency. *Hosp. Prac.*, **6**, 83–96
6. Van Lancker, J. L. and Tomura, T. (1974). Purification and some properties of a mammalian repair endonuclease. *Biochim. Biophys. Acta*, **353**, 99–114
7. Van Lancker, J. L. and Tomura, T. The enzymology of DNA repair and its relation to carcinogenesis. In: *Gene Expression and Carcinogenesis in Cultured Liver* (New York: Academic Press) (in press)
8. de Duve, C. (1973). The lysosome in retrospect. In: *Lysosomes in Biology and Pathology*, 3–40 (J. T. Dingle and H. B. Fell, editors) (New York: American Elsevier Publ. Co.)
9. de Duve, C. (1959). A new group of cytoplasmic particles. In: *Subcellular Particles*, 128 (T. Hayashi, editor) (New York: Ronald Press)
10. Bradley, H. C. (1938). Autolysis and atrophy. *Physiol. Rev.*, **18**, 173–196
11. Wilstätter, R. and Rohdewald, M. (1932). Über desmo-pepsin and desmo-kathepsin. I. Abhandlung: Zur kenntnis zellgebundener enzyme der gewebe und drüsen. *Z. Physiol. Chem.*, **208**, 258–272
12. Holtzer, R. L. and Van Lancker, J. L. (1962). Early changes in pancreas autolysis. *Amer. J. Pathol.*, **40**, 331–336

13. Van Lancker, J. L. and Holtzer, R. L. (1959a). The release of acid phosphatase and beta-glucuronidase from cytoplasmic granules in the course of autolysis. *Amer. J. Pathol.*, **35**, 563–573

14. Van Lancker, J. L. and Holtzer, R. L. Unpublished data

15. Vogt, M. T. and Farber, E. (1968). On the molecular pathology of ischemic renal cell death. Reversible and irreversible cellular and mitochondrial metabolic alterations. *Amer. J. Pathol.*, **53**, 1–26

16. Gottlieb, L. I. and Van Lancker, J. L. Unpublished data

17. Van Lancker, J. L. and Lentz, P. (1970). Study on the site of biosynthesis of glucuronidase and its appearance in lysosomes in normal and hypoxic rats. *J. Hist. Cytochem.*, **18**, 529–542

18. Van Lancker, J. L. (1960). Metabolic alterations after total body doses of x-radiation. I. The role of regenerating liver nuclei and cytoplasm in the inhibition due to x-radiation of incorporation of tritium-labeled thymidine into DNA. *Biochim. Biophys. Acta*, **45**, 57–62

19. Fausto, N., Smoot, A. O. and Van Lancker, J. L. (1964). Early effect of x-irradiation on *in vitro* DNA synthesis in mouse spleen. *Rad. Res.*, **22**, 288–304

20. Gottlieb, L. I., Fausto, N. and Van Lancker, J. L. (1964). Molecular mechanisms of liver regeneration. The effect of puromycin on deoxyribonucleic acid synthesis. *J. Biol. Chem.*, **239**, 555–559

21. Slater, T. F. and Greenbaum, A. L. (1965). Changes in lysosomal enzymes in acute experimental liver injury. *Biochem. J.*, **96**, 484–491

22. Slater, T. F. (1973). Lysosomes and experimentally induced tissue injury. In: *Lysosomes in Biology and Pathology*, 469–492 (J. T. Dingle and H. B. Fell, editors) (New York: American Elsevier Publ. Co.)

23. Novikoff, A. B. (1959). The proximal tubule cell in experimental hydronephrosis. *J. Biophys. Biochem. Cytol.*, **6**, 136–138

24. Ashford, T. P. and Porter, K. R. (1962). Cytoplasmic components in hepatic cell lysosomes. *J. Cell Biol.*, **12**, 198–202

25. Swift, H. and Hruban, Z. (1964). Focal degradation as a biological process. *Fed. Proc.*, **23**, 1026–1037

26. Van Lancker, J. L. (1964). Concluding remarks, Pathology Symposium–Lysosomes. *Fed. Proc.*, **23**, 1009–1052

27. Ericsson, J. L. E. (1973). Mechanism of cellular autophagy. In: *Lysosomes in Biology and Pathology*, 346–394 (J. T. Dingle and H. B. Fell, editors) (New York: American Elsevier Publ. Co.)

28. Fishman, W. H., Goldman, S. S. and DeLellis, R. (1967). Dual localization of β-glucuronidase in endoplasmic reticulum and in lysosomes. *Nature* (London), **213**, 457–460

29. Levy, M. R. and Elliott, A. M. (1968). Biochemical and ultrastructural changes in *Tetrahymena pyriformis* during starvation. *J. Protozool.*, **15**, 208–222

CHAPTER 4

Macromolecular syntheses and the maintenance of liver cell integrity*

E. Farber

The liver participates actively in the synthesis of a wide variety of proteins, not only for the maintenance and dynamic restructuring of its own cellular components but also for secretion into the blood. These latter proteins are diverse in nature and play important roles in many aspects of the metabolism in the whole organism, such as in lipid and protein metabolism, in blood coagulation, etc. as well as in maintaining the integrity of other organs (e.g. lung with alpha-l-antitrypsin). Since most if not all of these proteins are synthesised continually, since the liver adapts easily and readily to environmental perturbations by modulation at the level of transcription as well as translation, and since the turnover of various RNAs including messenger (mRNA), ribosomal (rRNA) and heterogeneous nuclear (HnRNA) is a continuous metabolic activity with half-lives of hours to a few days, the liver is obviously actively synthesising RNA virtually all the time. Thus, the syntheses of two of the major macromolecules, RNA and protein, are important and major metabolic activities of the liver on a continuing basis.

The synthesis of a third macromolecule, DNA, is also an important but sporadic activity associated with the stimulation of the liver cells to proliferate. Since hepatocyte proliferation is a common response seen in so many liver diseases, the synthesis of DNA becomes potentially an additional important metabolic focus for study of the molecular basis for cell injury.

Given the obvious importance of DNA, RNA and protein synthetic mechanisms in the economy of the liver and given the ubiquitous

* This investigation was supported in part by Public Health Service Research Grant No. AM-14882 from the National Institute of Arthritic, Metabolic and Digestive Diseases, CA-12218 and CA-12227 from the National Cancer Institute and the American Cancer Society (BC-7Q)

assumption, based almost entirely on intuition, that cell integrity generally, as exemplified by many studies in cancer chemotherapy, is closely tied to the operation of these mechanisms for macromolecular synthesis, it is not surprising that inhibition of these synthetic processes is invoked frequently as playing an important role in the pathogenesis of liver cell death. The observation that many hepatotoxins and other environmental disturbances (e.g. anoxia), some of which induce death of hepatocytes, are capable of inhibiting RNA and/or protein synthesis tends to favour the casual acceptance of the validity of this hypothesis.

However, a critical analysis of available data does not offer major support for such an hypothesis. Inhibition of transcription and of translation by a variety of agents, lasting in some instances many hours or days, can occur without any indication of hepatocyte death and necrosis. One of the purposes of this brief presentation is to summarise these data. In addition, some recent experimental data point to the possibility that protein synthesis may be involved in a positive manner in the *genesis* of liver cell death under some circumstances. These data and their implications will be presented briefly and discussed.

INHIBITION OF PROTEIN SYNTHESIS

There is an increasing number of hepatotoxic agents that inhibit hepatic protein synthesis[1-3]. These include CCl_4, thioacetamide, aflatoxin B_1, lasiocarpine, dimethylnitrosamine and a large group of other nitrosamines, ethionine and galactosamine. Since many of these agents disrupt protein synthesis early in their manifestations in the liver, it has been natural to assume that this metabolic disturbance may play an important role in the genesis of the subsequent cell death.

However, it is now evident that such an hypothesis does not hold up to careful scrutiny. Several situations are now known in which severe inhibition of protein synthesis can persist for hours or even days without leading to any sign of irreversible cell injury or death. This is most clearly seen with ethionine, in which inhibition of protein synthesis, along with apparently irreversible loss of function of ribosomes, can persist in the liver for from 24 to 48 hours, in the absence of liver cell death[4]. This is so despite the obvious damage to many cytoplasmic organelles. In addition, increasing understanding of liver damage induced by galactosamine[5,6] indicates that lower doses can induce a marked inhibition of protein synthesis for periods up to 24 hours or longer[7,8] without any evidence of liver cell death[9]. It is only with larger doses of galactosamine that liver cell death becomes evident[6,9].

Consistent with the conclusions derived from experiments with ethionine and galactosamine are those with antibiotics that inhibit protein synthesis. These include puromycin, cycloheximide and tenuazonic acid. Observations with puromycin and cycloheximide[10,11] as well as with tenuazonic acid[10,12] clearly show that severe inhibition of hepatic protein synthesis for several hours need not lead to death of hepatocytes. With puromycin, lack of liver cell necrosis occurs under conditions in which the pancreas shows acute acinar cell damage and necrosis in the same animal. Although each of these antibiotics induces structural and functional changes in the liver, no necrosis has been observed.

Thus, evidence with antibiotics inhibiting protein synthesis and with two hepatotoxic antimetabolites clearly shows that overall inhibition of protein synthesis in the liver is not by itself an important biochemical lesion in the pathogenesis of liver cell death and necrosis. Whether the interference with the synthesis of one or more specific and discrete proteins in the liver might be important in this context remains an interesting area for exploration. However, in the absence of data that incriminate some single protein, such a study of necessity would entail a large element of chance.

Also, since the known mechanisms of inhibition of protein synthesis vary considerably with each of the compounds (e.g. see Ref. 3), it is not likely that cell death is closely related to some one type of inhibition. For example, among the compounds mentioned, are some which induce dissociation of ribosomes on polysomes, some which preserve polysome structure, some appear to act primarily on initiation and some which act predominantly on elongation, some which act on free ribosomes and some on bound ribosomes. No apparent correlation can be discerned between some one type of inhibition and the subsequent induction of cell death. However, since it is only now becoming possible to analyse in great detail the molecular mechanism of inhibition in eukaryotic systems, this conclusion must await more detailed analyses of the effect of hepatotoxic agents on hepatic protein synthesis.

INHIBITION OF RNA SYNTHESIS

The arguments discussed above concerning the possible relationship of inhibition of protein synthesis to liver cell death also apply in principle to inhibition of RNA synthesis. Several hepatonecrogenic compounds, e.g. aflatoxin, α-amanitin, pyrrolizidine alkaloids, dimethylnitrosamine and D-galactosamine, are potent inhibitiors of RNA synthesis[10,13-16]. It is once again natural that this overall biochemical lesion be suggested as the basis for hepatic cell necrosis.

However, the suggestion of an active role for inhibition of RNA synthesis in the genesis of liver cell death is made untenable by studies with ethionine, methionine, actinomycin D, different doses of galacto-samine and toyocamycin[6,10,13,16,17]. With a variety of doses of actino-mycin[18], some inducing an inhibition of RNA synthesis of over 90% for as long as 24 hours, with ethionine[4] and with methionine in the guinea-pig[19] for periods up to 24 or 48 hours, and with subnecrogenic doses of D-galactosamine[16], severe inhibition of RNA synthesis can be induced in the liver without any evidence for liver cell death or necrosis. This concerns not only overall nuclear and cytoplasmic RNA but also selec-tive groups or classes of RNA, such as cytoplasmic RNA containing polyadenylic acid[20] and ribosomal RNA. Again, as with protein syn-thesis, it is possible that the highly selective inhibition of one class or one molecular species of RNA in the absence of any effect on other cellular RNA might play a mechanistic role in the development of cell death. However, the evidence with actinomycin D and toyocamycin does not favour such a view at this time.

INHIBITION OF DNA SYNTHESIS

Since the resting liver shows only very minimal DNA synthesis con-fined to a rare widely scattered cell, an interference with this metabolic pathway cannot be invoked in the induction of liver cell death in the normal host. However, even in the regenerating liver, inhibition of DNA synthesis, either directly[21,22] or via inhibition of protein syn-thesis[23] does not lead to any induction of liver cell death or necrosis.

POSSIBLE ROLE OF PROTEIN SYNTHESIS
IN CELL DEATH

Work several years ago suggested that necrosis of intestinal crypt cells induced by cytosine arabinoside, nitrogen mustard or X-irradiation may be mediated through one or more steps involving protein synthesis[24-26]. Recent work in our laboratory by Popp and Shinozuka[27] seems to implicate protein synthesis in the genesis of liver cell necrosis but not of balloon cells induced by CCl_4. This is in general a confirmation of the report of Flaks and Nicoll[28] on liver injury. Previous work[12] showed that two inhibitors of protein synthesis, cycloheximide or tenuazonic acid, could prevent irreversible damage of liver polyribosomes in rats treated with CCl_4 and dissociated the ribosome effects from the membrane lesions that seem to be essential for liver cell death. These newer data suggest that some aspect of the translation apparatus may be involved mechanistically in the genesis of liver cell death. However, according to these observations, an active system may favour and an inhibited one may protect against irreversible liver cell damage. It must be emphasised that the data are suggestive only. However, they are sufficiently provocative to warrant a more intensive investigation into this unorthodox approach to liver cell injury. Conceivably, the mechanism of induction of cell death involves several biochemical sequential steps, only one of which may be related to a labile protein or the induction of a protein, e.g. an enzyme[25,26].

GENERAL CONSIDERATIONS

Although the delineation of the sequences of biochemical or molecular events involved in the genesis of cell death remains a major challenge in modern hepatology, it appears that inhibition of synthesis of protein or RNA is not a major step. In anything, inhibition of protein synthesis may even be protective under some circumstances.

Although emphasis has been given in this presentation to protein, RNA and DNA as macromolecules, disturbances in the synthesis or metabolism of other types of macromolecules such as a wide variety of lipids, polysaccharides, including glycoproteins and glycolipids or even small molecular weight metabolites, could very well play key roles in the genesis of liver cell death. Some of these are particularly interesting in view of their importance in membrane structure and function.

It must also be stressed that hepatonecrogenic agents may initiate the process of cell death within minutes or a few hours after administration. This necessitates that the early biochemical events involve molecules that show an active metabolic turnover or synthesis or affect components that play a pivotal role in the organisation of some vital organelle such as the plasma membrane.

It is difficult to convince oneself that major progress towards understanding cell death will be achieved without a major commitment to biochemical and molecular approaches. However, equally important is the selection of a model. Hopefully, more reversible models such as with ethionine or galactosamine, might well enable new imaginative approaches to be made in this fundamental area of liver disease.

REFERENCES

1. Smuckler, E. A. and Barker, E. A. (1966). Effects of drugs on amino acid incorporation in the liver. *Proc. Eur. Soc. Study Drug Toxicity*, **7**, 83–112
2. Smuckler, E. A. and Arcasoy, M. (1969). Structural and functional changes of the endoplasmic reticulum of hepatic parenchymal cells. *Int. Rev. Exp. Pathol.*, **7**, 305–418
3. Farber, E. (1972). The pathology of translation. In: *The Pathology of Transcription and Translation*, 123–158 (E. Farber, editor) (New York: Marcel Dekker)
4. Shinozuka, H., Reid, I. M., Shull, K. H., Liang, H. and Farber, E. (1970). Dynamics of liver cell injury and repair. I. Spontaneous reformation of the nucleolus and polyribosomes in the presence of extensive cytoplasmic damage induced by ethionine. *Lab. Invest.*, **23**, 253–267
5. Decker, K. and Keppler, D. (1972). Galactosamine induced liver injury. In: *Progress in Liver Diseases*, 183–199, **Vol. IV** (H. Popper and F. Schaffner, editors) (New York: Grune and Stratton)
6. Shinozuka, H., Farber, J. L., Konishi, Y. and Anukarahanonta, T. (1973). D-galactosamine and acute liver cell injury. *Fed. Proc.*, **32**, 1516–1526
7. Anukarahanonta, T., Shinozuka, H. and Farber, E. (1973). Inhibition of protein synthesis in rat liver by D-galactosamine. *Res. Commun. Chem. Pathol. Pharmacol.*, **5**, 481–491
8. Anukarahanonta, T. (1973). Studies on inhibition of protein synthesis in the rat liver following D-galactosamine administration (University of Pittsburgh: Ph.D. Thesis)
9. Farber, J. L., Gill, G. and Konishi, Y. (1973). Prevention of galactosamine-induced liver cell necrosis by uridine. *Amer. J. Pathol.*, **72**, 53–60
10. Farber, E. (1971). Biochemical pathology. *Ann. Rev. Pharmacol.*, **11**, 71–96

11. Verbin, R. S. (1968). The effects of cycloheximide, an inhibitor of protein synthesis, on cell structure, ultrastructure and function. (University of Pittsburgh: Ph.D. Thesis)
12. Farber, E., Liang, H. and Shinozuka, H. (1971). Dissociation of effects on protein synthesis and ribosomes from membrane changes induced by carbon tetrachloride. *Amer. J. Pathol.*, **64**, 601–617
13. Farber, J. (1972). Pathology of RNA. In: *Pathology of Transcription and Translation*, 55–72 (E. Farber, editor) (New York: Marcel Dekker)
14. Fiume, L. (1972). Pathogenesis of the cellular lesions induced by α-amanitin. In: *Pathology of Transcription and Translation*, 105–122 (E. Farber, editor) (New York: Marcel Dekker)
15. Keppler, D. O. R., Pausch, J. and Decker, K. (1974). Selective uridine triphosphate deficiency induced by D-galactosamine in liver and reversed by pyrimidine nucleotide precursors. Effect on ribonucleic acid synthesis. *J. Biol. Chem.*, **249**, 211–216
16. Konishi, Y., Shinozuka, H. and Farber, J. L. (1974). The inhibition of rat liver nuclear RNA synthesis by galactosamine and its reversal by uridine. *Lab. Invest.*, **30**, 751–756
17. Shinozuka, H. (1972). Response of nucleus and nucleolus to inhibition of RNA synthesis. In: *Pathology of Transcription and Translation*, 73–103 (E. Farber, editor) (New York: Marcel Dekker)
18. Goldblatt, P. J., Sullivan, R. J. and Farber, E. (1969). Morphologic and metabolic alterations in hepatic cell nucleoli induced by varying doses of actinomycin D. *Cancer Res.*, **29**, 124–135
19. Cox, R., Martin, J. T. and Shinozuka, H. (1973). Studies on acute methionine toxicity. II. Inhibition of ribonucleic acid synthesis in guinea-pig liver by methionine and ethionine. *Lab. Invest.*, **29**, 54–59
20. Konishi, Y. and Farber, J. L. (1974). Personal communication
21. Schwartz, H. S., Garofalo, M., Sternberg, S. S. and Philips, F. S. (1965) Hydroxyurea: inhibition of deoxyribonucleic acid synthesis in regenerating liver of rats. *Cancer Res.*, **25**, 1867–1870
22. Farber, E. and Baserga, R. (1969). Differential effects of hydroxyurea on survival of proliferating cells *in vivo*. *Cancer Res.*, **29**, 136–139
23. Verbin, R. S., Sullivan, R. J. and Farber, E. (1969). The effects of cycloheximide on the cell cycle of regenerating rat liver. *Lab. Invest.*, **21**, 179–192
24. Lieberman, M. W., Verbin, R. S., Landay, M., Liang, H., Farber, E., Lee, T.-N. and Starr, R. (1970). A probable role for protein synthesis in intestinal epithelial cell death induced *in vivo* by cytosine arabinoside, nitrogen mustard or X-irradiation. *Cancer Res.*, **30**, 942–951
25. Farber, E., Verbin, R. S. and Lieberman, M. W. (1971). Cell suicide and cell death. In: *Mechanisms of Toxicity*, 163–170 (W. N. Aldridge, editor) (London: Macmillan and Co.)
26. Lieberman, M. W. (1972). DNA metabolism, cell death and cancer chemotherapy. In: *Pathology of Transcription and Translation*, 37–53 E. Farber, editor) (New York: Marcel Dekker)

27. Popp, J. A., Shinozuka, H. and Farber, E. (1974). Possible role of protein synthesis in the pathogenesis of cell necrosis. *Amer. J. Pathol.*, **74**, 58A
28. Flaks, B. and Nicoll, J. W. (1974). Modification of toxic liver injury in the rat. I. Effect of inhibition of protein synthesis on the action of 2-acetylaminofluorene, carbon tetrochloride, 3'-methyl-4-dimethyl-aminoazobenzene and dimethylnitrosamine. *Chem.-Biol. Interactions*, **8**, 135–150

CHAPTER 5

Quantitative aspects of biochemical mechanisms leading to cell death

K. DECKER

Cells and organisms die by the action of built-in mechanisms of self-destruction or as a result of damages inflicted from without. The former include the process of ageing and have to be regarded as physiological and necessary in terms of biological evolution. The latter processes leading to cell death are triggered by external factors, such as bacteria, viruses, toxic substances, malnutrition, physical damage and other environmental influences. If the organism cannot defend itself successfully against these agents, they will start to disturb molecular events within the cells and will interfere with the proper course of enzymic processes and the turnover of cellular structures. Among the events which can alter the steady states of metabolic fluxes and the turnover of cellular components are inadequate or defective protein synthesis, faulty mechanisms of enzyme regulation and disturbed activity correlations of enzymes. It is the rationale and also the justification of a biochemical approach to pathology that diseases originate in cellular metabolism and are thus amenable to biochemical and biophysical analysis.

The analytical methodology for studies of pathologic processes must account for the dynamic state of cellular matter and, therefore, has to deal with the distribution and change of substances in the space-time co-ordinates of metabolism (Table 5.1). Considering the complexity of these parameters, it is obvious that neither the biochemical nor the morphologic approach alone will suffice to describe the physiologic state of the cell and the pathologic deviations thereof. For this reason, biochemists and morphologists must join forces if ever they want to understand what goes on in a living cell.

It must be pointed out, however, that it is not sufficient to deal with

Table 5.1   DIMENSIONS OF CELLULAR METABOLISM

Space	*Time*

Concentrations
    of matter
	Activities
	    of enzymic processes

Compartmentation
    of reactions
	Regulation
	    of enzymic processes

Structures
    of matter
	Fluxes
	    of metabolites

Specificities
    of reactions
	Turnover
	    of matter

cellular metabolism and structure in a qualitative way. Statements such as, 'the concentration is increased', 'the activity is reduced', 'the nuclear material is less dense', 'the endoplasmic reticulum appears enlarged', are of limited value in elucidating the state of a cell or the direction and progress of an alteration. We must realise that quantitative analyses are required and that this applies not only to critical concentrations of matter. As we recognise the involvement of the factor *time* in the dynamic state of the cell and in the turnover of its constituents, the kinetic parameters of metabolism become of crucial importance in studies both of physiologic and pathologic conditions. It is not even enough to measure the extent to which concentrations or activities of cellular components rise or fall; it is also essential to know, over which periods of time these metabolic alterations persist.

Let me now elaborate these proposals to some extent by using as a model the liver injury that can be induced by administration of D-galactosamine[1]. This experimental liver damage—which we call galactosamine hepatitis for simplicity's sake, if not for better reasons—has over the years been extensively studied by many people, including my own group (for review see Refs. 2 and 3); I shall, therefore, not dwell on the details of this model in this presentation. D-galactosamine induces a potentially reversible liver cell injury, the severity and duration of which can be experimentally controlled by the amount of D-galactosamine, the schedule of its application and by several countermeasures. The sequence of events which is elicited by D-galactosamine is given in shorthand in Figure 5.1. It is important, however, to realise that two metabolic routes are involved in the development of the primary biochemical lesion: the conversion of D-galactosamine by the galactose pathway and the *de novo* UTP synthesis via orotate (Figure 5.2).

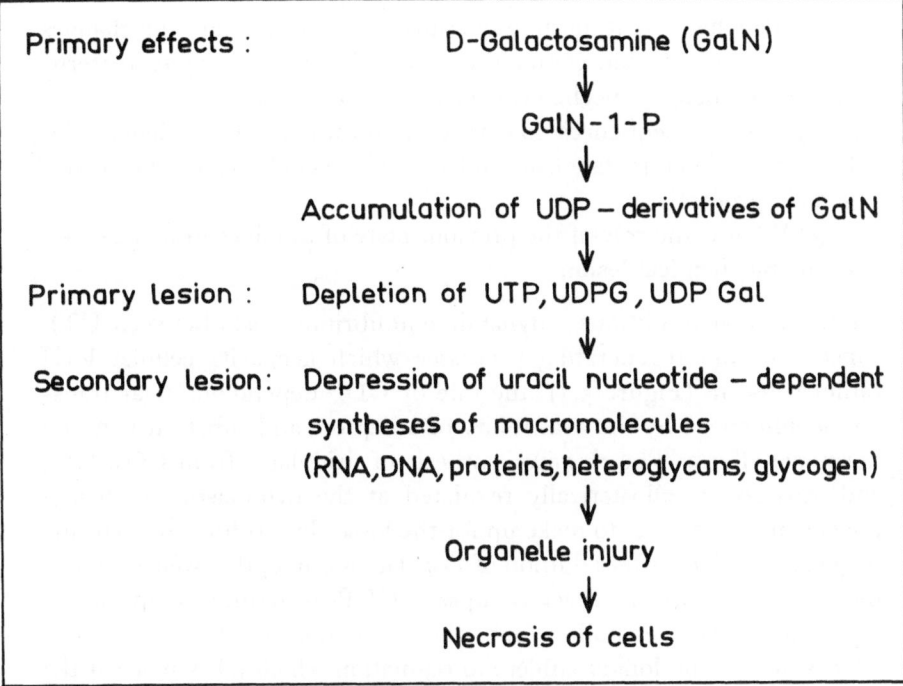

FIGURE 5.1 D-galactosamine-induced sequence of events in liver cells

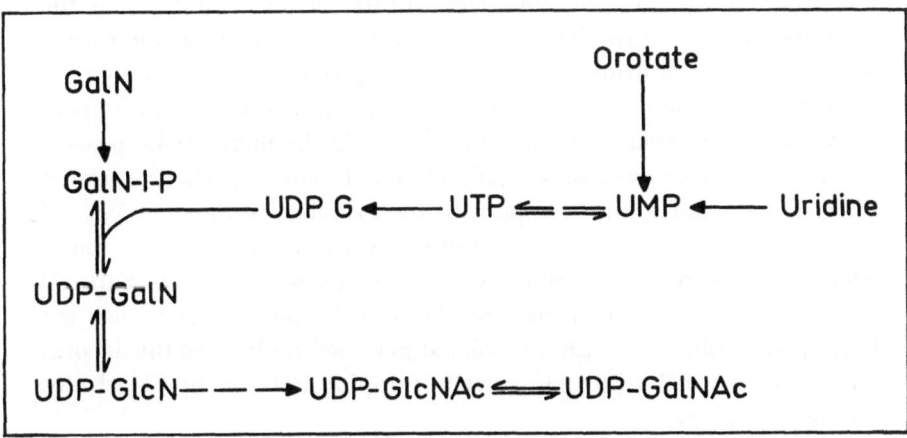

FIGURE 5.2 Hepatic D-galactosamine metabolism and its dependence on uracil nucleotide biosynthesis

With this background in mind we will ask the following questions:

(*a*) To what extent, both in quantity and duration, are the changes of uridine nucleotide contents determined by the activity patterns and the regulatory mechanisms of these pathways?

(*b*) What consequences do extent and duration of these deficiencies have on cellular metabolism and on the reversibility of the pathogenetic process?

(*c*) What is the role of the previous state of the liver in its response to the biochemical lesion?

Under normal conditions a dynamic equilibrium exists between UTP consuming and regenerating processes which keeps its cellular level rather constant (Figure 5.3): the rate of UDP-dependent sugar transfers is influenced by the availability of acceptors and substrates and by hormonal effects. The *de novo* synthesis of uridylates from CO_2, NH_3 and aspartate is allosterically regulated at the cytoplasmic carbamyl phosphate synthetase[4] to make up for the losses by uridine and cytosine degradation. Soon after addition of D-galactosamine, this well-balanced metabolic network is severely upset. UDP-hexosamines appear as unphysiological metabolites and the formation of UDP-N-acetyl-hexosamines is no longer subject to regulation which takes place at the fructose-6-phosphate level and is bypassed here; as a result, these compounds accumulate excessively thereby depleting the limited pools of UTP, UDP, UMP, UDPG and UDPGal. The liver cell responds to this situation with an immediate release of the feedback inhibition of the *de novo* synthesis of uridylates which could be measured as an increase of the total amount of uridylate derivatives (Figure 5.4) and as a more than tenfold stimulation of CO_2-incorporation into the uridylate pool (Table 5.2). However, the quantitative data of the fluxes of D-galactosamine conversion and of the stimulated *de novo* synthesis make it clear, that the latter cannot cope with the uridylate trapping activity of the enzymes of the galactose pathway. A similar situation is found after D,L-ethionine poisoning, which has been shown by Farber's group and by others to result in adenosine trapping (for review see Ref. 5). Data obtained with the isolated perfused rat liver in this laboratory[6] compare well with the uridylate trapping induced by D-galactosamine treatment.

It is obvious from these findings that activity patterns of competing metabolic pathways are responsible for the changes in metabolite levels

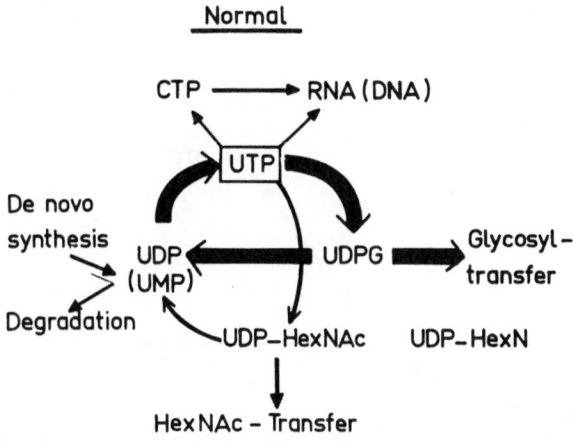

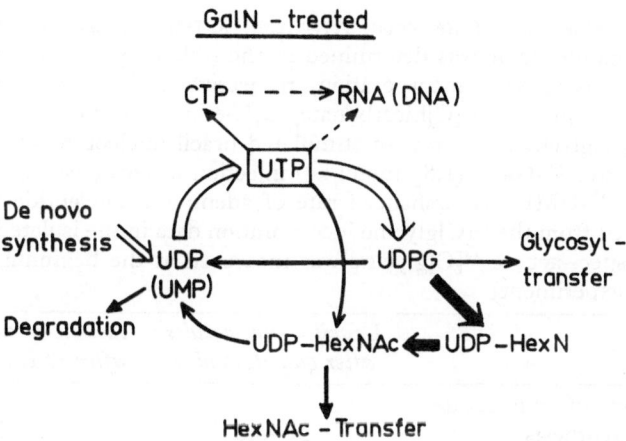

FIGURE 5.3 Schematic presentation of the dynamic equilibrium of UTP consuming and regenerating processes in normal and galactosamine-treated livers

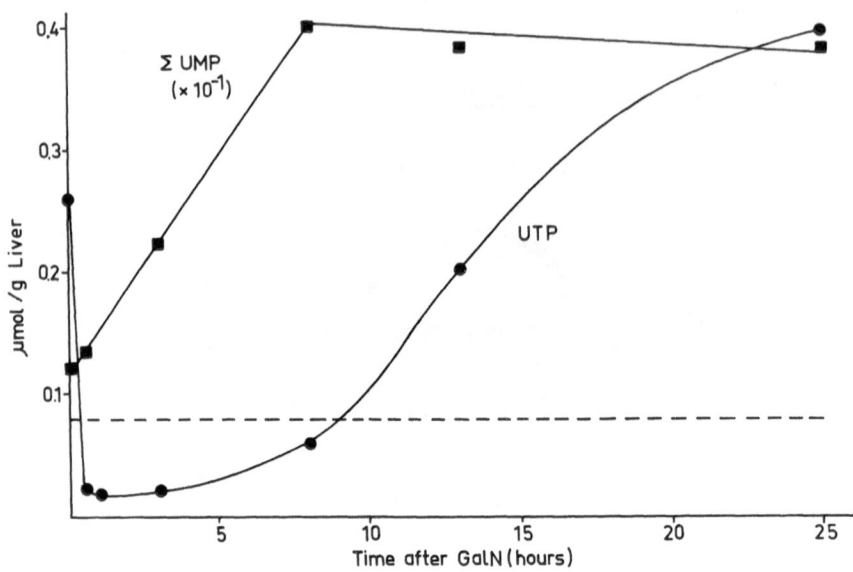

FIGURE 5.4   Stimulated uridylate synthesis following UTP deficiency
Σ-UMP represents the sum of acid-soluble uracil 5′-nucleotides, determined as
5′-UMP after enzymic hydrolysis

Table 5.2 STIMULATED *de novo* SYNTHESIS AFTER NUCLEOTIDE TRAPPING.
The stimulation factor was determined in the isolated perfused rat liver by
$^{14}CO_2$ and ^{14}[C]glycine incorporation, respectively. D-GalN (2 mM) was
added 30 min prior to ^{14}[C]bicarbonate, D,L-ethionine (0.9 mM) one hour
prior to ^{14}[C]glycine. The rate of stimulated uracil nucleotide synthesis was
measured after D-GalN (1.85 mmol/kg) injection *in vivo* (see Figure 5.4) as
increase of Σ-UMP; the enhanced rate of adenine 5′-nucleotide formation
was obtained from the ^{14}[C]glycine incorporation data in the isolated perfused
liver (the spec. act. of ^{14}[C]glycine was measured at the beginning and the
end of the experiment)

	Uracil 5′-nucleotides after galactosamine	*Adenine-5′-nucleotides after D,L-ethionine*
Stimulation of nucleotide *de novo* synthesis	13-fold	14-fold
Rate of stimulated synthesis (nmol/min × g)	5.7	2.6
Rate of trapping (nmol/min × g)	28.4	7.7
Ratio of activities $\dfrac{\text{trapping}}{\text{synthesis}}$	5	3

and for all the consequences of this deviation. The different suscept-
ibilities of several animals to D-galactosamine were also traced to
different activity correlations[3]. It is, of course, necessary to determine
these activity correlations quantitatively under conditions which
approach the *in vivo* situation as closely as possible.

The dissimilarity of the D,L-ethionine and the D-galactosamine
model as far as the further pathologic sequences of events are concerned
is due mainly to two factors: one is the difference of the metabolic
processes in which uracil and adenine nucleotides, respectively, are
involved. The other has to do with the absolute levels of the respective
triphosphates. Their reduction to about 20% of normal means an UTP
content of 50, but an ATP content of about 500 nmol/g! Since the
K_m values of most ATP- and UTP-dependent reactions are in the
order of $1-5 \times 10^{-4}$ M, it is obvious that this reduction affects the
UTP-dependent processes more than those working with ATP.

In this context, let me add a word to the limits of the use of Atkinson's
energy charge concept[7] which has proved its merit in a number of
metabolic situations. The ratio of the adenosine phosphates plays a
regulatory role in those ATP-dependent reactions which are near
equilibrium *in vivo*[8]; also, competitive and especially allosteric effects of
any one of the adenosine phosphates depend on the adenylate energy
charge. However, for ATP-dependent processes which are irreversible
in the intracellular milieu—and many biosynthetic processes belong to
that group—only the local concentration of ATP and its affinity to the
respective enzyme are of importance. For example, D-galactosamine
treatment reduces the UTP level but does not change significantly the
uridylate energy charge. Nevertheless, RNA synthesis and glycogen
formation via UDPG are strongly depressed. On the other hand,
ethionine poisoning of the liver lowers both the ATP content and the
adenylate energy charge resulting, for instance, in a reduction of
gluconeogenesis and of urea synthesis; however, an increase of the
energy charge above the normal level does not enhance gluconeogenesis
for which an ATP half-saturation content of 590 nmol/g was measured
in the isolated perfused liver[6]. It appears that the level of ATP saturation of the limiting kinase is responsible for the ATP dependency of
glucose synthesis.

The depression of the UTP content of the liver (and concomitantly
the UDP, UMP, UDPG, and UDPGal level) itself is necessary but not
sufficient to explain the pathologic consequences of the D-galactosamine

treatment. We know experimental and physiological situations in which the UTP content drops below the critical 80 nmol/g, but which are not accompanied by irreversible cell damage. One of them is the uridine reversal of the D-galactosamine-induced UTP deficiency[9] (Figure 5.5). Due to the high hepatic activity of uridine kinase, administration of this nucleoside to D-galactosamine-treated rats raises the content of UTP (and of course also of other uridylates) within 20 min above the threshold level and within 70 min up to the normal value. It depends entirely on the time interval between the D-galactosamine and the uridine injection whether liver injury will develop 24 hours later[3]; uridine will protect young adult rats completely if administered as late as three hours after D-galactosamine but if given five hours after the amino sugar it will be without any protective effect. This means, that the UTP level must be below the threshold concentration for a minimum length of time in order to provoke irreversible cell damage. We call this trough in the concentration–time diagram of a substance the Metabolite Deficit Period.

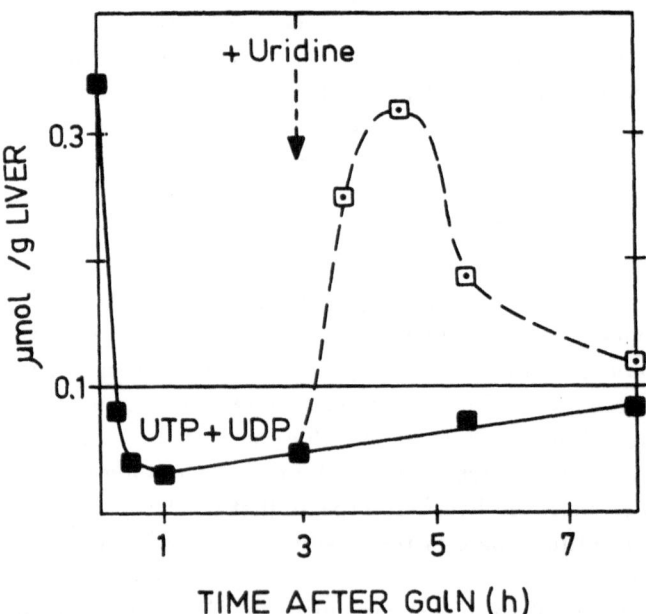

FIGURE 5.5   Effect of uridine administration on uridine phosphate contents of rat liver. 1.85 mmol GalN/kg body wt. injected at zero time, 3 mmol uridine/kg three hours later

The involvement of the time factor in the pathogenicity of a meta-bolic aberration has several implications: It provides the cell with a safe area for physiologically occurring deviations from the normal steady state, e.g. after feeding, heavy exercise etc. Furthermore, the dynamic state of the cell constituents requires that the turnover of each molecule, i.e. the relative velocities of its synthesis and its breakdown are adjusted to result in a steady-state concentration compatible with and necessary for cell viability and function. If only one leg of this cycle is disturbed, the substance will either accumulate or become deficient. Both can be detrimental to the cell as witnessed by several storage diseases on one hand and by fatal deficiencies on the other. If the liver is depleted of UTP, UDPG and UDPGal, then, RNA synthesis[9], glycogen synthesis[10] and maybe some other glycosylations[11] are strongly reduced and so will be the contents of many macromolecules derived from or dependent on these processes.

In most cases, a cell can bear a certain irregularity of synthesis and sometimes it can adjust the degradative processes to the changed syn-thetic rates, e.g. during starvation[12]. But there is a 'point of no return' for every cell constituent beyond which the deficiency results in an irreparable damage. This point of irreversibility depends, as we have seen, on the relation of the velocities of synthesis and degradation. The pathologic consequences of a Deficit Period, as I have defined it, will therefore be influenced by the rate of breakdown of the most critical cell constituent. This correlation has been most clearly established in comparative studies of D-galactosamine action on adult, neonatal and regenerating rat liver[13,14]; it was observed that neonatal and partially hepatectomised rats do not respond to comparable D-galactosamine doses with the hepatitis-like liver injury seen in adult animals. This D-galactosamine refractory state of the liver correlates with phases of active cell proliferation. It is known that under these conditions the rates of degradative processes are significantly reduced[15]. One would, therefore, assume that during proliferation and net synthesis of cellular matter the Deficit Period established for livers of normal adult animals does not retard the synthetic processes long enough, to reach the point of irreversibility (Figure 5.6). This interpretation implies that an *extension* of the Deficit Period *will* result in hepatic injury; exactly that was observed after repeated D-galactosamine administration to hepa-tectomised animals[14].

The impact of enzyme activity correlations and of the Metabolite

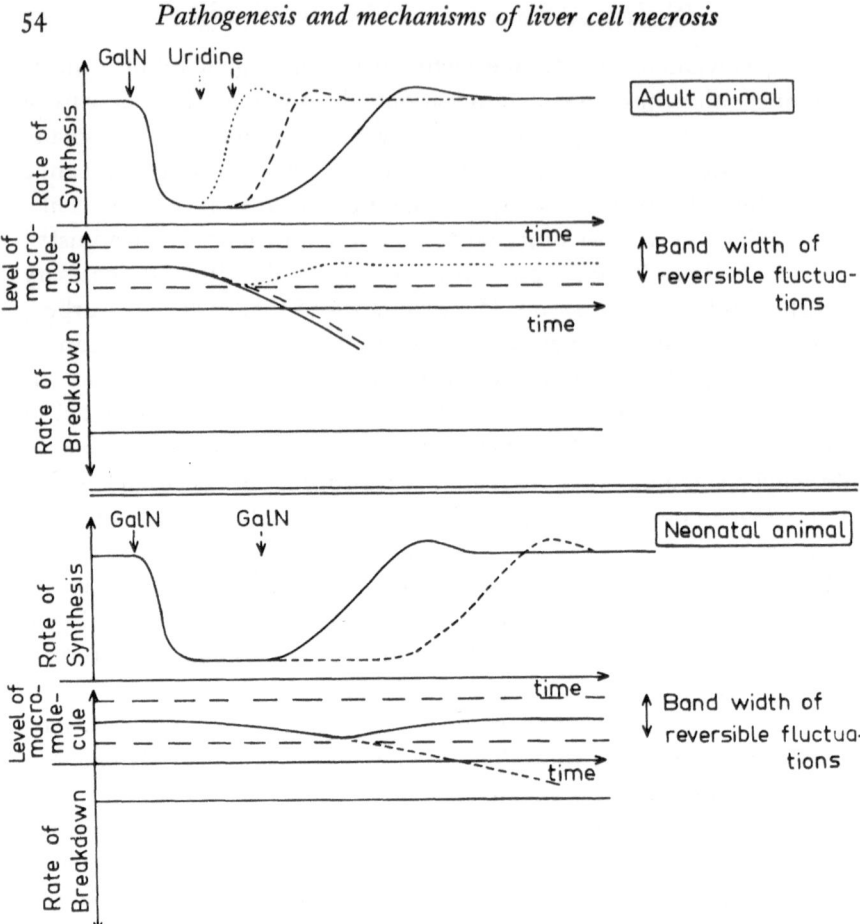

FIGURE 5.6   Scheme of the interdependence of the Metabolite Deficit Period and the turnover of cell constituents. Solid lines: effects of a single injection of D-galactosamine. Dotted lines: effects of uridine given *ca*. three hours after GalN. Broken lines: effects of uridine given *ca*. five hours after GalN (upper part); effects of second GalN injection (lower part)

Deficit Period on cell viability became clearly evident from these observations. It could also be demonstrated in a variety of other metabolic situations where rates of syntheses and metabolite levels were altered for certain periods of time[3]. Every one of these investigations emphasised the importance of quantitative analyses of concentrations, of reaction rates under *in vivo* conditions, and of the time course of the alterations under study. I do not doubt that the analytical principles outlined here will be applicable to many other pathological processes and necessary for the elucidation of biochemical sequences leading to cell necrosis and cell death. But it will be necessary to conduct quantitative measurements on all relevant levels of experimentation including histochemistry, autoradiography and even light and electron microscopy. In short, we are urged to proceed to quantitative pathology.

REFERENCES

1. Keppler, D., Lesch, R., Reutter, W. and Decker, K. (1968). Experimental hepatitis induced by D-galactosamine. *Exp. Molec. Pathol.*, **9**, 279–290
2. Decker, K. and Keppler, D. (1972). Galactosamine-induced liver injury. In: *Progress in Liver Diseases*, **Vol. 4**, 183–199 (H. Popper and F. Schaffner, editors) (New York: Grune and Stratton)
3. Decker, K. and Keppler, D. (1974). Galactosamine hepatitis. Key role of the nucleotide deficiency period in the pathogenesis of cell injury and cell death. *Rev. Physiol. Biochem. Pharmacol.*, **Vol. 71**, 77–106 (Berlin, Heidelberg, New York: Springer Verlag)
4. Pausch, J., Wilkening, J., Nowack, J. and Decker, K. (1975) Control of pyrimidine biosynthesis in the isolated perfused liver. Feedback inhibition of glutamine-dependent carbamoyl phosphate synthetase. *Eur. J. Biochem.*, **53**, 349–356
5. Farber, E. (1973). ATP and cell integrity. *Fed. Proc.*, **32**, 1533–1539
6. Wilkening, J., Nowack, J. and Decker, K. (1975). The dependence of glucose formation from lactate on the adenosine triphosphate content in the isolated perfused rat liver. *Biochim. Biophys. Acta*, **392**, 299–309
7. Atkinson, D. E. and Walton, G. M. (1967). Adenosine triphosphate conservation in metabolic regulation. *J. Biol. Chem.*, **242**, 3239–3241
8. Stubbs, M., Veech, R. L. and Krebs, H. A. (1972). Control of the redox state of the nicotinamide-adenine dinucleotide couple in rat liver cytoplasm. *Biochem. J.*, **126**, 59–65
9. Keppler, D., Pausch, J. and Decker, K. (1974). Selective uridine triphosphate deficiency induced by D-galactosamine in liver and reversed by pyrimidine nucleotide precursors. Effect on ribonucleic acid synthesis. *J. Biol. Chem.*, **249**, 211–216
10. Keppler, D. and Decker, K. (1969). Studies on the mechanism of galactosamine hepatitis: Accumulation of galactosamine-1-phosphate and its inhibition of UDP-glucose pyrophosphorylase. *Eur. J. Biochem.*, **10**, 219–225
11. Bauer, C., Lukaschek, R. and Reutter, W. (1974). Studies on the Golgi apparatus. Cumulative inhibition of protein and glycoprotein secretion by D-galactosamine. *Biochem. J.*, **142**, 221–230
12. Schimke, R. T. and Doyle, D. (1970). Control of enzyme levels in animal tissues. *Ann. Rev. Biochem.*, **39**, 929–976

13. Reutter, W., Bauer, C. and Lesch, R. (1970). On the mechanism of action of galactosamine: Different response to D-galactosamine of rat liver during development. *Die Naturwissenschaften*, **57**, 674–675

14. Reutter, W., Bauer, C., Bachmann, W. and Lesch, R. (1975). The galactosamine-refractory regenerating rat liver. In: *Liver Regeneration after Experimental Injury*, 259–272 (R. Lesch and W. Reutter, editors) (New York: Stratton Intercontinental Medical Book Corp.)

15. Scornik, O. A. (1972). Decreased *in vivo* disappearance of labelled liver protein after partial hepatectomy. *Biochem. Biophys. Res. Commun.*, **47**, 1063–1066

CHAPTER 6

Pathogenesis of hepatic necrosis caused by amanitin-albumin conjugate

L. Fiume

The peptides amanitins are the most powerful toxins of the toadstool *Amanita phalloides*[1]. Their cytopathic effect is due to inhibition of eucaryotic RNA-polymerase B (for reviews see Refs. 2 and 3). The low molecular weight of these toxic peptides (about 900) accounts for their lack of antigenic power. In order to obtain an immune response against these toxins, some years ago an attempt was made to render β-amanitin antigenic by conjugating it with rabbit serum albumin[4]. The water soluble carbodiimide ethyl-CDI was employed as the coupling agent. An unexpected increase was found in the toxicity of β-amanitin after conjugation. The LD_{50} of β-amanitin is 0.4 μmol/kg in the mouse and after conjugation this decreases several times. Mice injected with a lethal dose of the conjugate died of an hepatic necrosis morphologically different from that observed following α-amanitin or β-amanitin administration. In mice killed by amanitin–albumin conjugates, ascites is often observed and the livers appear greatly enlarged and dark red. Histologic examination shows that sinusoidal spaces are extremely dilated. On the contrary in mice killed by free amanitin, liver congestion is rare and ascites is never observed.

A study of the early ultrastructural changes induced in mouse liver by amanitin–albumin conjugate explained these differences and showed that the conjugate brings about hepatic necrosis by a different mechanism from that of free amanitin[5].

Before describing the ultrastructural changes produced in the liver by the conjugate, I will give a brief description of the lesions caused by free amanitins. When injected into the commonly used laboratory animals, amanitins cause necrosis of the liver and, with the exception of the rat[6], of the kidney. In the liver only hepatocytes are damaged, while sinusoidal cells appear unaffected even after the administration of high doses. The first ultrastructural changes in hepatocytes are observed in the nuclei. Changes in cytoplasmic organelles appear much later. Damage of the nucleus can be summed up as follows[7]: (1) chromatin condensation, (2) break-up of nucleoli, with separation of fibrils from granules, (3) temporary increase in number of perichromatin granules and (4) accumulation of interchromatinic granules at the centre of nucleus (Figure 6.1).

Now I will deal with the morphologic changes detected in mouse liver at various time intervals after injection with 2 LD_{50} of an amanitin–bovine–albumin conjugate[5]. This conjugate had a molar ratio of amanitin to albumin of 1.9. Its LD_{50} per 10 g body weight was 2.5 μg. Since this amount of conjugate contains 70 pmol of amanitin, and the LD_{50} per 10 g body weight of free β-amanitin is 4000 pmol, the toxicity of β-amanitin increased 57 times after conjugation to albumin. The mice killed by 1 or 2 LD_{50} of this conjugate died in 3–5 days. One or three hours after administration of the conjugate no appreciable changes were visible in hepatocytes or sinusoidal cells. After six hours the typical nuclear lesions of amanitin were observed in sinusoidal cells (Figure 6.2). In these cells the proportion of condensed chromatin increased while the nucleoplasm was less electron-dense. The nucleoli appeared to be fragmented with segregation of fibrillar and granular components. A large number of perichromatin and interchromatin granules were seen at varying distances from the nucleolar fragments. At this time (six hours) no lesions were seen in hepatocytes.

After 24 hours the sinusoidal spaces had become appreciably larger; most of the sinusoids did not contain endothelial or Kupffer cells any more; the sinusoids were directly bounded by the surface of hepatocytes, the microvilli of which jutted out directly into the lumen. At this time (24 hours) no glycogen is left in hepatocytes and many lipid droplets had appeared while the nuclei appeared to be intact.

After 48 hours the sinusoidal spaces appeared even more conspicuously enlarged than before. No sinusoidal cells could be observed under electron microscope (Figure 6.3). Severe fatty degeneration was found in the vast majority of hepatocytes, whose nuclei, however, appeared basically unchanged.

After 72 hours in some areas the sinusoids showed marked ectasia and were full of blood cells. The fatty degeneration of hepatocytes was even more severe; some appeared to be necrotic. Large cytoplasmic vacuoles

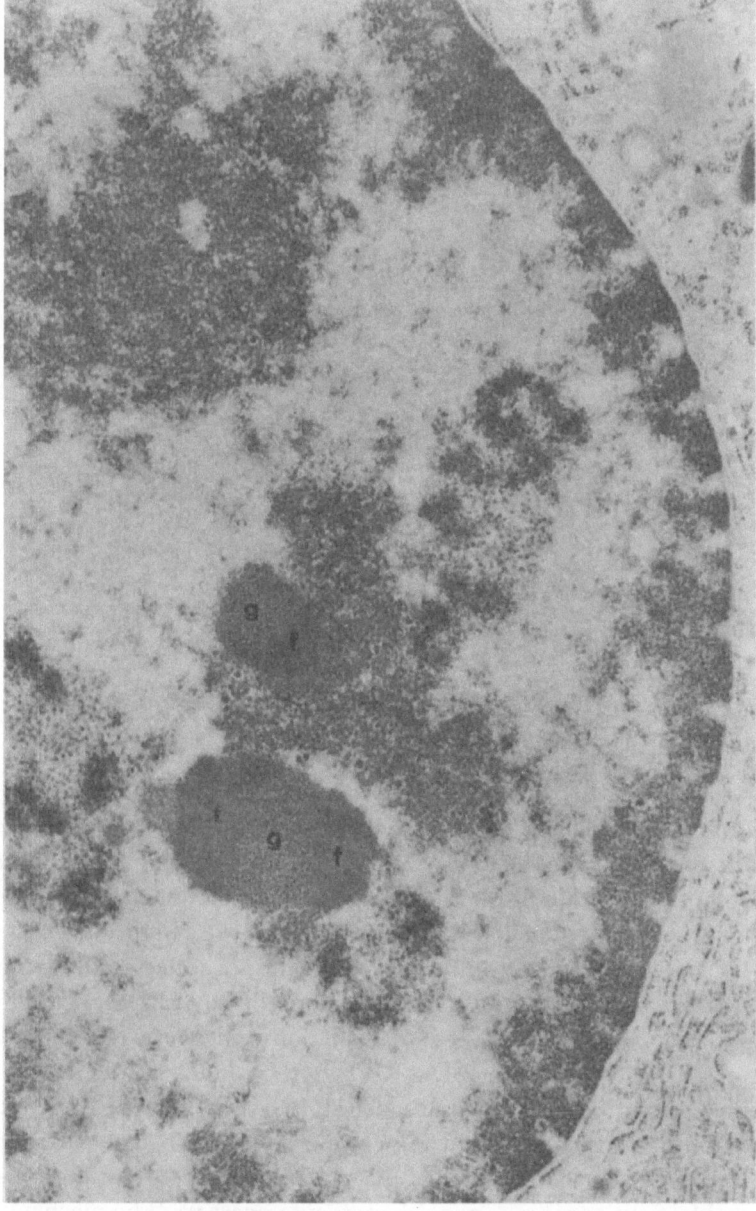

FIGURE 6.1 Nucleus of a mouse hepatocyte three hours after intraperitoneal injection of α-amanitin (5 μg/10 g body wt.). The quantities of condensed chromatin have risen. Two nucleolar fragments can be seen. They show separation of fibrillar (f) and granular (g) components into distinct areas (× 32 400)

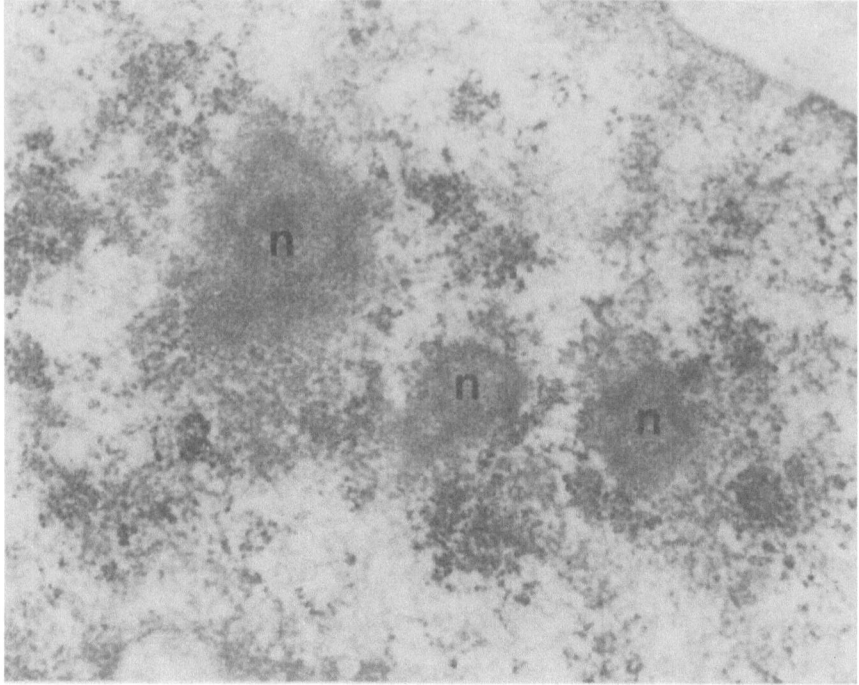

FIGURE 6.2   Nucleus of a mouse liver sinusoidal cell six hours after intraperitoneal injection of amanitin–albumin conjugate. Three nucleolar fragments (n) are visible (× 60 000)

were seen in some hepatocytes; they were usually near the nucleus and sometimes deformed it. Vacuole-containing hepatocytes were damaged in other ways too. Their nuclei had shrunk; larger quantities of condensed chromatin were present and nucleoli were abnormally compact. No fragmentation of nucleoli was however observed (Figure 6.4).

In conclusion amanitin–albumin conjugate produced the typical lesions of amanitin in sinusoidal cells (endothelial cells and Kupffer cells). No lesions characteristic of amanitin poisoning were ever observed in hepatocytes, at least when only 2 LD_{50} of the conjugate were injected. In hepatocytes non-specific nuclear lesions were preceded by fatty degeneration and vacuolation of the cytoplasm which began to develop only after most sinusoidal cells had disappeared. Therefore, the damage of sinusoidal cells appears to cause hepatocyte necrosis. The mechanism of this necrosis is not clear, but we might suppose that the disappearance of sinusoidal cells increases the leakage of the fluid component of the blood from sinusoidal spaces and that the impairment of hepatic circu ·

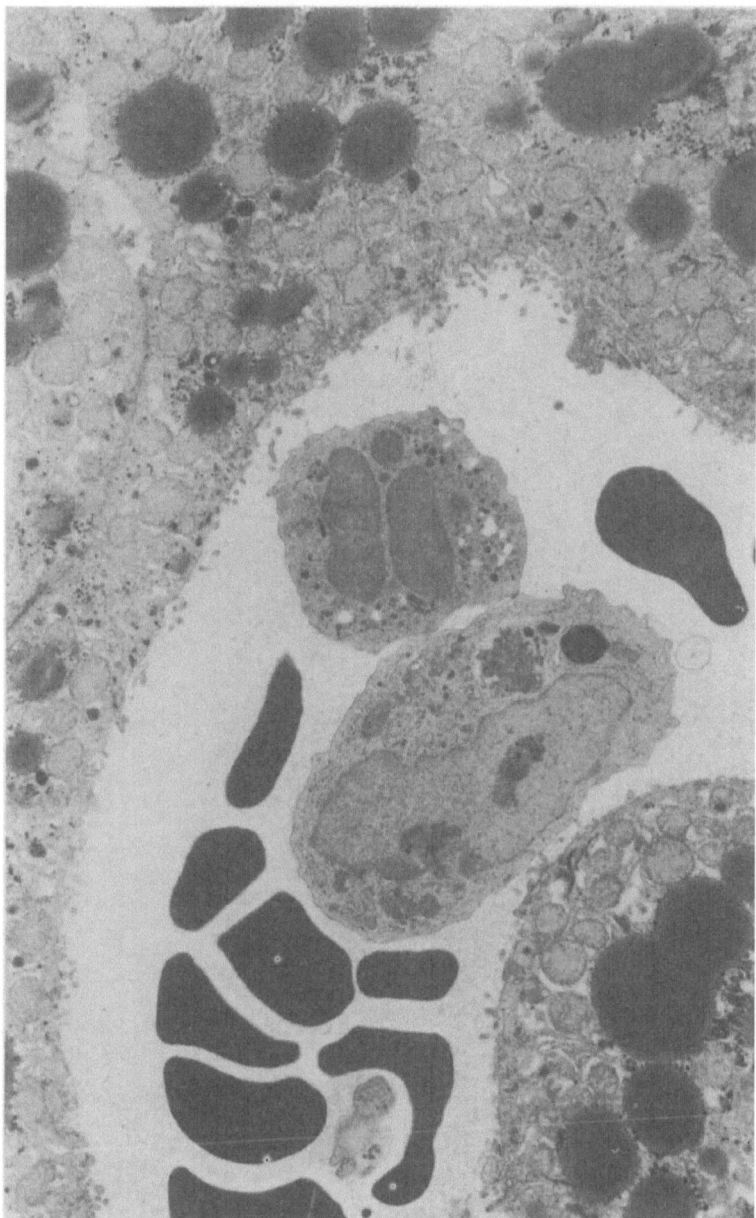

FIGURE 6.3 Mouse killed 48 hours after amanitin–albumin conjugate injection. The sinusoidal surface of the hepatocytes directly limits the sinusoidal lumen (× 5400)

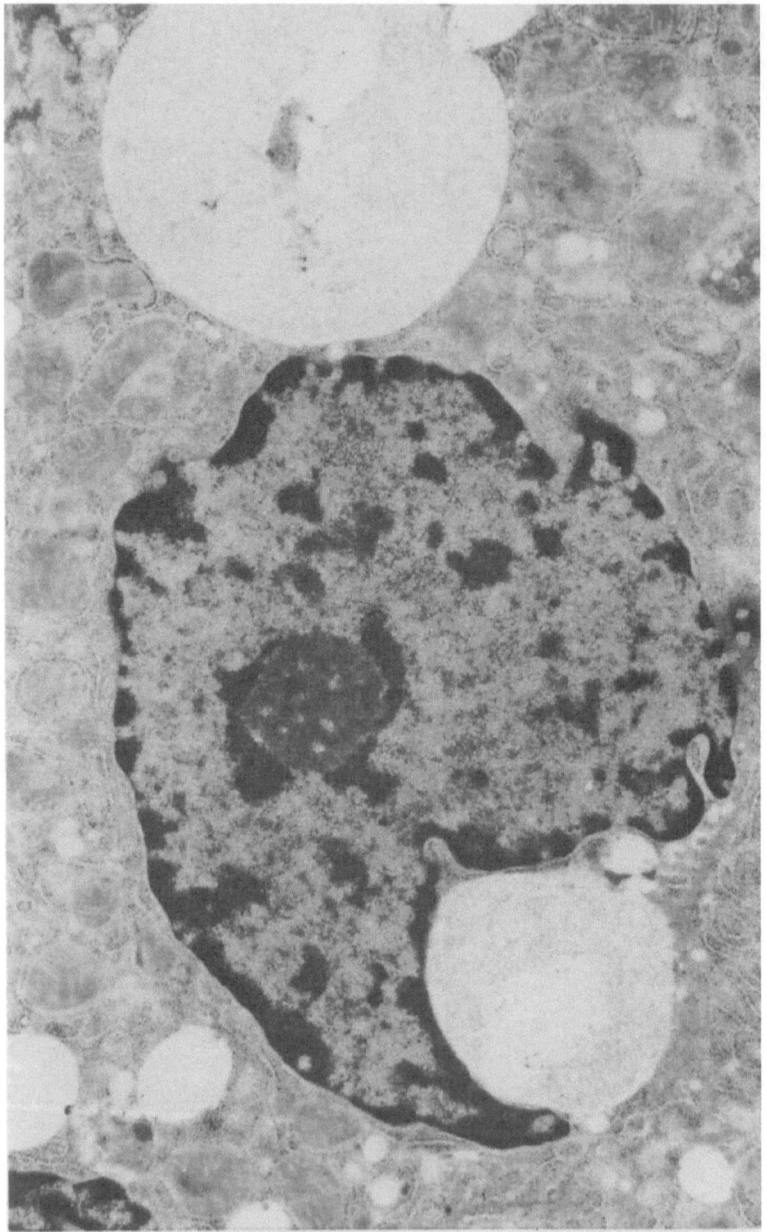

FIGURE 6.4 Hepatocyte of a mouse killed 72 hours after conjugate injection. In the cytoplasm large vacuoles and lipid droplets are visible. In the nucleus there is no fragmentation of nucleolus (× 19 800)

lation resulting from the thickening of the blood contributes to cause the necrosis of hepatocytes. The finding that in the livers of the animals killed by the conjugate, sinusoidal spaces were constantly filled with blood cells is consistent with a local haemoconcentration.

It is well known that proteins injected into animals are taken up by the cells of the reticuloendothelial system by pinocytosis[8]. In the liver both Kupffer and endothelial cells are involved in protein uptake[9]. When a protein is administered by intravenous or intraperitoneal route the largest amount of it is taken up by the liver sinusoidal cells[8]. It is likely that liver sinusoidal cells are the target of amanitin–albumin conjugate because this conjugate, like all other foreign proteins, is taken up by these cells.

This conclusion was supported by experiments *in vitro* which showed that the sensitivity of macrophages to amanitin–albumin conjugate was much higher than that of other kinds of cells[10,11]. Amanitin–albumin conjugate may exert its toxic activity directly because it inhibits RNA-polymerase B *in vitro*[5] or by releasing amanitin after penetration into the cells. The second mechanism is more likely because it is known that proteins which have penetrated into the cells by pinocytosis are digested by lysosomal enzymes[8].

These results indicate that the amanitin–albumin conjugate may be a tool to selectively kill those cells which display a high uptake of proteins.

Lastly I wish to reinforce another point. The liver sinusoidal cells remain unaffected after the administration of free amanitin, even in large amounts; the finding that these cells are damaged by amanitin–albumin conjugate indicates that they are susceptible to the action of amanitin but that the toxin is unable to penetrate them unless coupled to a protein and so forced to enter by pinocytosis.

This conclusion suggests a possible use of conjugates in biological research.

There are substances such as toxins and drugs, which have biological activity only in some cells. Sometimes it is difficult to assess whether they enter only the cells in which they are active or whether only within these cells do they find the target of their action. For some of these substances this problem might be solved by conjugating them to a protein and by testing whether in cells with a high protein uptake the conjugates produce the same effects as are caused by free substances in target cells.

One example. Amanitin kills the cells of proximal convoluted tubules

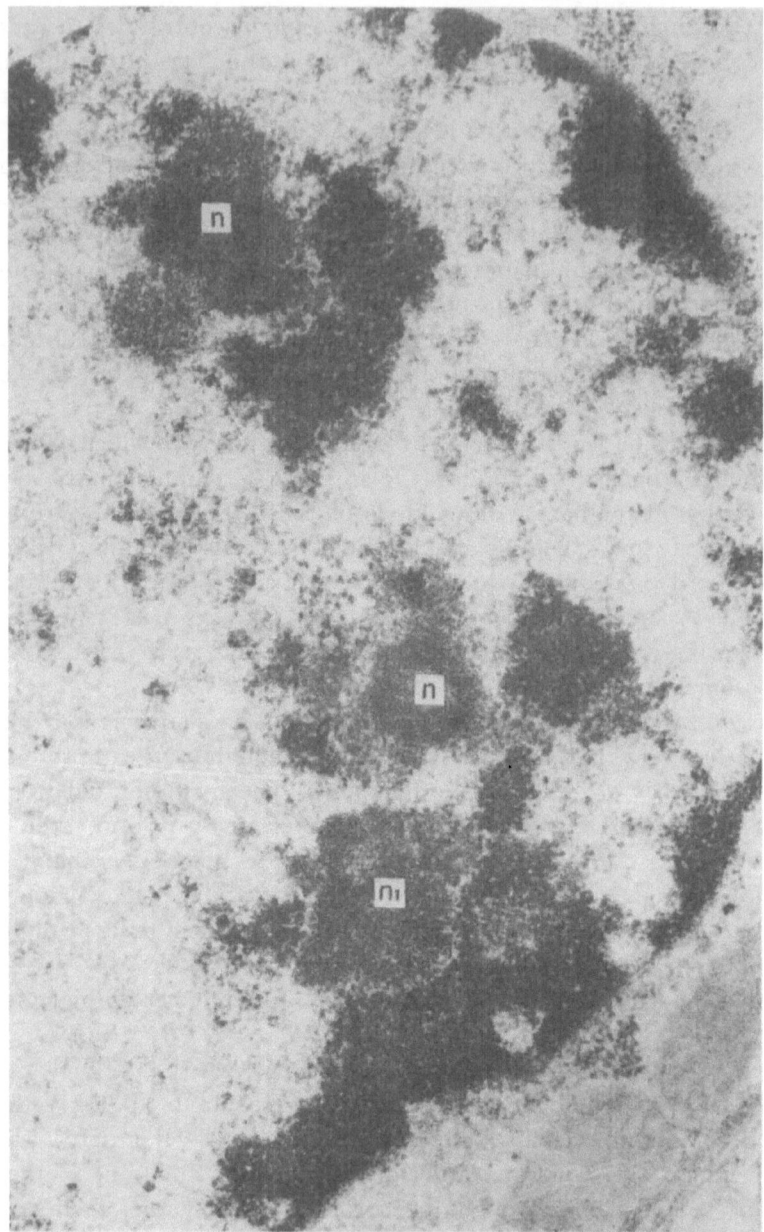

FIGURE 6.5   Nucleus of an epithelial cell in a proximal convoluted tubule of rat kidney 48 hours after injection of amanitin–albumin conjugate (0.5 mg/100 g body wt.). The chromatin is condensed. Fragments of nucleolus are visible (n). One of them (n₁) shows separation of fibrillar and granular components into distinct areas (× 54 000)

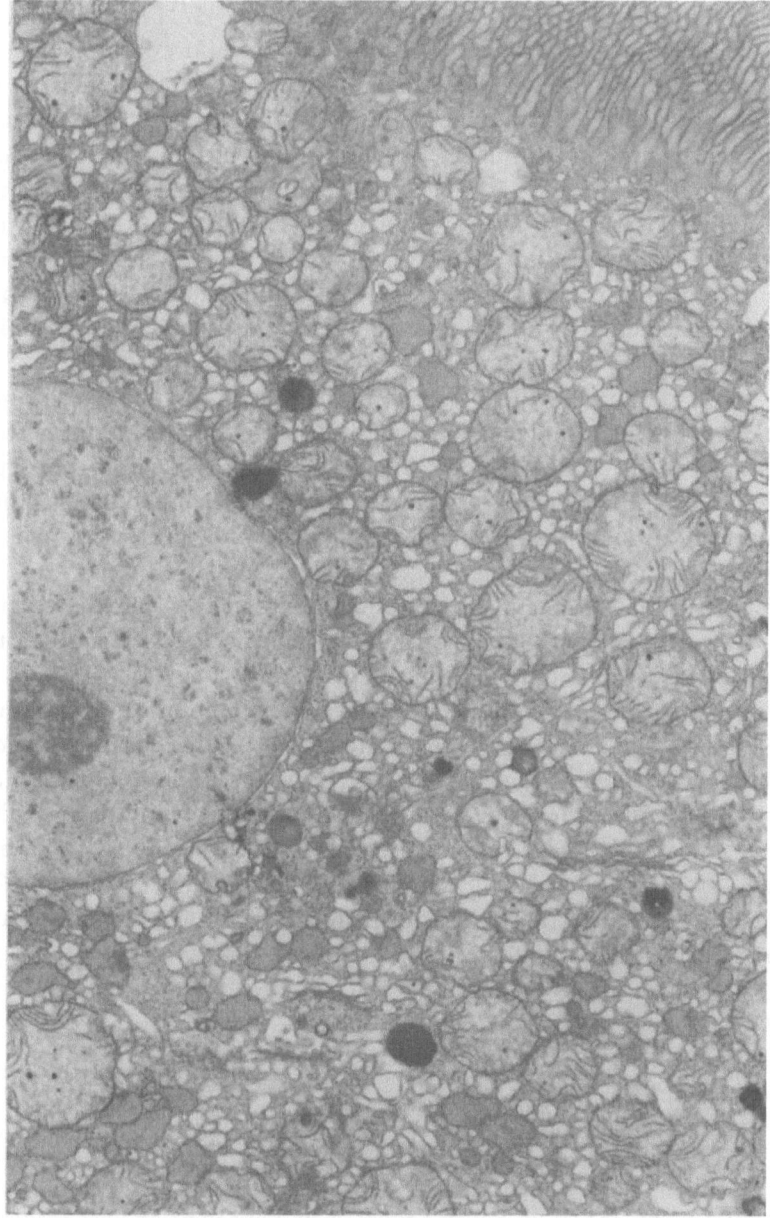

FIGURE 6.6 Epithelial cell in a proximal convoluted tubule of mouse kidney 24 hours after injection of phalloidin–albumin conjugate (80μg/10 g body wt.). The cisternae of the endoplasmic reticulum form vesicles (× 10 800)

of mouse kidney but it has no effect in the same cells in rat kidney[6]. This absence of lesions might be due to the failure of amanitin to penetrate the cells. Since the proximal convoluted tubule cells of rat kidney have been found to take up albumin[12,13], we tested the effect of an amanitin–albumin conjugate in these cells. We found that the conjugate produces the lesions typical of amanitin in these cells[14] (Figure 6.5). This observation indicates that the absence of lesions in the proximal convoluted tubule cells of rat kidney after amanitin administration is due to the inability of the toxin to enter these cells. When amanitin is coupled to albumin and forced to enter by pinocytosis, the typical lesions do appear.

A second example. Phalloidin is another toxic peptide in *Amanita phalloides*[1]. Rats and mice injected with this toxin die in 2–4 hours from hepatic necrosis. Dilatation of the endoplasmic reticulum with the appearance of large vacuoles in cytoplasm are the first ultrastructural changes in hepatocytes. Hepatocytes are the only cells damaged by phalloidin in mice and in rats.

Two possible explanations why phalloidin damages hepatocytes and not other cells are: (1) phalloidin enters only hepatocytes and (2) the target of this toxin is only found in hepatocytes.

We conjugated phalloidin to bovine serum albumin and administered the conjugate to mice[15]. We found the typical lesions of phalloidin in those cells which have a high protein uptake, such as liver sinusoidal cells and proximal convoluted tubule cells of kidney (Figure 6.6). This result indicates that at least for these cells (i.e. liver sinusoidal cells and kidney proximal convoluted tubule cells) the absence of lesions after phalloidin administration is due to inability of the free toxin to enter into the cells.

REFERENCES

1. Wieland, T. (1968). Poisonous principles of mushrooms of the genus *Amanita*. *Science*, **159**, 946–952
2. Fiume, L. and Wieland, T. (1970). Amanitins. Chemistry and action. *FEBS Letters*, **8**, 1–5
3. Chambon, P. (1974). Eucaryotic RNA-polymerases. In: *The Enzymes*, **Vol. 10**, 261–331 (P. B. Boyer, editor) (New York and London: Academic Press)
4. Cessi, C. and Fiume, L. (1969). Increased toxicity of β-amanitin when bound to a protein. *Toxicon*, **6**, 309–310
5. Derenzini, M., Fiume, L., Marinozzi, V., Mattioli, A., Montanaro, L.

and Sperti, S. (1973). Pathogenesis of liver necrosis produced by amanitin-albumin conjugates. *Lab. Invest.*, **29**, 150–158

6. Fiume, L., Marinozzi, V. and Nardi, F. (1969). The effects of amanitin poisoning on mouse kidney. *Brit. J. Exp. Pathol.*, **50**, 270–276

7. Marinozzi, V. and Fiume, L. (1971). Effects of α-amanitin on mouse and rat liver cell nuclei. *Exp. Cell Res.*, **67**, 311–322

8. Unanue, E. R. (1972). The regulatory role of macrophages in antigenic stimulation. *Adv. Immunol.*, **15**, 95–165

9. Kruse, H. and McMaster, P. D. (1949). The distribution and storage of blue antigenic azoproteins in the tissues of mice. *J. Exp. Med.*, **90**, 425–445

10. Barbanti-Brodano, G. and Fiume, L. (1973). Selective killing of macrophages by amanitin–albumin conjugates. *Nature New Biology*, **243**, 281–283

11. Fiume, L. and Barbanti-Brodano, G. (1974). Selective toxicity of amanitin–albumin conjugates for macrophages. *Experientia*, **30**, 76–77

12. Smetana, H. (1947). The permeability of the renal glomeruli of several mammalian species to labelled proteins. *Amer. J. Pathol.*, **23**, 255–267

13. Schiller, A. A., Schayer, R. W. and Hess, E. L. (1953). Fluorescein-conjugated bovine albumin. Physical and biological properties. *J. Gen. Physiol.*, **36**, 489–506

14. Bonetti, E., Derenzini, M. and Fiume, L. (1974). Lesions in the cells of proximal convoluted tubules in rat kidney induced by amanitin–albumin conjugate. *Virchows Arch.* (Abt. B.), **16**, 71–78

15. Barbanti-Brodano, G., Derenzini, M. and Fiume, L. (1974). Toxic action of phalloidin–albumin conjugate on cells with a high protein uptake. *Nature* (London), **248**, 63–65

CHAPTER 7

Amanitin poisoning in the dog

H. Faulstich and U. Fauser

So far, most experimental investigations concerning amanitin poisoning
have been done in the mouse or in the rat. In order to obtain conditions
which could be better compared to human intoxication, we chose the
dog for experiments. Among the amatoxins available, there are two
compounds, which can be radioactively labelled: ^{14}[C]O-methyl-γ-
amanitin and ^{3}[H]demethyl-O-methyl-γ-amanitin. Both these compounds exhibit shortcomings in *in vivo* experiments. O-methyl-γ-
amanitin is as toxic as α-amanitin, the label, but undergoes microsomal
oxidation. The second compound is probably stable under *in vivo*
conditions but is 15 times less toxic, and, as we know from the experiments of Chambon's laboratory[1], binds 10 times less effectively to
RNA-polymerase. We decided upon the first, more toxic compound.

With ^{14}[C]methyl-γ-amanitin we measured a rapid decrease in the
serum concentrations of the toxin in three dogs. The concentration
falls to zero after 5–6 hours[2]. Correspondingly the toxin is rapidly
excreted by the urine. After six hours 85–90% of the dose is excreted,
showing that the toxin (MW 918) is dialysed very well. In an artificial
dialysis system we measured 30% of the dialysis rate of urea. The
excreted amount of toxin in a dog, which had died with 0.12 mg/kg
body wt., enabled us to estimate the amount of amanitin, which could
maximally be absorbed by the liver. We calculated a lethal concentration
of 30 ng/g liver, which is two orders of magnitude lower than the value
for the phallotoxins[3].

Some dogs had a bile fistula (choledochus drainage); consequently
we could monitor radioactivity in the bile. The greater part of the
radioactivity in the bile was the metabolised label; about 40%, however,
was the unchanged toxin. This means that methyl-γ-amanitin, one of
the toxins with the highest affinity for RNA-polymerase, had passed the
liver cells without binding to the enzyme. This is in good agreement

with the observation that all dogs with a bile fistula survived doses which were 60% higher than the lethal dose in the dog. It may be concluded, thus, that the enterohepatic circulation is important for the course of intoxication. The lethal dose in the dog was determined to be 0.06–0.07 mg/kg body wt., which is the lowest dose known so far for mammals. The dogs developed all symptoms, which were also known from human intoxications with Amanita mushrooms.

We classified the dogs into four classes, which were characterised by the time of death and by the different symptoms. The first symptom, leading to death within 36 hours, was observed preferentially with higher doses and is characterised by hypoglycaemia with only a few necrotic cells in the liver. The phase of *hypo*glycaemia was preceded by a phase of *hyper*glycaemia within the first 12 hours of intoxication. The source of this high blood glucose value was glycogen, as already stated by O. Wieland and co-workers[4] in 1952 for the amanitin poisoned mouse. In the group of dogs, which died within the first 36 hours, the phase of hyperglycaemia was followed by a phase of hypoglycaemia with blood glucose values < 20 mg/100 ml serum while the dogs surviving this phase, never had values of blood glucose below 50 mg/ 100 ml serum. A second symptom was observed, when the lifetime of the hypoglycaemic dogs was prolonged by glucose infusions. By this the dogs survived 56 hours; the prognosis, however, could not be improved and all the dogs died. They developed a severe liver necrosis and a liver dystrophy and died in deep coma. The third symptom leading to death within about 80 hours was liver necrosis in combination with a fatal disturbance of blood coagulation. General bleeding occurred in various organs like the gut, the myocardium, the kidneys and the lungs. Less severe bleedings of this type were also observed in some dogs of the hypoglycaemic group. A fourth symptom, finally, was uraemia. These dogs lived longest; about 140 hours. Uraemia was observed only twice; in a dog, which was poisoned with 0.07 mg of amanitin/kg body wt., and in another dog, in which a fresh, cooked mushroom of 50 g was given orally. Further evidence for the classification into four clinical symptoms was given histologically.

The liver of the hypoglycaemic dogs was totally depleted of glycogen. A great part of the nuclei, however, appeared unaffected (Figure 7.1). In the group of dogs treated with glucose, besides the total destruction of the liver there was evidence for the infiltration of lymphoid cells into the liver (Figure 7.2). In the third group of dogs, which had died from

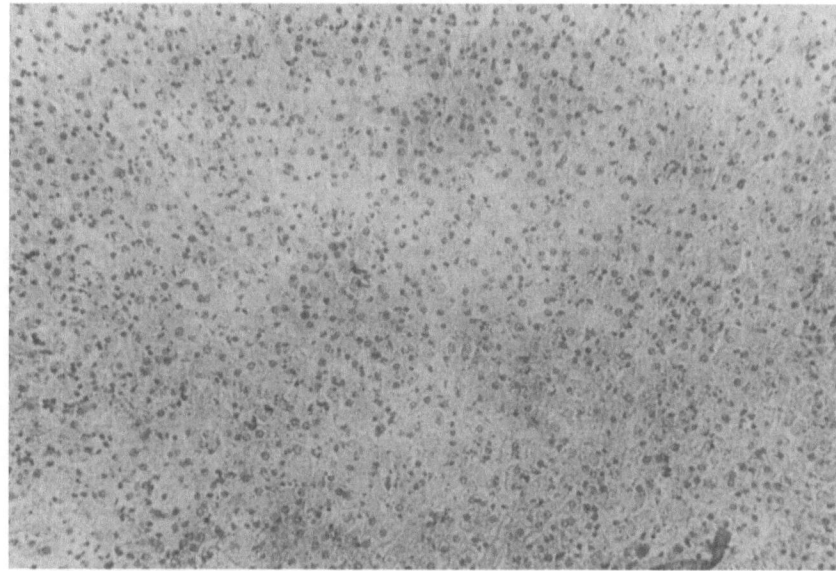

FIGURE 7.1   Liver of a dog, which had died from hypoglycaemia. Glycogen stain (not visible). Nuclei widely intact

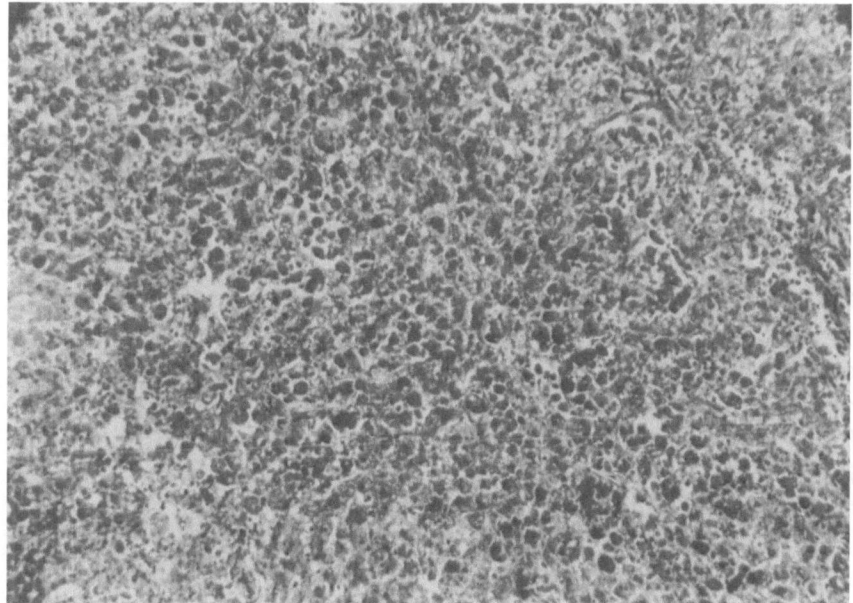

FIGURE 7.2   Liver of a dog, which had died in liver coma. Hematoxilin-eosin stain. Nearly all hepatocytes damaged, beginning infiltration of lymphoid cells

internal bleeding, the liver showed also necrosis of single cells and cell areas with mostly pycnotic nuclei (Figure 7.3). In this group the factors of the blood clotting system as well as the platelets and the fibrinogen had declined to almost zero.

The two dogs, which had also survived this critical phase and had died from uraemia, showed regeneration of the liver function as determined by a normal blood clotting system. Also the structure of the liver had normalised histologically. The tubuli in the kidney, however, were necrotic, causing severe uraemia in these two dogs, which led to death

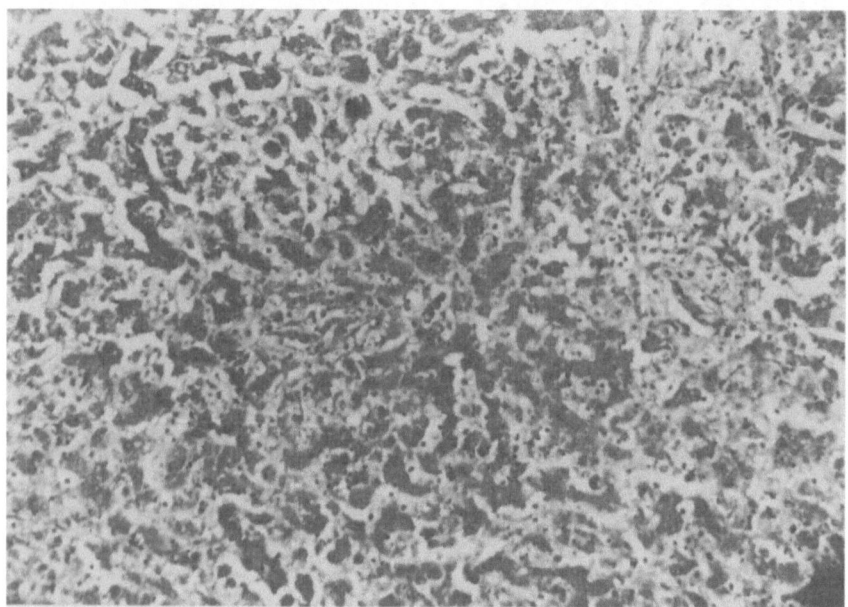

FIGURE 7.3   Liver of a dog, which had died in liver coma. Hematoxilin-eosin stain. Nearly all hepatocytes damaged, heavy infiltration of lymphoid cells

after six days (Figure 7.4). This was also proved by the high values of creatinine and urea in the serum. Death after six days is also known from human intoxication. Uraemia in man, however, is mostly described in combination with severe liver dystrophy.

In summary, then, I would like to conclude with three statements:

1. The amatoxins can pass the liver cell without being resorbed, and only very small amounts are necessary for liver destruction.
2. Among the symptoms observed, the early hypoglycaemia is a

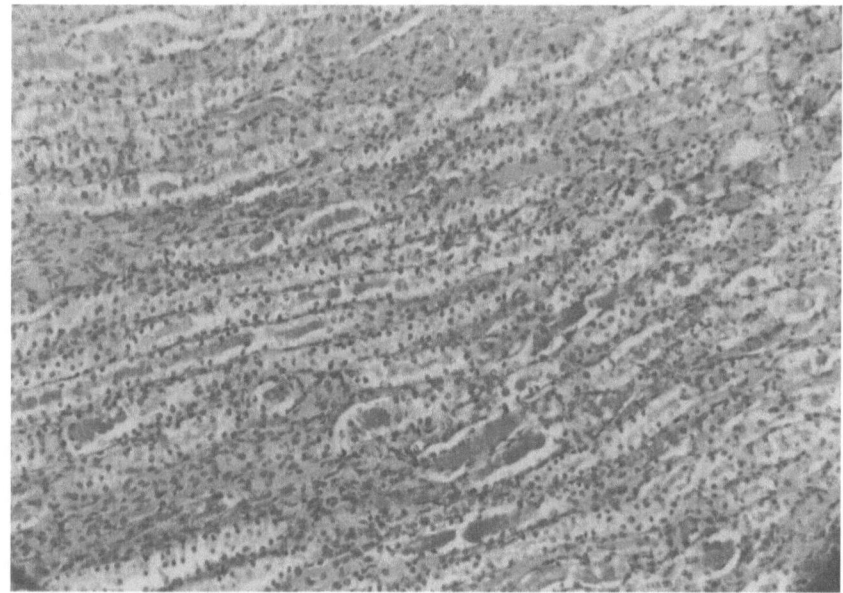

FIGURE 7.4   Kidney of a dog, which had died with uraemia. Hematoxilin-eosin stain. Necrosis of kidney cells

critical phase only in the dog, not in human intoxications. Disturbance of blood coagulation and liver necrosis are similar to human intoxication.

3. The liver dystrophy in the amanitin-poisoned dog balanced with glucose is, as far as we know, a first model for a liver dystrophy, which may perhaps become useful for clinical research. However, since only the dogs treated with glucose developed a dystrophy of the liver, the routine treatment of mushroom intoxicated humans with glucose needs a revaluation.

REFERENCES

1. Cochet-Meilhac, M. and Chambon, P. (1974). Animal DNA-dependent RNA polymerases. 11. Mechanism of the inhibition of RNA polymerases B by amatoxins. *Biochim. Biophys. Acta*, **353**, 160–184
2. Faulstich, H. and Fauser, U. (1974). Untersuchungen zur Frage der Hämodialyse bei der Knollenblätterpilzvergiftung. *Dtsch. Med. Wschr.*, **98**, 2258–2259
3. Wieland, Th., Faulstich, H., Jahn, W., Govindan, V. M., Puchinger, H.,

Kopitar, Z., Schmaus, H. and Schmitz A. (1972). Über Antamanid XIV: Zur Wirkungsweise des Antamanids. *Hoppe Seyler's Z. Physiol. Chem.*, **353**, 1337–1345

4. Wieland, O., Fischer, H. E. and Reiter, E. (1952). Über den Wirkungsmechanismus des Knollenblätterpilzgiftes α-Amanitin. *Arch. Exp. Pathol. Pharmakol.*, **215**, 75–84

CHAPTER 8

Pathogenesis of frog virus 3 induced hepatitis in mice

M. Elharrar, A. Bingen, J. L. Gendrault and A. Kirn

Cellular death in the course of a virus infection is usually related to the multiplication of the virions in the cells but it is not actually established whether it is the synthesis of the structural components or that of specific cytotoxic proteins which are involved in the cytopathic effect. At the same time, the significance of the cut-off of the cellular metabolism and its role in the process of cell necrosis are not yet clearly understood. The acute degenerative hepatitis induced by frog virus 3 (FV 3) in mice provides evidence that necrosis of hepatocytes can be induced by structural viral proteins and that the switch off of the cellular metabolism may be related to this necrosis.

FROG VIRUS 3

Frog virus 3 (FV 3) is a polyhedral deoxyribovirus which has been primarily isolated from a renal carcinoma of *Rana pipiens*[1]. Similar virus strains have been isolated from healthy frogs and tumours could not be induced by inoculation of embryos and larvae[2]. FV 3 grows in the cytoplasm of amphibian, bird and mammalian cells provided that the temperature is less than 30 °C. Figure 8.1 shows a pseudocrystalline structure consisting of the assembly of virus particles in the cytoplasm of a BHK cell. Though most of the virions remain in the cell until its necrosis, some particles leave the cell by budding at the cytoplasmic membrane[3]. In the course of this process, the portion of the membrane surrounding the virion acquires viral specific antigens[4]. At 37 °C the multiplication of FV 3 is completely blocked and no detectable viral material is synthesised[5]. However, under these conditions, the

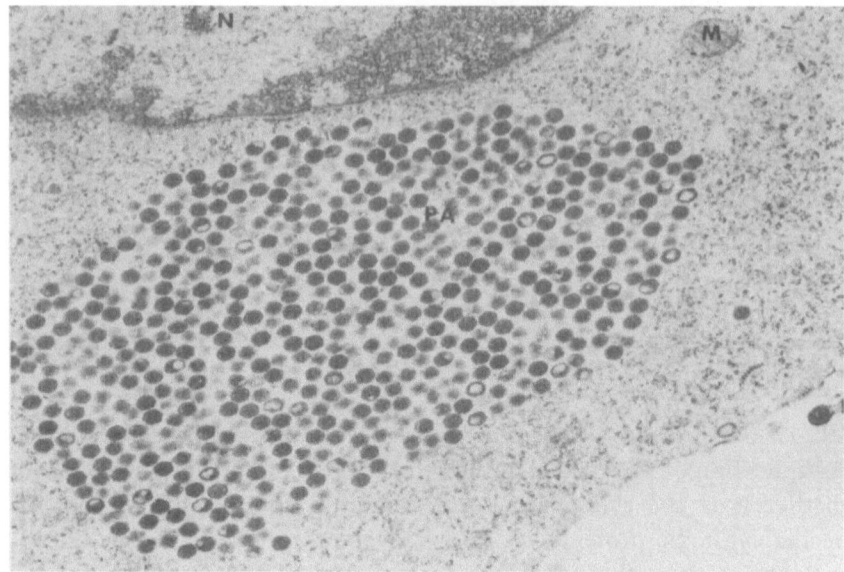

FIGURE 8.1   Baby hamster kidney cells (BHK$_{21}$ strain) infected with FV 3 and incubated at 26 °C for 10 hours. In the cytoplasm many particles at the same degree of maturation are packed into a pseudocrystalline structure (Fixation: glutaraldehyde. Postfixation: osmium tetroxide. Staining: uranyl-acetate and lead citrate, × 18 000)

macro-molecular metabolism of the infected cells is completely shut-off[6].

THE DEGENERATIVE HEPATITIS INDUCED BY FV 3 IN MICE

Intraperitoneal or intravenous inoculation of FV 3 into mice produces an acute degenerative hepatitis which leads to the death of the animal within 24 hours[7,8]. This hepatitis is of toxic origin since the virus does not multiply in the mice and since the same effect may be obtained with inactivated virus[9]. When the distribution of 20 lethal doses (LD) of radioactive virus was studied in the bodies of the mice it could be determined that 73% of the label found in the organs was associated with the liver six hours after inoculation[10]. It has been calculated that the lethal dose found in the liver corresponded to 1.75 μg of FV 3 proteins. The correlation between the outbreak of the hepatitis and the presence of the virus in the liver could be established by challenging immunised animals with lethal doses of radioactive FV 3. In immunised mice the penetration of the virus into the liver was inhibited, parenchymal damage did not occur and the animals survived[10].

EARLY MORPHOLOGICAL LESIONS INDUCED BY FV 3

Except for an acute stasis of the proximal segment of the intestine and of the spleen, FV 3 poisoning produces mainly damage of the liver characterised by massive parenchymal necrosis of the hepatocytes. Electron microscopic observations show that the primary lesions appear in the nuclei of the hepatocytes[11]. Nuclear damage can be summed up as followed:

1. modification in the shape of the nuclei and important chromatin condensation;
2. increase in the number of perichromatin granules and accumulation of interchromatin granules in dense clusters at the centre of the nucleus;
3. appearance in the nucleoplasm, which had lost its fibrillar material, of nuclear bodies composed of small filaments;
4. increase of the fibrillar material of the nucleolus.

It should be emphasised that, when the nuclear lesions were complete, the cytoplasm remained completely free of changes (Figure 8.2).

CHROMATIN

As early as one hour after the infection with 20 LD the nuclei lose their spherical shape and present a very irregular outline without any visible damage to the nuclear membrane. The condensation of the chromatin around the inner membrane of the nucleus is the most striking phenomenon (Figure 8.3); it increases as time progresses. Another noticeable change is the increase in the number of perichromatin granules.

NUCLEOPLASM

Accumulation of interchromatin granules in dense clusters at the centre of the nucleus is a very constant and early change noticed in all the damaged nuclei (Figures 8.2 and 8.3). The use of the 'regressive

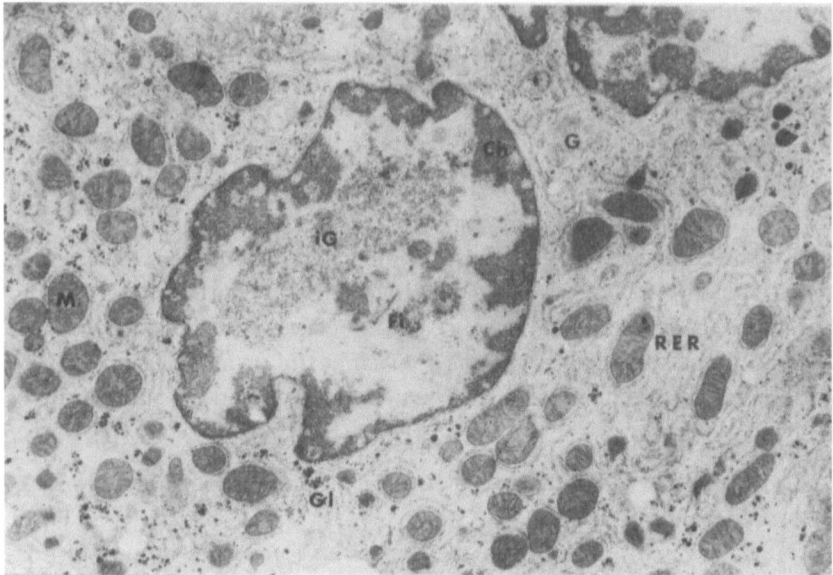

FIGURE 8.2   Mouse hepatocyte nucleus four hours after IP inoculation of 20 LD of FV 3. The nucleus presents an irregular shape and an important margination of the perinuclear chromatin. In the nucleoplasm a dense cluster of interchromatin granules is noticeable. The surrounding cytoplasm does not present any visible change; the mitochondria and the endoplasmic reticulum have retained their structural integrity (× 11 000)

coloration' of Bernhard[12] showed that the fibrillar material of the nucleoplasm had completely disappeared[11]. Another remarkable change is the appearance of filamentous nuclear bodies. These inclusions, which show no preferential localisation in the nucleoplasm, appear to be composed of numerous filaments ranging from 7–8 nm in diameter (Figure 8.4). The filaments are arranged roughly parallel to one another with spaces of 10 nm between them. Histochemical methods showed that these inclusions were of a proteinous nature[13]. The significance of these filamentous bodies is as yet completely unknown.

NUCLEOLUS

The alterations of the nucleolus appear as late as the damage of the chromatin and of the nucleoplasm appears early. Figure 8.2 shows an hepatocyte nucleus four hours after the administration of 20 LD which presents all the changes described above but whose nucleolus does not

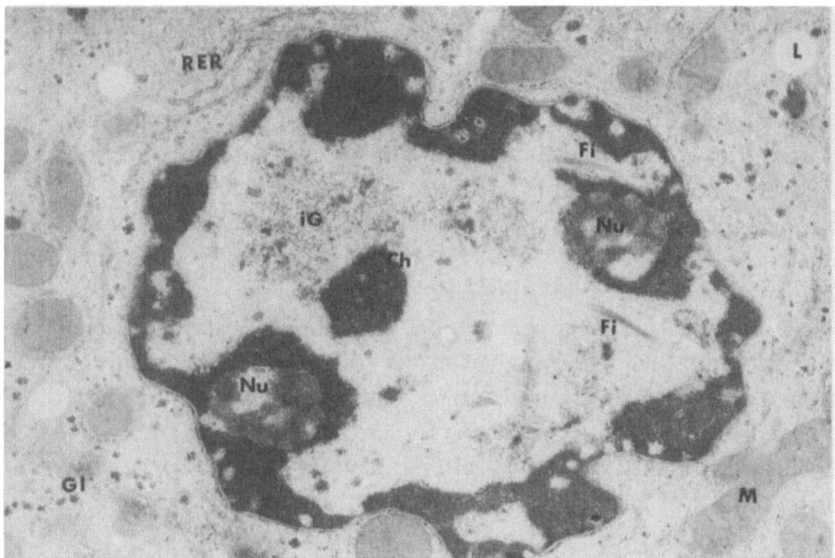

FIGURE 8.3 Mouse hepatocyte-nucleus four hours after IP inoculation of 20 LD of FV 3. The most striking nuclear changes are summed up in this picture: irregular shape of the nucleus, margination of the chromatin, assembling of the interchromatin granules in dense clusters and appearance of two filamentous inclusions near the nucleolus which does not present any particular changes (× 11 000)

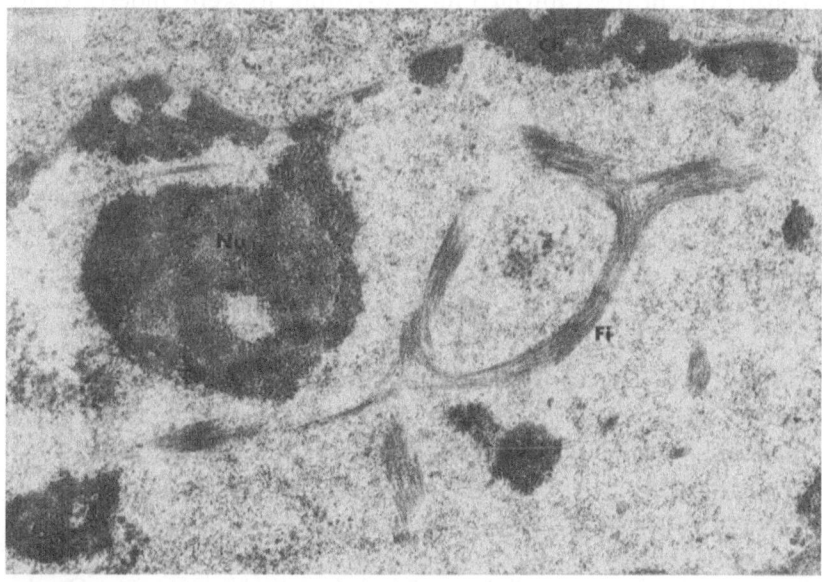

FIGURE 8.4 Nuclear inclusions in an hepatocyte nucleus of a FV 3 infected mouse. The inclusions whose shape and size are variable are composed of numerous filaments of 7 to 8 nm in diameter (× 28 600)

reveal any particular lesion. The first recognisable damage in hepatocyte nucleoli from infected mice is a slight increase of the fibrillar
material. Later on, relatively speaking, in the course of the infection, the
nucleolus shows noticeable changes essentially characterised by the
disappearance of the granular material whereas the fibrillar component
remains present (Figure 8.5). It should be stressed that nucleolar
fragmentation is only rarely observed.

The kinetic of the appearance of the above described lesions is
dependent on the dose of virus used. When a lower inoculum was
employed (1 LD) the same changes could be demonstrated but they
appeared later. In these conditions the first noticeable alterations of the
nucleus were visible 5–7 hours after infection. Just as it was observed
with a high dose of virus, so the nuclear lesions were complete before
the cytoplasm showed any alteration with 1 LD.

BIOCHEMICAL CHANGES INDUCED BY FV 3

Since the morphological observations demonstrated nuclear damage in
the hepatocytes of FV 3 infected mice, experiments were undertaken to
determine the underlying biochemical changes. It could be established
that DNA, RNA and, to a lesser extent, protein synthesis were rapidly
inhibited a few hours after infection[14]. As for the RNA synthesis, a
50% inhibition of ^{3}[H]orotic acid incorporation in the liver was noticed
three hours after the inoculation of 20 LD. There was no preferential
inhibition of the ribosomal or the messenger RNA synthesis as could be
demonstrated by studying:

1. the incorporation in RNA isolated from liver polysomes
2. the incorporation in the nucleolar and nucleoplasmic fractions[14].

In hepatocyte nuclei from infected mice, the activity of RNA polymerases was notably inhibited: four hours after infection there was a
60% inhibition of RNA· polymerases A and a 50% inhibition of RNA-
polymerases B activity. The shut-off of the activity of polymerases B
corresponded to the disappearance of molecules able to bind amanitin;
as shown in Table 8.1, five hours after the infection there was a 72%
inhibition of the fixation of ^{3}[H]O-methyl-demethyl-γ-amanitin. On the
other hand, only 39% of active polymerases B could be solubilised from
the hepatocyte nuclei from infected mice at the fifth hour. These results

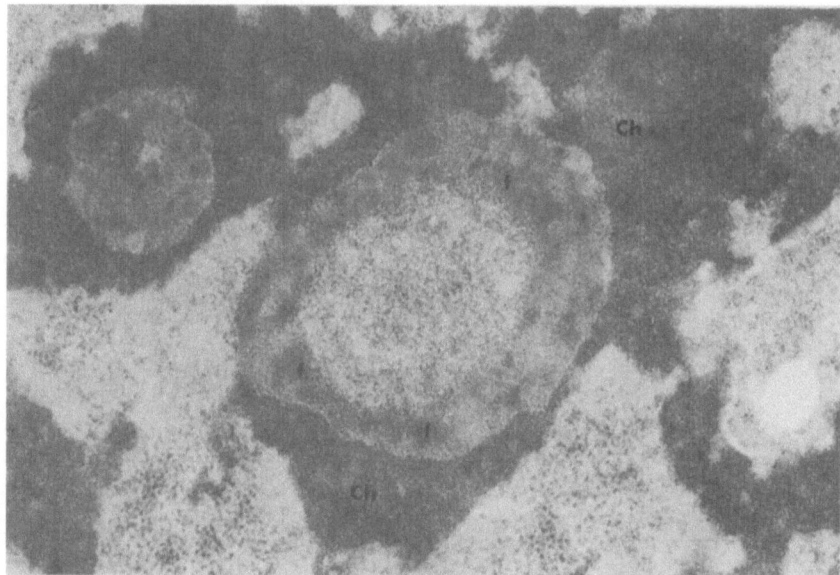

FIGURE 8.5 Nucleolus of a mouse hepatocyte seven hours after the inoculation of 20 LD of FV 3. The ring-shaped nucleolus is composed entirely of its fibrillar material ($\times$ 29 000)

Table 8.1 BINDING OF AMANITIN AND SOLUBILISATION OF ACTIVE ENZYME MOLECULES AS A MEASUREMENT OF THE AMOUNT OF POLYMERASE B IN THE LIVER NUCLEI OF CONTROLS AND OF MICE INFECTED WITH 20 LD OF FV$_3$. The amount of $^3[H]$O-methyl-demethyl-γ-amanitin bound to RNA-polymerase B was determined in the nuclei of liver from control and infected mice by $(NH_4)_2SO_4$ precipitation method[20]. For RNA-polymerase activity, the reaction mixtures were based on those used by Jacob *et al.* to study soluble nuclear enzymes[21]

System	*Fixation of* $^3[H]$O-methyl-demethyl-γ-amanitin cpm per 800 μg of nuclear proteins	*RNA-polymerase activity of solubilised enzyme μmol AMP incorporated/mg protein/15 min*
Control	6.292	642
Mice infected for 5 hours	1.754 (27.8%)	251 (39%)

provide good evidence of a direct or indirect action of FV 3 infection on the amount of RNA-polymerases B molecules. However until now it has not been possible to establish whether the inhibition of the poly-merases activity is responsible for the shut-off of the RNA synthesis.

Using the system consisting of isolated liver nuclei which it was possible to stimulate with exogenous primer DNA[15], it could be demonstrated that in the case of nuclei from infected mice there was a smaller amount of active DNA-polymerase (Table 8.2). However the DNA-

Table 8.2 DNA-POLYMERASES ACTIVITY IN THE LIVER OF CONTROLS AND OF MICE INFECTED WITH 20 LD OF FV 3. In the case of the whole nuclei, the assay conditions were based on those of Probst[23]. For the soluble DNA-polymerase found in the supernatant 105 000 g of the cytoplasmic fraction the assay conditions were those used by Montecuccoli *et al.*[22]

| System | Incorporation of $^3[H]dTTP$ pmol/mg protein | | | |
| | Nuclei | | Cytoplasmic fraction | |
	Endogenous primer	Exogenous primer	Native DNA	Denatured DNA
Control	33.9	110.13	11.2	18.0
Mice infected for 5 hours	10.47 (30.8%)	44.46 (40.3%)	11.8 (105%)	19.6 (108%)

polymerase activity checked in the cytoplasmic fraction of the liver cells of infected mice was as high as that measured in non-infected animals whether native or denatured DNA was used as a primer (Table 8.2). Similar results were found for another cytoplasmic enzyme involved in nucleic acid synthesis, thymidine kinase whose activity remained unaffected until the seventh hour after infection.

These results demonstrate that the biochemical changes induced in the liver of FV 3 infected animals affect principally the nuclei of the hepatocytes and correspond closely to the morphological observations.

TOXIC CONSTITUENTS OF THE VIRUS PARTICLE

The shut-off of the macromolecular metabolism produced by FV 3 in tissue cultures can be related to a toxic component of the virion. Thus, Aubertin *et al.*[16] have obtained a soluble viral extract (SVE) by solubilisation of purified virus particles with NP 40 and LiCl. Treatment of KB or BHK cells with SVE produces an inhibition of host DNA, RNA and protein synthesis quite comparable to that produced by the whole particles. It should be stressed that in isolated nuclei proceeding from SVE-treated KB cells there was also a drastic inhibition of the activity of the polymerases[17]. For polymerase B, at least, the inhibition of the activity could be related to a decrease in the number of active molecules. Thus, three hours after the treatment of the cells with SVE only 46% of the active molecules of polymerase B could be solubilised; on the other hand there was a 40% diminution of the binding of radioactive amanitin (A. M. Aubertin, personal communication). The toxic factor has been shown to be a specific viral protein since its effects, which could be neutralised by an FV 3 antiserum are destroyed by trypsin digestion[16].

In order to identify the liver-damaging factor with the cut-off protein of Aubertin, a system consisting of suspended liver slices was established[18]. Slices proceeding from the livers of control mice incorporated ³[H]uridine for more than two hours. However when the livers had been previously perfused with SVE, the incorporation in the slices was completely blocked 30 min after incubation and histological changes of the nuclei, similar to the lesions found *in vivo*, could be noticed. This effect was also neutralised by FV 3 antiserum. These experiments bear evidence that the proteins which are responsible for the cut-off effect in tissue culture are those which produce liver damage *in vivo*.

CONCLUSIONS

Frog virus 3 liver damage represents a new model of hepatotoxicity. It demonstrates that in mice, viral proteins are capable of producing lesions accompanied by biochemical perturbations leading to the death of the animals. There are strong analogies with the action of other liver toxics such as α-amanitin or aflatoxin B₁. Compared with α-amanitin[19] most of the ultrastructural changes in FV 3 intoxication of mice are similar, except for the appearance of the intranuclear filamentous inclusions and the relatively late nucleolar changes. This would indicate that condensation of the chromatin is not sufficient to produce a breakup of nucleoli[19]. The mechanism of action of the toxic proteins on the hepatocytes is not yet clearly established but it seems evident that the target is the nucleus. It has been shown *in vitro* that FV 3 proteins are able to bind to DNA[17]. Substances binding to DNA are known to produce chromatin condensation. The question whether an interaction of the cut-off protein with DNA is sufficient to explain all the morphological and biochemical changes can not yet be answered.

ABBREVIATIONS

N   : Nucleus
M   : Mitochondria
PA   : Pseudocrystalline area
Ch   : Chromatin
Nu   : Nucleolus
iG   : Interchromatin granules
Fi   : Filamentous inclusion
RER: Rough-endoplasmic reticulum
GP   : Glycogen particle
G   : Golgi apparatus
f   : fibrillar material of the nucleolus

REFERENCES

1. Granoff, A., Came, P. F. and Rafferty, K. A. (1965). The isolation and properties of viruses from *Rana pipiens*: their possible relationship to the renal adenocarcinoma of the leopard frog. *Ann. N.Y. Acad. Sci.*, **126**, 237–255

2. Tweedell, K. and Granoff, A. (1968). Viruses and renal carcinoma of *Rana pipiens*. V. Effect of Frog Virus 3 on developing frog embryos and larvae. *J. Nat. Cancer Inst.*, **40**, 407–410

3. Bingen-Brendel, A., Tripier, F. and Kirn, A. (1971). Etude morphologique séquentielle du développement du FV_3 sur cellules BHK_{21}. *J. de Microscopie*, **11**, 249–258

4. Tripier, F., Braunwald, J. and Kirn, A. (1974). Budding of Frog Virus 3: studies by immunological and cytochemical methods in electron mioroscopy. *Intervirology* **3**, 305–318

5. Granoff, A. (1969). Viruses of amphibia. *Current Topics Microbiol. Immunol.*, **50**, 107–137

6. Guir, J., Braunwald, J. and Kirn, A. (1971). Inhibition of host-specific DNA and RNA synthesis in KB cells following infection with Frog Virus 3. *J. Gen. Virol.*, **12**, 293–301

7. Kirn, A. (1971). Pouvoir léthal pour la souris du virus 3 de la grenouille (FV_3). *C.R. Acad. Sci. (Paris)*, **Serie D, 272**, 2504–2506

8. Kirn, A., Gut, J. P., Bingen, A. and Hirth, C. (1972). Acute hepatitis produced by FV_3 in mice. *Arch. Ges. Virusforsch.*, **36**, 394–397

9. Bingen-Brendel, A., Batzenschlager, A., Gut, J. P., Hirth, C., Vetter,

J. M. and Kirn, A. (1972). Etude histologique et virologique de l'hépatite dégénérative aiguë provoquée par le FV₃ (Frog Virus 3) chez la souris. *Ann. Inst. Pasteur*, **122**, 125–142

10. Kirn, A., Gut, J. P., Steffan, A. M. and Gendrault, J. L. (1973/74). Immunization of mice against the toxic hepatitis produced by FV₃: inhibition of virus penetration into the liver. *Intervirology*, **2**, 244–252

11. Bingen, A. and Kirn, A. (1973). Modifications ultrastructurales précoces des noyaux des hépatocytes de souris au cours de l'hépatite dégénérative aiguë provoquée par le FV₃. *J. Ultrastructure Res.*, **45**, 343–355

12. Bernhard, W. (1968). Une méthode de coloration régressive a l'usage de la Microscopie Electronique. *C. R. Acad. Sci. (Paris)*, **Serie D, 267**, 2170–2173

13. Bingen, A. and Kirn, A. (1975). Fibrillar bodies in hepatocyte nuclei during the course of the toxic hepatitis produced by Frog Virus 3 in mice. *J. Ultrastructure Res.* **50**, 167–173

14. Elharrar, M., Hirth, C., Blanc, J. and Kirn, A. (1973). Pathogénie de l'hépatite toxique de la souris provoquée par le FV₃ (Frog Virus 3). Inhibition de la synthèse des macromolécules du foie. *Biochim. Biophys. Acta*, **319**, 91–102

15. Elharrar, M. and Kirn, A. (1974). Inhibition of DNA synthesis by isolated liver nuclei from Frog Virus 3 infected mice. *Biochem. Biophys. Res. Commun.*, **57**, 801–807

16. Aubertin, A. M., Hirth, C., Travo, C., Nonnenmacher, H. and Kirn, A. (1973). Preparation and properties of an inhibitory extract from Frog Virus 3 particles. *J. Virol.*, **11**, 694–701

17. Aubertin, A. M. (1973). Réplication du génome du FV₃ (Frog Virus 3). Inhibition de la synthèse des acides nucléiques par un constituant de la particule virale. (Université Louis Pasteur, Strasbourg: Thèse de Doctorat d'Etat de Sciences)

18. Gendrault, J. L., Steffan, A. M. and Kirn, A. (1973/74). Inhibition of *in vitro* synthesis in mouse liver perfused with Frog Virus 3 and solubilized FV₃ proteins. *Intervirology*, **2**, 366–370

19. Fiume, L. (1972). Pathogenesis of the cellular lesions produced ⸢by⸣ α-amanitin. In: *The Pathology of Transcription and Translation*, 105–122 (E. Farber, editor) (New York: Marcel Dekker Inc.)

20. Cochet-Meilhac, M., Nuret, P., Courvalin, J. C. and Chambon, P. (1974). Animal DNA-dependent RNA polymerases. Determination of cellular number of RNA polymerase B molecules. *Biochim. Biophys. Acta*, **353**, 185–192

21. Jacob, S. T., Sajdel, E. M. and Munro, H. N. (1970). Different responses of soluble whole nuclear RNA polymerase and soluble nucleolar RNA polymerase to divalent cations and to inhibition by α-amanitin. *Biochem. Biophys. Res. Commun.*, **38**, 765–770

22. Montecuccoli, G., Novello, F. and Stirpe, F. (1973). Effect of α-amanitin

poisoning on the synthesis of deoxyribonucleic acid and of protein in regenerating rat liver. *Biochim. Biophys. Acta*, **319**, 199–208

23. Probst, G. S., Bikoff, E., Keller, S. J. and Meyer, R. R. (1972). DNA biosynthesis in nuclei. Characterization of DNA synthesis by isolated rat liver nuclei using endogenous DNA as primer. *Biochim. Biophys. Acta*, **281**, 216–227

CHAPTER 9

Consequences of uridine triphosphate deficiency in liver and hepatoma cells*

D. KEPPLER

A sequence of events caused by an acute injury leading to cellular death and subsequently to necrosis can be analysed best if the following prerequisites are given:

1. The injurious agent or the toxin under study causes a selective primary lesion rather than a variety of initial effects.
2. The primary lesion can be reversed at any time before the 'point of no return'[1] is reached.

The galactose analogues D-galactosamine (GalN)[2,3] and 2-deoxy-D-galactose[4] would be agents fulfilling these prerequisites perfectly if the subsequent necrosis of hepatocytes were exclusively a consequence of UTP deficiency. The arguments supporting this statement[5,6] had been incomplete and controversial until recently. A pathogenetic role of toxic GalN metabolites[7-10] as well as the consequences of UDP-glucose and UDP-galactose deficiency have been considered[3,7,11,12]. This paper summarises our recent work on the consequences of UTP deficiency in liver and ascites hepatoma cells and presents the evidence supporting my conclusion that GalN-induced cell death is a result of UTP deficiency.

GalN selectively depletes the UTP pool to less than 10% of normal without reducing the hepatic contents of ATP, GTP, or CTP[5]. GalN action, however, requires the formation of GalN metabolites[3,6,7,11]. It has been essential therefore to rule out a specific pathogenetic function of the metabolites of GalN. This has been achieved by use of

* This investigation was supported by grants from the Deutsche Forschungsgemeinschaft, Bonn-Bad Godesberg ('Forschergruppe Leberrkrankheiten' and 'SFG 46', Freiburg)

2-deoxy-D-galactose which does not share any common metabolites with GalN.

This analogue, however, also induces hepatic UTP deficiency[4]. All of the morphologic lesions induced by 2-deoxy-D-galactose + 6-azauridine in rats[13,14] have also been observed after administration of GalN. Further evidence against a significant role of GalN metabolites in the pathogenesis of hepatocellular necrosis came from our uridine reversal studies[15]. Reversal of UTP deficiency as late as three hours after GalN administration prevented the increase in plasma enzyme activities and the development of hepatocellular necrosis (Table 9.1).

Table 9.1   PREVENTION OF GALN-INDUCED LIVER INJURY BY URIDINE. Plasma enzyme activities (mU/ml) and bilirubin (mg/100 ml) were determined 24 hours after a single dose of GalN (1.85 mmol/kg). Uridine (4 mmol/kg) was injected intraperitoneally at 3, 5 and 8 hours after GalN. Mean values $\pm$ standard deviation from fed, female rats of the Wistar strain, weighing 150–170 g[16]

	Control	Galactosamine + Uridine	Galactosamine
Sorbitol dehydrogenase	3 ± 2	4 ± 1	139 ± 56
Glutamate dehydrogenase	3 ± 1	5 ± 1	129 ± 48
Alanine transaminase	42 ± 8	45 ± 9	720 ± 304
Aspartate transaminase	38 ± 5	75 ± 10	659 ± 279
Total bilirubin	< 0.2	0.1	1.2 ± 0.4
Direct reacting bilirubin (%)	—	—	$71 \pm 9\%$

Combined administration of GalN and uridine results, however, not only in a prevention of liver injury[3,6,15-17] but also in a formation of all metabolites of GalN in high amounts[18].

In this context the attention should be drawn to the influence of uridine, cytidine, orotate and RNA as components of food which will markedly influence the content of hepatic UTP and the severity of GalN-induced injury.

DEPRESSION OF MACROMOLECULAR SYNTHESES

The depression of the hepatic UTP content from 0.26 to 0.02 μmol/g corresponds to estimated intracellular concentrations of 0.35 and

0.03 mM, respectively[5,15]. UTP-dependent reactions with K_m values for UTP in this concentration range will be slowed down after administration of GalN or 2-deoxy-D-galactose. *RNA-polymerases* are affected directly since K_m values of about 0.05 mM UTP have been determined for rat liver nuclear RNA-polymerases[19]. K_m values for UTP of 0.016 and 0.029 mM have been measured with calf thymus RNA-polymerases[20]. The depression of RNA synthesis should be an immediate consequence of hepatic UTP deficiency since cytoplasmic and nuclear ribonucleoside phosphates equilibrate rapidly[21]. It is consistent that the *in vivo* RNA synthesis was depressed to 21% of normal as early as 30–60 min after GalN administration (Figure 9.1). The instant reversal of UTP deficiency by uridine[15] was associated with an immediate increase in [14][C]guanosine incorporation into RNA[5]. This system[5,15] provides for the first time a means to inhibit RNA synthesis *in vivo* for defined periods of time. The conclusion that the depression of RNA synthesis is due to substrate deficiency[5,10,22] is further supported by studies *in vitro*. The template activity of chromatin, the activity of partially purified RNA-polymerase, and the ability of isolated nuclei to incorporate labelled ribonucleoside phosphates into RNA have been found perfectly normal in preparations from rat livers two hours after a dose of GalN administered *in vivo*[10,22]. The ultrastructural demonstration of extensive nucleolar fragmentation soon after the administration of GalN or 2-deoxy-D-galactose[4,14,23] is in line with the biochemical evidence for an inhibition of RNA synthesis. Uridine prevents and reverses the fragmentation of nucleoli caused by both analogues[14,23]. The inhibition of RNA synthesis by GalN-induced selective UTP deficiency differs from the types of inhibition established previously. The advantage of reversibility is evident in comparison with actinomycin D and α-amanitin. However, UTP deficiency is a less specific mechanism with regard to the synthesis of different RNA species by different RNA polymerases.

Protein synthesis inhibition is another consequence of GalN action[10,18,24–27]. The depressed incorporation of amino acids into proteins can be prevented and reversed by means of uridine[10,27,28]. It is not clear whether GalN-induced inhibition of protein synthesis is a direct consequence of UTP deficiency[27] or whether it is due to the strong depression of RNA synthesis. The close relation observed between the level of UTP and the rate of RNA synthesis (Figure 9.1) cannot be demonstrated for the rate of protein synthesis. The latter

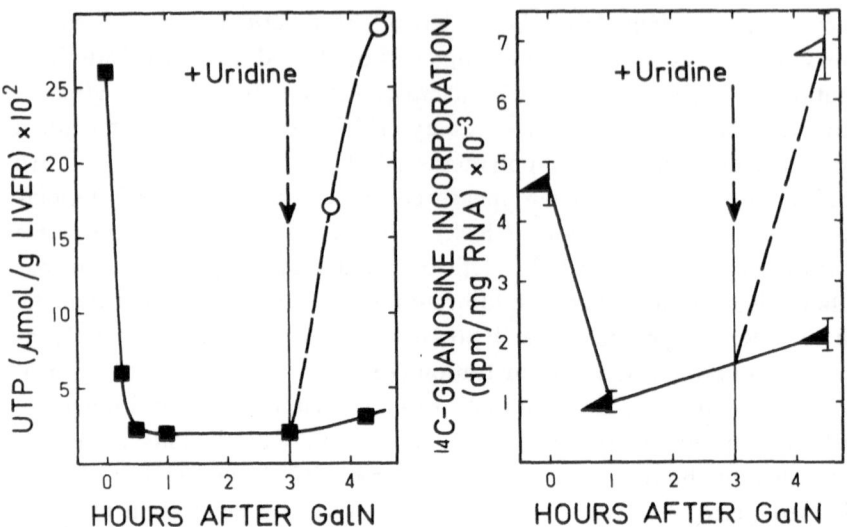

FIGURE 9.1   GalN-induced depression of hepatic *in vivo* RNA synthesis and its reversal by uridine (right). The rapid induction of UTP deficiency and its reversal (left) parallel the incorporation of ^{14}C]guanosine into RNA isolated from liver. Details of this experiment were described previously[5]

reaches its minimum after 2–6 hours[27,28] whereas the minimum of the UTP content is measured less than one hour after the administration of GalN. The time course of the events suggests that protein synthesis inhibition is not directly related to UTP deficiency and may well be a consequence of the depressed synthesis of RNA.

The onset of *DNA synthesis* is delayed when GalN is given in the prereplicative phase after partial hepatectomy[29]. This effect is consistent with the dependence of DNA synthesis on protein synthesis[30,31] but also with the effect of other RNA synthesis inhibitors, particularly actinomycin D, on the cell cycle[30,32]. So far, no evidence is available that GalN-induced depletion of uridine phosphate pools would lead to an early deficiency of TTP. However, GalN-induced inhibition of RNA synthesis may serve as the link between UTP deficiency and inhibition of initiation of DNA replication. Recent studies have demonstrated that RNA synthesis is required also in mammalian cells for the formation of RNA–DNA complexes with the RNA serving as primer for newly synthesised DNA strands[33,34]. Rutter *et al.* have implicated RNA-polymerase III in this specific role for initiation of DNA replication[35]. This process would thus depend directly on the concentration of UTP.

INDUCTION OF UTP DEFICIENCY IN UDP-HEXOSE DEFICIENT HEPATOMA CELLS

In the liver injury induced by GalN or 2-deoxy-D-galactose it is important to differentiate between the consequences of UTP deficiency and
the associated depression of UDP-glucose and UDP-galactose levels.
Two hepatoma cell lines originally derived from liver have been found
which are characterised by a high content of UTP and a genetically
determined selective deficiency of UDP-glucose and UDP-galactose[36].
These UDP-hexose levels are comparable to those found in liver after
GalN treatment[11]. The AS-30D ascites hepatoma line[37] has kept the
capacity to metabolise D-galactose. Incubation of AS-30D cells at
37 °C in a medium[36] containing D-galactose ($>$ 1 mM) resulted in an
elimination of galactose of 9 μmol/hour/g wet cells. This amounts to
50% of the galactose elimination rate of rat liver *in vivo*[38] and exceeds
greatly the maximal rate observed with rat liver slices[39]. GalN which is
metabolised mainly by enzymes of the galactose pathway[6] was used
therefore to depress the UTP content of ascites hepatoma cells[36]. However, even with a GalN concentration of 2 mM no severe depression of
the UTP content could be induced (Figure 9.2). UTP levels between
0.2 and 0.3 μmol/g correspond to the control range in rat liver and were
insufficient to produce marked effects on macromolecular syntheses.
This resistance of hepatoma cells to GalN action was not due to a low
rate of formation of GalN metabolites (Figure 9.3) as compared to
liver[7,11,18,41]. However, the uridylate trapping[11] by formation of UDP-
aminosugars derived from GalN at a rate of about 1.1 μmol/hour/g cells
(Figure 9.3) was efficiently compensated by an increased *de novo*
synthesis of uridylate. The sum of all acid soluble uracil nucleotides
increases at a rate of 1.2 μmol/hour/g cells (Figure 9.4) when the UTP
level was close to 0.2 μmol/g. This increase was completely suppressed
(Figure 9.4) by an inhibition of the *de novo* synthesis of uridylate at the
orotidine-5'-monophosphate decarboxylase step by means of 6-azauri-
dine[43]. The rate of net *de novo* synthesis of uridylate in the hepatoma
cells (Figure 9.4) was more than threefold higher than the rate observed
in liver[11]. This high capacity of the hepatoma cells to compensate the
GalN-induced trapping of uridylate explains the lack of a severe depletion of the UTP pool. This finding may also serve as an explanation for
the resistance of solid hepatomas to GalN action[44].

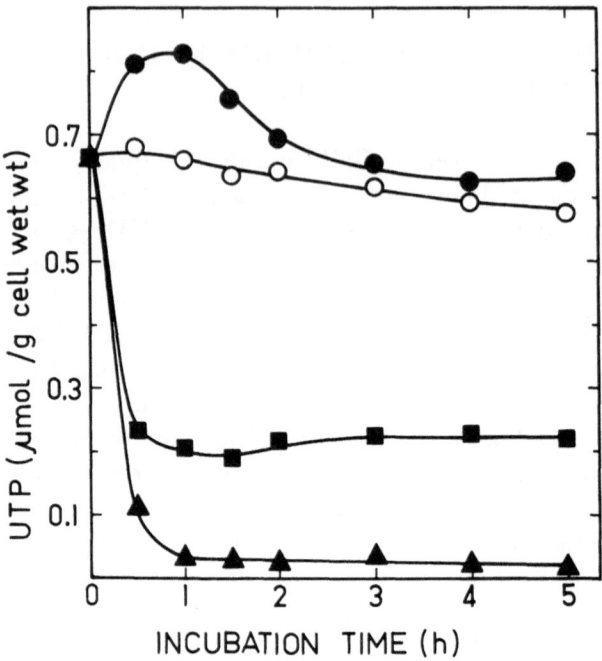

FIGURE 9.2 UTP contents of hepatoma cells in suspension. AS-30D rat ascites hepatoma cells[37] were studied from transplant generation 315 to 330. The cells were incubated on a gyratory shaker at 37 °C at a cell concentration of about 2.5 × 10⁶/ml in standard medium[36]. Nucleotide contents of hepatoma cells were analysed as described previously[36]. UTP was determined enzymatically[40]. ○—control cells; ■—2 mM GalN; ▲—2 mM GalN + 1 mM 6-azauridine; ●—2 mM GalN + 1 mM 6-azauridine + 1 mM uridine. Each point is the mean from 3–4 analyses in different suspensions; standard deviations are below 20%

It follows from the observations mentioned above that GalN-induced uridylate trapping will cause severe UTP deficiency in the hepatoma cells when combined with a blockage of the *de novo* synthesis of uridylate. 6-azauridine together with GalN caused a depression of the UTP content to less than 5% of the controls (Figure 9.2). This depletion of the UTP pool could be reversed within 15 min by addition of uridine to the medium (Figure 9.5). The rate of uptake and phosphorylation of uridine by the UTP-deficient hepatoma cells amounted to 6 μmol/hour/g cells. This rate is more than threefold higher than in rat liver[5] and indicates an active salvage pathway of these hepatoma cells. Induction of UTP deficiency in AS-30D cells did not affect significantly the low levels of UDP-glucose (Figure 9.5) and UDP-galactose. The low UDP-

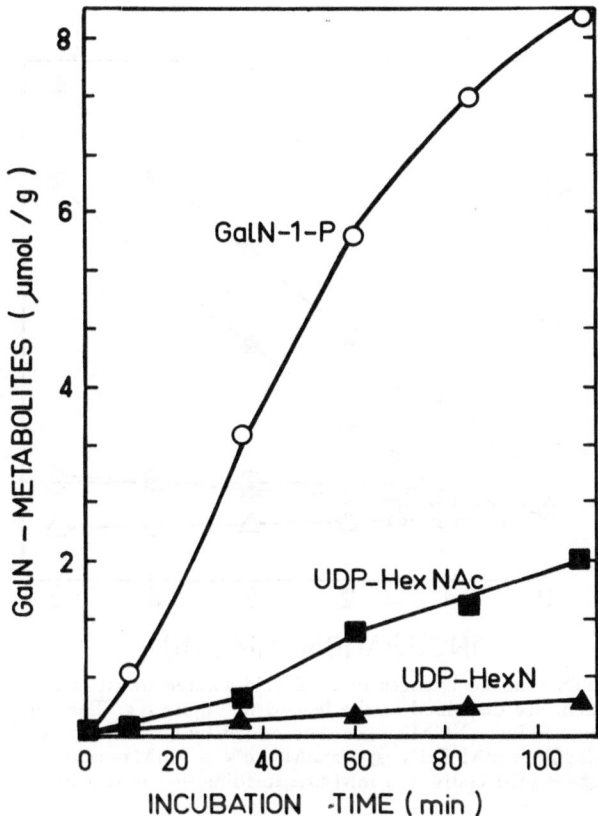

FIGURE 9.3   Formation of galactosamine metabolites in AS-30D hepatoma cells. The cells were incubated as described in the legend to Figure 9.2 in the presence of 2 mM GalN. Addition of [1-^{14}C]GalN resulted in a specific radioactivity of 0.35 Ci/mol. Metabolites formed from GalN were determined by radioactivity analysis after paper chromatography of the acid-soluble supernatants[41]. ○—GalN-1-phosphate; ■—UDP-N-acetylhexosamines (= UDP-N-acetylglucosamine + UDP-N-acetylgalactosamine); ▲—UDP-hexosamines (UDP-galactosamine + UDP-glucosamine)

glucose content could be increased, however, when UTP-deficient cells were treated with uridine (Figure 9.5).

CONSEQUENCES OF THE DEPLETION OF THE UTP POOL OF HEPATOMA CELLS

UDP-hexose-deficient ascites hepatoma cells provide a system to discriminate between the consequences of UDP-hexose and UTP

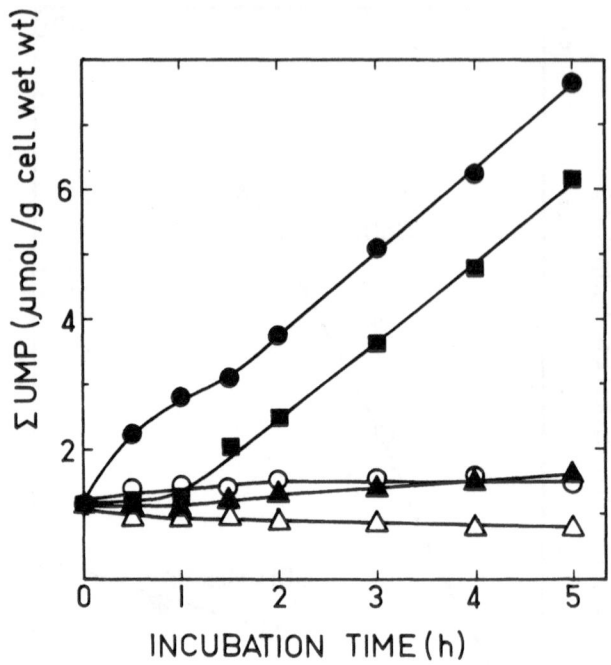

FIGURE 9.4   GalN-induced changes in total acid-soluble uracil nucleotides. Details of this experiment are described in the legend to Figure 9.2. The sum of all acid-soluble uracil nucleotides (ΣUMP) was determined by specific enzymatic analysis[42]. ○—control cells; ■—2 mM GalN; ▲—2 mM GalN + 1 mM 6-azauridine; △—1 mM 6-azauridine; ●—2 mM GalN + 1 mM 6-azauridine + 1 mM uridine

deficiency. Depletion of the cellular UTP pool *in vitro* lead to a loss of *transplantability* and growth of the AS-30D ascites hepatoma *in vivo* (Table 9.2). Intracellular accumulation of GalN metabolites (Figure 9.3) and a limited depression of the UTP content by GalN alone (Figures 9.2 and 9.5) did not affect transplantability and growth of these cells *in vivo* (Table 9.2). Prevention or reversal by uridine of UTP deficiency induced by GalN + 6-azauridine (Figures 9.2 and 9.5) argues against an effect of 6-azauridine or its intracellular metabolite 6-azaUMP[45] on transplantability (Table 9.2).

GalN at a concentration of 0.5 mM allowed exponential *cell growth* in suspension culture at a rate similar to control cells (Figure 9.6). Purine nucleotide contents and the adenylate energy charge remained within the control range at this low concentration of GalN. This is in contrast to the non-selective depression of nucleotide contents by high GalN concentrations[36]. Inhibition of *de novo* pyrimidine biosynthesis by

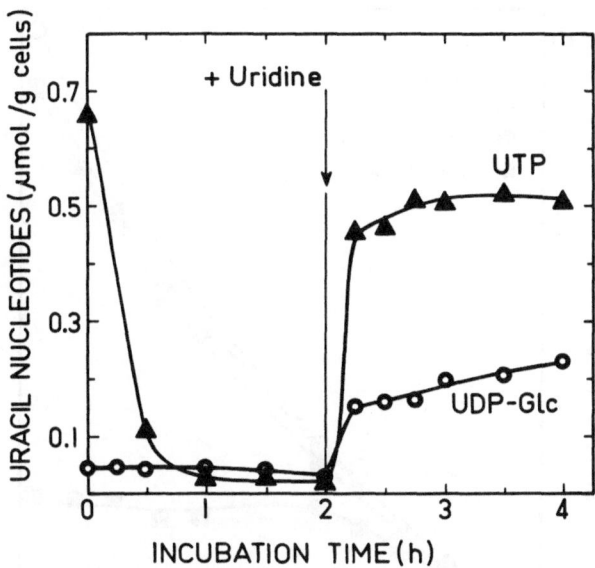

FIGURE 9.5 Reversal of UTP deficiency by uridine. AS-30D cells were incubated as described in the legend to Figure 9.2. UTP deficiency was induced by addition of 2 mM GalN + 1 mM 6-azauridine at zero time; 1 mM uridine was added at two hours. UTP[40] and UDP-glucose[42] contents were analysed as described earlier[36]

Table 9.2 INHIBITION OF TRANSPLANTABILITY AND ASCITES HEPATOMA GROWTH IN RATS BY UTP DEFICIENCY. AS-30D cells were collected on the seventh day after transplantation, washed and incubated[36] as described in the legend to Figure 9.2. The concentration of GalN in the medium was 2 mM; 6-azauridine and uridine were 1 mM each. The cells were collected by centrifugation (120 g, 5 min) after an incubation for six hours, and resuspended in cold Swim's S-77 medium supplemented with 25 mM Na_2HPO_4 and 2 mM glutamine, pH 7.4, at a cell concentration of 10^8/ml. Female Sprague-Dawley rats, weighing 210 ± 30 g, and 82 ± 8 days of age were injected intraperitoneally with 3 × 10^7 cells per animal. The mean survival time of animals with hepatoma cell growth was 23 days. Ascites tumour growth is expressed by the number of tumour-bearing animals as compared to the number of rats injected with hepatoma cells

Treatment	Ascites tumour growth	Survival (%)
Control	15/16	6
GalN	13/14	7
GalN + 6-azauridine	0/14	100
GalN + 6-azauridine + uridine	12/12	0

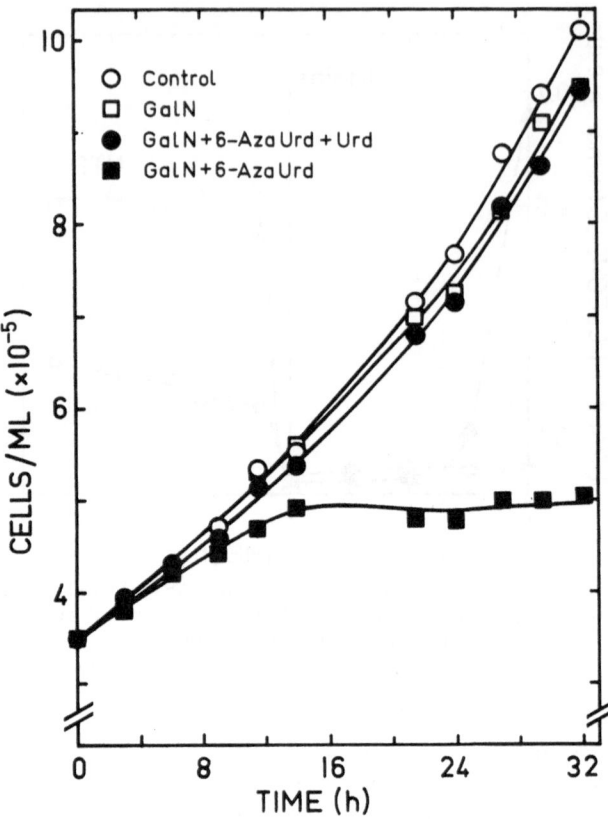

FIGURE 9.6 Inhibition of hepatoma cell growth in suspension culture by UTP deficiency. AS-30D cells were collected under sterile conditions on the sixth day after transplantation and suspended at a cell concentration of about 4×10^5/ml in Swim's 67-G medium (containing 4% pancreatic autolysate) supplemented with 2 mM glutamine and 2% ascitic fluid sterilised by filtration of rat AS-30D ascites hepatoma fluid. The cells were grown at 37 °C on a gyratory shaker at 120 rpm under 5% CO_2/air. The concentrations of GalN, 6-azauridine and uridine were 0.5 mM each

addition of 6-azauridine together with the GalN-induced uridylate trapping resulted in a selective depletion of the UTP pool to less than 0.03 μmol/g of cells and lead subsequently to a complete inhibition of hepatoma cell growth (Figure 9.6). The delay in the inhibition of cell proliferation by GalN + 6-azauridine depends largely on the presence of small amounts of uridine and cytidine in the culture medium. As shown in Figure 9.4, 6-azauridine caused a slow decrease of uracil nucleotides with time. The effect of 6-azauridine on UTP contents and growth of the hepatoma cells was limited and small as compared to the combined action of GalN + 6-azauridine.

The inhibition of hepatoma cell growth by UTP deficiency (Figure 9.6) had no significant influence on the amount of DNA or protein per weight or number of cells. In the culture medium used, a growth rate in the normal range could be restored when uridine was added to a suspension after an incubation for nine hours in the presence of GalN + 6-azauridine as described in the legend to Figure 9.6. UTP deficiency for prolonged periods of time resulted in a loss of cell clusters and an increasing number of necrotic hepatoma cells became evident upon examination by phase contrast microscopy. The GalN concentration required together with 6-azauridine to cause necrosis of the hepatoma cells was 10–200 times lower than the concentrations employed in studies with Sarcoma-180 and Ehrlich ascites carcinoma cells[46].

SEQUENCE OF EVENTS CAUSED BY UTP DEFICIENCY AND LEADING TO CELL DEATH

The conclusion that the cell injury induced by galactose analogues[2-4] is due to UTP deficiency as the selective primary biochemical lesion is based on the following observations. (a) A specific pathogenetic function of GalN metabolites has been ruled out[4,6,13,15,16,18]; (b) only the depletion of the UTP pool leads to growth inhibition and cell death in UDP-glucose and UDP-galactose deficient hepatoma cells (Figures 9.2, 9.5 and 9.6); (c) an increase of the UDP-galactose content in liver by administration of D-galactose[47] is incapable of preventing the development of GalN-induced injury[12] at a time when the uridine reversal of UTP deficiency[6,15] is fully effective (Table 9.1); (d) the depletion of the UTP pool is highly selective with regard to the other ribonucleoside triphosphates[5].

The primary biochemical lesion[48,49] is followed by a cascade of secondary metabolic alterations[50]. The duration of the reversible part of the sequence[51] caused by UTP deficiency and leading to hepatocellular death has been determined by reversal of UTP deficiency at various times after GalN administration[6]. The secondary events related to cell death must occur during the reversible phase and persist beyond the point of lost reparability. Depression of RNA synthesis is an immediate consequence of the depletion of the UTP pool[5,22]. This type of RNA synthesis inhibition should have effects that differ from those of RNA synthesis inhibitors which are unable to cause liver cell necrosis[32]. The time course of events suggests that the inhibition of regular protein synthesis[27,28] is secondary to the early depression of RNA synthesis[5]. Further studies are required to identify the injury to a vital cell component or organelle which is caused by UTP deficiency and is mediated by the specific disturbance in macromolecular syntheses.

The galactose analogues cause a primary biochemical lesion which is selective and reversible. This tool can be used for studies on the reversible part of the sequence leading to cell death in liver. With the malignant hepatoma cells we can extend the period of UTP deficiency beyond the point of lost reparability and thereby induce necrosis.

ACKNOWLEDGMENT

The excellent technical assistance by Mrs Ute Stumpp-Grigat is gratefully acknowledged.

REFERENCES

1. Majno, G., La Gattuta, M. and Thompson, T. E. (1960). Cellular death and necrosis: Chemical, physical and morphologic changes in rat liver. *Virchows Arch. Pathol. Anat.*, **333**, 421–465
2. Keppler, D., Lesch, R., Reutter, W. and Decker, K. (1968). Experimental hepatitis induced by D-galactosamine. *Exp. Molec., Pathol.*, **9**, 279–290
3. Decker, K. and Keppler, D. (1972). Galactosamine induced liver injury. In: *Progress in Liver Diseases*, **Vol. 4**, 183–199 (H. Popper and F. Schaffner, editors) (New York: Grune and Stratton)
4. Keppler, D. and Hübner, G. (1973). Liver injury induced by 2-deoxy-D-galactose. *Exp. Molec. Pathol.*, **19**, 365–377
5. Keppler, D., Pausch, J. and Decker, K. (1974). Selective uridine triphosphate deficiency induced by D-galactosamine in liver and reversed by pyrimidine nucleotide precursors. Effect on ribonucleic acid synthesis. *J. Biol. Chem.*, **249**, 211–216
6. Decker, K. and Keppler, D. (1974). Galactosamine hepatitis: Key role of the nucleotide deficiency period in the pathogenesis of cell injury and cell death. *Rev. Physiol. Biochem. Pharmacol.*, **71**, 77–106
7. Keppler, D. and Decker, K. (1969). Studies on the mechanism of galactosamine hepatitis: Accumulation of galactosamine-1-phosphate and its inhibition of UDP-glucose pyrophosphorylase. *Eur. J. Biochem.*, **10**, 219–225

8. Reutter, W., Bauer, Ch. and Lesch, R. (1970). On the mechanism of action of galactosamine: Different response to D-galactosamine of rat liver during development. *Naturwissenschaften*, **57**, 674–675
9. Bauer, Ch. and Reutter, W. (1973). Inhibition of uridine diphospho-glucose dehydrogenase by galactosamine-1-phosphate and UDP-galactosamine. *Biochim. Biophys. Acta*, **293**, 11–14
10. Shinozuka, H., Farber, J. L., Konishi, Y. and Anukarahanouta, T. (1973). D-galactosamine and acute liver cell injury. *Fed. Proc.*, **32**, 1516–1526
11. Keppler, D., Rudigier, J., Bischoff, E. and Decker, K. (1970). The trapping of uridine phosphates by D-galactosamine, D-glucosamine, and 2-deoxy-D-galactose. A study on the mechanism of galactosamine hepatitis *Eur J. Biochem.*, **17**, 246–253
12. Reutter, W., Bauer, Ch., Bachmann, W. and Lesch, R. (1973). Über die primäre und sekundäre biochemische Antwort der Leber nach Gabe von D-Galaktosamin beim Zustandekommen der Galaktosaminhepatitis. *Verh. Dtsch. Ges. Inn. Med.*, **79**, 927–930
13. Decker, K., Keppler, D., Rudigier, J. and Domschke, W. (1971). Cell damage by trapping of biosynthetic intermediates. The role of uracil nucleotides in experimental hepatitis. *Hoppe Seyler's Z. Physiol. Chem.*, **352**, 412–418
14. Shinozuka, H. (1974). Ultrastructural study of liver cell injury due to UTP deficiency. *Virchows Arch. Abt. B. Zellpath.*, **15**, 119–130
15. Keppler, D. and Decker, K. (1971) Der Wirkungsmechanismus von D-Galaktosamin in der Leber. *Verh. Dtsch. Ges. Inn. Med.*, **77**, 1182–1185
16. Keppler, D. (1973). Hépatite expérimentale à la D-galactosamine. *Ann. Gastroenterol. Hépatol.*, **9**, 211–221
17. Farber, J. L., Gill, G. and Konishi, Y. (1973). Prevention of galacto-samine-induced liver cell necrosis by uridine. *Amer. J. Pathol.*, **72**, 53–62
18. Reynolds, R. D. and Reutter, W. (1973). Inhibition of induction of rat liver tyrosine aminotransferase by D-galactosamine. Role of uridine triphosphate. *J. Biol. Chem.*, **248**, 1562–1567
19. Chambon, P. (1972). Personal communication
20. Gissinger, F., Kedinger, C. and Chambon, P. (1974). Animal DNA-dependent RNA polymerases. X. General enzymatic properties of purified calf thymus RNA polymerases A I and B. *Biochimie*, **56**, 319–333
21. Siebert, G. (1972). The biochemical environment of the mammalian nucleus. *Sub-Cell. Biochem.*, **1**, 277–292
22. Konishi, Y., Shinozuka, H. and Farber, J. L. (1974). The inhibition of rat liver nuclear ribonucleic acid synthesis by galactosamine and its reversal by uridine. *Lab. Invest.*, **30**, 751–756
23. Shinozuka, H., Martin, J. T. and Farber, J. L. (1973). The induction of fibrillar nucleoli in rat liver cells by D-galactosamine and their subsequent re-formation into normal nucleoli. *J. Ultrastruct. Res.*, **44**, 279–292
24. Reutter, W., Keppler, D., Lesch, R. and Decker, K. (1969). Zum Glykoproteidstoffwechsel bei der Galaktosamin-induzierten Hepatitis. *Verh. Dtsch. Ges. Inn. Med.*, **75**, 363–365

25. Monier, D. and Wagle, S. R. (1971). Study of protein synthesis in galactosamine hepatitis. *Fed. Proc.*, **30**, 405
26. Koff, R. S., Fitts, J. J. and Sabesin, S. M. (1971). D-galactosamine hepatotoxicity. II. Mechanism of fatty liver production. *Proc. Soc. Exp. Biol. Med.*, **138**, 89–92
27. Anukarahanouta, T., Shinozuka, H. and Farber, E. (1973). Inhibition of protein synthesis in rat liver by D-galactosamine. *Res. Commun. Chem. Pathol. Pharmacol.*, **5**, 481–491
28. Bauer, Ch. H., Lukaschek, R. and Reutter, W. G. (1974). Studies on the Golgi apparatus. Cumulative inhibition of protein and glycoprotein secretion by D-galactosamine. *Biochem. J.*, **142**, 221–230
29. Lesch, R., Bachmann, W. and Reutter, W. (1973). The alteration of the regenerative activity and the cell cycle of partially hepatectomised rat liver following administration of D-galactosamine. *Cell Tissue Kinet*, **6**, 315–323
30. Baserga, R. (1972). Pathology of DNA. In: *The Pathology of Transcription and Translation*, 1–19 (E. Farber, editor) (New York: Marcel Dekker)
31. Farber, E. (1972). The pathology of translation. In: *The Pathology of Transcription and Translation*, 123–158 (E. Farber, editor) (New York: Marcel Dekker)
32. Farber, J. (1972). Pathology of RNA. In: *The Pathology of Transcription and Translation*, 55–72 (E. Farber, editor) (New York: Marcel Dekker)
33. Fox, R. M., Mendelsohn, J., Barbosa, E. and Goulian, M. (1973). RNA in nascent DNA from cultured human lymphocytes. *Nature New. Biol.*, **245**, 234–237
34. Neubort, S. and Bases, R. (1974). RNA–DNA covalent complexes in HeLa cells. *Biochim. Biophys. Acta*, **340**, 31–39
35. Rutter, W. J., Hager, G., Holland, M., Goldberg, M., Masiarz, F., Thompson, E. A. and Brakel, C., (1974). RNA polymerases and transcriptive specificity in eukaryotic cells. *Abstr. 11th Int. Cancer Congr., Florence 1974, Symposium on Transcriptional and Translational Control*, **1**, 130 (Amsterdam: Excerpta Medica Publ.)
36. Keppler, D. and Smith, D. F. (1974). Nucleotide contents of ascites hepatoma cells and their changes induced by D-galactosamine. *Cancer Res.*, **34**, 705–711
37. Smith, D. F., Walborg, E. F. Jr and Chang, J. P. (1970). Establishment of a transplantable ascites variant of a rat hepatoma induced by 3'-methyl-4-dimethylaminoazobenzene. *Cancer Res.*, **30**, 2306–2309
38. Keiding, S. (1974). Effect of ethanol and fructose on galactose elimination in rat. *Scand. J. Clin. Lab. Invest.*, **34**, 91–96
39. Tygstrup, N., Schmidt, A. and Thieden, H. I. D. (1971). The galactose utilization rate in liver slices from man and rat and its relation to the lactate/pyruvate ratio of the medium. *Scand. J. Clin. Lab. Invest.*, **28**, 27–31
40. Keppler, D., Gawehn, K. and Decker, K. (1974). Uridin-5'-triphosphat, Uridin-5'-diphosphat, Uridin-5'-monophosphat. In: *Methoden der*

Enzymatischen Analyse, 2222–2228 (H. U. Bergmeyer, editor) (Weinheim: Verlag Chemie)

41. Bauer, Ch., Bachmann, W. and Reutter, W. (1972). Studies on galactosamine hepatitis: determination of galactosamine metabolites in the developing rat liver. *Hoppe-Seyler's Z. Physiol. Chem.*, **353**, 1053–1058
42. Keppler, D., Rudigier, J. and Decker, K. (1970). Enzymic determination of uracil nucleotides in tissues. *Anal. Biochem.*, **38**, 105–114
43. Creasey, W. A. and Handschumacher, R. E. (1961). Purification and properties of orotidylate decarboxylases from yeast and rat liver. *J. Biol. Chem.*, **236**, 2058–2063
44. Reutter, W., Bauer, Ch., Kreisel, W. and Lesch, R. (1971). Galactosamine hepatitis in fast growing liver tissues: studies on newborn, partially hepatectomized and hepatoma bearing rats. *Digestion*, **4**, 173
45. Korbecki, M. and Plagemann, P. G. W. (1969). Competitive inhibition of uridine incorporation by 6-azauridine in uninfected and mengovirus-infected Novikoff hepatoma cells. *Proc. Soc. Exp. Biol. Med.*, **132**, 587–595
46. St-Arneault, G., Walter, L. and Bekesi, J. G. (1971). Cytotoxic effects of exogeneous D-galactosamine on experimental tumors. *Int. J. Cancer*, **7**, 483–490
47. Keppler, D., Rudigier, J. and Decker, K. (1970). Trapping of uridine phosphates by D-galactose in ethanol-treated liver. *Fed. Eur. Biochem. Soc. Lett.*, **11**, 193–196
48. Peters, R. A. (1963). *Biochemical Lesions and Lethal Synthesis* (New York: Macmillan)
49. Keppler, D. (1972). Biochemische Läsion als Ursache experimenteller Erkrankungen. *Umschau*, **72**, 771
50. Van Lancker, J. L. (1970). Hydrolases and cellular death. In: *Metabolic Conjugation and Metabolic Hydrolysis*, 355–418 (W. H. Fishman, editor) (New York, London: Academic Press)
51. Trump, B. F., Laiho, K. A., Mergner, W. J. and Aristala, A. U. (1974). Studies on the subcellular pathophysiology of acute lethal cell injury. *Beitr. Pathol.*, **152**, 243–271

CHAPTER 10

Ribosomes in dying liver cells

A. Bernelli-Zazzera

The cells that I will describe are dying because blood flow has been interrupted: the left lateral and median liver lobes have been made ischaemic by clamping their blood vessels. According to the duration of the interruption of blood supply we can distinguish between: (1) Short-duration ischaemia, lasting 15–30 min and producing slight and easily reversible cellular damage. (2) Long-duration reversible ischaemia, lasting about 60 min and leading to severe but essentially reversible cell damage; no widespread necrosis occurs. (3) Long-duration irreversible ischaemia, lasting 120 min. The term irreversible does not refer to the interruption of the blood flow, which is re-established by removing the clamp after this time, but to the consequence to the tissue, where signs of widespread necrosis become evident later[1].

Ribosomes are affected by ischaemia in many ways. First of all their number decreases in the post mitochondrial supernatant (PMS). Equal amounts of PMS obtained from liver cells made ischaemic for increasing time-periods, centrifuged over continuous sucrose gradients, yield patterns of progressively reduced area, which represents the amount of ribosomal RNA present in the PMS (Table 10.1). This loss of ribosomes has been further confirmed by chemical determinations of RNA in the different subcellular fractions. Concurrently with the reduction in area there is a change in shape of the patterns, with a reduction of the polysomal shoulder and a percentage increase, relative to the total RNA content, of the area of dimers and monomers (Table 10.1). The shift of the ribosomal population towards less aggregated forms has been confirmed with preparations of purified polysomes, i.e. polysomes sedimented, washed and resuspended to a constant concentration of RNA[2]. Evidence of disappearance of the large polysomes comes also from observations in the electron microscope, either with ribosomal suspensions or with tissue slices. Further analysis of the state

Table 10.1 REDUCTION IN AREA OF THE POLYSOMAL SIZE–DISTRIBUTION PATTERNS AND CHANGES IN THE POLYSOMES/MONOSOMES RATIO IN POST-MITOCHONDRIAL SUPERNATANT FROM ISCHAEMIC LIVERS (Calculated from data by Ragnotti et al.[2], by courtesy of *Exp. Molec. Pathol.* and Cajone et al., (1971). State and function of liver polysomes during recovery from ischemia. *Exp. Molec. Pathol.*, **14**, 392–403, by courtesy of Academic Press)

Duration of ischaemia	o (control)	30 min	60 min	120 min
Area	100	78	42	33
Area in cycloheximide protected animals	100	82	79	55
% monosomes	22	25	28	42
polysomes/monosomes ratio	3.5	3.0	2.6	1.4
% monosomes in C-ribosomes	25	29	35	40

of ribosomal aggregation carried out with suspensions of free and membrane-bound ribosomes, has shown that the most relevant changes occur in the ribosomes obtained from the membranes. This is in good agreement both with the results of chemical determinations carried out with these two ribosome fractions and with recent experiments on the relationships between ribosomes and membranes in ischaemic livers[3]. In these experiments we were able to show that membranes from rough endoplasmic reticulum (RER), isolated from ischaemic liver cells and previously stripped of their ribosomes bind less added ribosomes than their normal counterparts during incubation *in vitro*: the defect in the binding capacity is correlated with the severity of the injury suffered by the liver (Table 10.2). Rough membranes from ischaemic livers are also less efficient in retaining their native ribosomes in the presence of increasing concentrations of KCl: on the contrary, the puromycin-dependent release of ribosomes is higher in normal than in ischaemic

Table 10.2 BINDING OF NORMAL RIBOSOMES TO CONDITIONED ROUGH MEMBRANES FROM NORMAL AND ISCHAEMIC LIVERS (Calculated from data by Cajone et al.[3], by courtesy of *Biochem. Soc. Trans.*)

Duration of ischaemia	o (control)	30 min	60 min	120 min
% binding	100	44	29	21

preparations, in agreement with the fact that the number of ribosomes engaged in protein synthesis is reduced in ischaemic livers, as we shall see later. Rough membranes from ischaemic livers are less 'heavy' than normal and float in the centrifuge tube while normal rough membranes sediment as a compact layer[4]. All these results point to the existence of loosened relationships between membranes and ribosomes in ischaemic livers.

Concomitantly with these effects on the composition of the ribosomal population, the capacity for protein synthesis decreases in various cellular or cell-free preparations from ischaemic livers; tissue slices, PMS, microsomes, isolated ribosomes[2,5] (Table 10.3). The inefficiency

Table 10.3 REDUCTION IN PROTEIN SYNTHESIS BY VARIOUS PREPARATIONS FROM ISCHAEMIC LIVERS (Calculated from data by Ragnotti *et al.*[2], by courtesy of *Exp. Molec. Pathol.* and Cajone and Schiaffonati[5], by courtesy of *Brit. J. Exp. Pathol.*)

Duration of ischaemia	*0 (control)*	*30 min*	*60 min*	*120 min*
Liver slices + amino acids	100	21	7	3
Liver slices (endogenous amino acids)	100	32	14	8
Postmitochondrial supernatant	100	47	37	15
C-ribosomes + ischaemic cell-sap	100	80	63	44
C-ribosomes + normal cell-sap	100	98	83	66

of the protein-synthesising machinery is particularly pronounced in complex systems such as liver slices, suggesting that ischaemia can affect many different subcellular structures (e.g. plasma membrane, mitochondria etc.) and many different steps in protein synthesis; but the defect of aggregation of the ribosomes is likely to play an important role, in view of the well-known relationship between polysome structure and amino acid incorporation activity.

By application of the peptidyl puromycin technique—which measures peptide bond formation, an integral part of the activity of the ribosome— we have been able to show that there is an actual decrease in the number of active particles, rather than a proportionate loss of functional capacity of all the ribosomes[6]. What then is the mechanism of formation of these inactive ribosomal monomers? Of the possible mechanisms of poly-somal breakdown two in particular might operate in ischaemic liver cells: (1) the messenger strand, linking the ribosomes together, could be cut by ribonuclease action (let's remember that mRNA is more sensitive to ribonuclease than ribosomal RNA). This process has been called 'random fragmentation'[7]; (2) the ribosomes could separate from intact messenger strands, because chain completion can still go on, while chain initiation is inhibited, or at least more inhibited than chain completion. This metabolic release has been called 'n-1 process' because ribosomes get free one at a time[7]. Three kinds of evidence are in favour of the second hypothesis (n-1 process).

1. Cycloheximide, an inhibitor known to interfere with the flow of ribosomes along the messenger strand, when injected into the animals just before the onset of liver ischaemia preserves the area of the poly-some size–distribution patterns and prevents the disappearance of the polysomal shoulder. This protection should not be active against 'random fragmentation' (Table 10.1).

2. Recovery of the area and shape of the tracings and of the capacity for protein synthesis after long-duration reversible ischaemia occurs promptly upon re-establishment of the blood supply; this seems to suggest that mRNA is present in the cytosol, ready to accept mono-somes for a new readout cycle. Recovery of the patterns does not occur after long-duration irreversible ischaemia where the situation further deteriorates with time. (Figure 10.1; Table 10.4).

Table 10.4 RECOVERY OF PROTEIN SYNTHESIS BY POSTMITOCHONDRIAL SUPERNATANTS FROM ISCHAEMIC LIVERS, AFTER RE-ESTABLISHMENT OF THE BLOOD SUPPLY (Calculated from data by Cajone *et al.* (1971). State and function of liver polysomes during recovery from ischemia. *Exp. Molec. Pathol.*, **14**, 392–403, by courtesy of Academic Press)

Restoration of the blood supply	0 (end of ischaemia)	2 hours	4 hours
Duration of ischaemia			
0 (control)	100	—	—
30 min	47	81	96
60 min	37	69	88
120 min	15	13	17

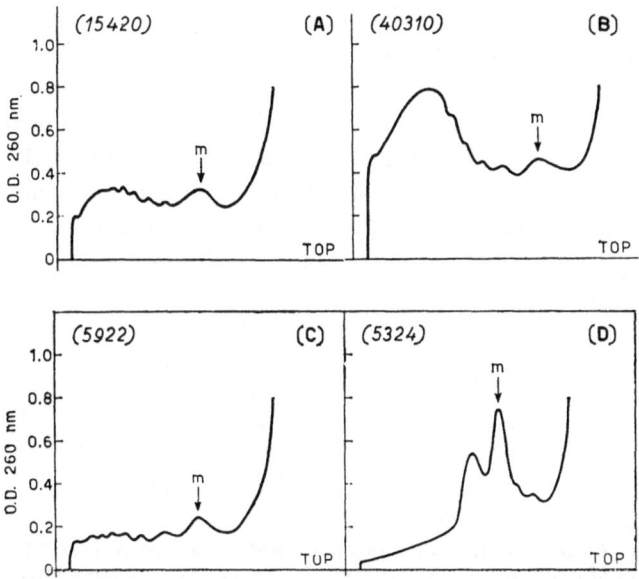

FIGURE 10.1   Polysomal patterns and protein synthesis (in parenthesis: cpm/mg RNA) in rat liver after restoration of the blood supply. A: 60-min ischaemia. B: 60-min ischaemia, two hours after the restoration. C: 120-min ischaemia. D: 120-min ischaemia, two hours after the restoration (From Cajone *et al.* (1971). State and function of liver polysomes during recovery from ischemia. *Exp. Molec. Pathol.*, **14**, 392-403, by courtesy of Academic Press)

3. The pretreatment of the animals with actinomycin D, which prevents the synthesis of new mRNA, does not interfere with the reconstitution of the polysomal patterns after long-duration reversible ischaemia (Figure 10.2). All this does not mean that initiation is the only step affected by ischaemia: it only shows that initiation is more affected than elongation and termination. Indeed, there is also evidence that the readout process is slowed down. First of all, the fact that protein synthesis is inhibited with PMS and isolated ribosomes in reconstructed systems; under these conditions it is generally maintained that initiation occurs minimally or not at all[8,9], and any observed impairment in synthesis must be due to an interference with the completion of initiated peptide chains. Then, there is the more direct observation that poly-somes of definite chain length (tetrasomes and pentasomes) from ischaemic livers carry out the readout process more sluggishly than their normal counterparts[6].

The discussion about the possibility and the ways of recovery brings us to an important point: what is the relevance of the inhibition of protein synthesis to the pathogenesis of cell death? The need for caution in assigning pathogenetic significant to one or other of the metabolic alterations found in dying liver cells has been stressed many times and by many authors[1,10,11]; therefore I will not try to interpret cell death by ischaemia as the result of an impairment in protein synthesis and polysomal aggregation, but I will only discuss the possible role of these factors in the onset of the irreversibility of cell injury.

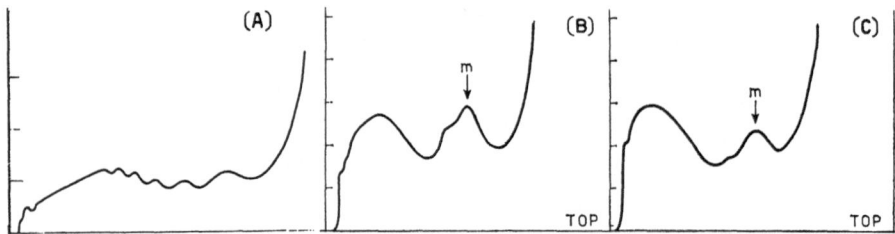

FIGURE 10.2   Recovery of the polysomal pattern after long-term reversible ischaemia. A: at the end of ischaemia. B: Actinomycin D-treated rat, two hours after restoration of the blood supply. C: non-ischaemic (control) treated with actinomycin (From Cajone *et al.* (1971). State and function of liver polysomes during recovery from ischaemia. *Exp. Molec. Pathol.*, **14**, 392–403, by courtesy of Academic Press)

Impairment of protein synthesis occurs early after the onset of ischaemia, more with some preparations (e.g. liver slices), less with others (e.g. polysomes of definite chain length): but on the whole the decay of this activity is progressive with time and there is no clear break between reversible or irreversible ischaemia. The main difference between these two conditions is the possibility—or the lack of possibility—of recovery. The lack of recovery after long-duration irreversible ischaemia may depend on many factors, some intrinsic and some extrinsic to the machinery for protein synthesis. I will briefly point out some of them, but others could also play a significant role.

1. Damage to the monomers. Native monomers, isolated from livers subjected to irreversible ischaemia, incubated with an exogenous messenger such as poly-U, synthesise polyphenylalanine at a rate considerably lower than normal; those isolated from short-duration ischaemia are as active as the normal ones. The persistence beyond a certain time in monomer form, and the exclusion from the functional activity, could prevent the reconstitution of the polyribosomes and hamper the resumption of protein synthesis. Initiation with poly-U has some peculiar features: therefore this observation is only a strong

suggestion—rather than a proof—that the re-entry of the monomers in the ribosomal cycle is considerably impaired after long-duration irreversible ischaemia.

2. Deficiency of mRNA. The prompt reconstitution of the polysomal patterns after reversible ischaemia, even in the presence of actinomycin D, implies the existence of intact mRNA; but mRNA strands could be broken down if they were left for a long time in the cytosol unprotected by attached ribosomes. This is a possibility but we do not have any experimental evidence about it.

3. Lack of energy. Protein synthesis is energy-dependent, and in particular it has been said that chain initiation requires a much higher energy of activation than chain extension. Ischaemia causes a decrease in the oxidative and glycolytic activities of the liver cells[1,12,13]. Mitochondria lose respiratory control and show a lowered ADP/O ratio; ATP content and the energy-charge of liver cells drop, with a con-current profound decrease of the [NAD$^+$]/[NADH] ratio, both in the cytoplasm and mitochondria[14]. All these changes are prompt and deep after the interruption of blood supply and do not become appreciably more severe by prolonging blood deprivation. But the persistence beyond a certain time of a low energy-state and redox-state, together with the incapacity of mitochondria to resume their normal function after irreversible ischaemia, could hamper the recovery of protein synthesis.

4. Depletion of cell-sap factors. Many enzymes and factors necessary for protein synthesis associate temporarily with the ribosomes during certain steps of the ribosomal cycle, but are essentially contained in the cell-sap. We have shown that cell-sap from ischaemic livers has a reduced capacity of supporting protein synthesis in reconstructed systems *in vitro*[2]. Cell-sap is now under investigation in our laboratory; in some preliminary experiments we have seen that it contains a reduced equipment of transfer RNAs, that the formation of the charged RNA is impaired, and the binding of the aminoacyl-RNA to the 40S-messenger complex is also deficient. Cell-sap factors may become critically insufficient after long-duration irreversible ischaemia.

Most of these remarks are only working hypotheses. But on the whole it seems that ischaemia interferes with many cellular functions just as it affects many different cellular structures[15]. Each of these injuries may not be lethal in itself, but when they all occur together the disorganisation of the structural–functional pattern of the cell may become too severe to be repaired: the 'point of no return'[16] is reached, the cell dies and the process proceeds to its conclusion with the appearance of microscopic and macroscopic signs of necrosis at a later stage.

REFERENCES

1. Bernelli-Zazzera, A. and Gaja, G. (1964). Some aspects of glycogen metabolism following reversible or irreversible liver ischemia. *Exp. Molec. Pathol.*, **3**, 351–368
2. Ragnotti, G., Cajone, F. and Bernelli-Zazzera, A. (1970). Structural and functional changes in polysomes from ischemic livers. *Exp. Molec. Pathol.*, **13**, 295–306
3. Cajone, F., Schiaffonati, L. and Bernelli-Zazzera, A. (1973). The binding of ribosomes to rat liver endoplasmic-reticulum membranes *in vitro*: effects of ischaemia. *Biochem. Soc. Trans.*, **1**, 945–947
4. Cajone, F., Schiaffonati, L., Piccoletti, R. and Bernelli-Zazzera, A. (1974). Ribosome–membrane relationships in ischemic livers. *Exp. Molec. Pathol.*, **21**, 40–50
5. Cajone, F. and Schiaffonati, L. (1974). Effects of amino acids on protein synthesis by cellular and subcellular preparations from ischaemic livers. *Brit. J. Exp. Pathol.* (in press)
6. Bernelli-Zazzera, A., Cajone, F., Simonetta, M., Schiaffonati, L. and Piccoletti, R. (1972). Further studies on ribosomal damage in liver ischemia. *Exp. Molec. Pathol.*, **17**, 121–131
7. Noll, H. (1969). Polysomes: analysis of structure and function. In: *Techniques in Protein Biosynthesis*, **2**, 101–179 (P. N. Campbell and J. R. Sargent, editors) (London: Academic Press)
8. Falvey, A. K. and Staehelin, T. (1970). Structure and function of mammalian ribosomes. II. Exchange of ribosomal subunits at various stages of *in vitro* polypeptide synthesis. *J. Molec. Biol.*, **53**, 21–34
9. Henshaw, E. C., Hirsch, C. A., Morton, B. E. and Hiatt, H. H. (1971). Control of protein synthesis in mammalian tissues through changes in ribosome activity. *J. Biol. Chem.*, **246**, 436–446
10. Ashworth, C. T., Werner, D. J., Glass, M. D. and Arnold, N. J. (1965). Spectrum of fine structural changes in hepatocellular injury due to thioacetamide. *Amer. J. Pathol.*, **47**, 917–951
11. Vogt, M. and Farber, E. (1968). On the molecular pathology of ischemic renal cell death. Reversible and irreversible cellular and mitochondria metabolic alterations. *Amer. J. Pathol.*, **53**, 1–24
12. Gaja, G., Bernelli-Zazzera, A. and Sorgato, G. (1965). Glycolysis in dying liver cells. *Exp. Molec. Pathol.*, **4**, 275–281
13. Ragnotti, G., Gaja, G. and Bernelli-Zazzera, A. (1968). Decline and restoration of glycolysis in homogenates. *Exp. Molec. Pathol.*, **9**, 148–159
14. Gaja, G., Ferrero, M. E., Piccoletti, R. and Bernelli-Zazzera, A. (1973).

Phosphorylation and redox states in ischemic liver. *Exp. Molec. Pathol.*, **19**, 248–265

15. Bassi, M. and Bernelli-Zazzera, A. (1964). Ultrastructural cytoplasmic changes of liver cells after reversible and irreversible ischemia. *Exp. Molec. Pathol.*, **3**, 332–350

16. Majno, G., La Gattuta, M. and Thompson, T. E. (1960). Cellular death and necrosis: chemical, physical and morphologic changes in rat liver. *Virchows Arch. Pathol. Anat.*, **333**, 421–465

Histotopochemistry of glycogen and glycogen enzymes after allyl formate poisoning

D. Sasse

Liver poisons can be useful in that they give the anatomist the opportunity to study the functional structure of liver parenchyma.

In 1917 Piazza[1] was the first to describe allyl formate as a hepatotoxic substance which attacks the periportal region of the liver parenchyma. The damage begins with capillary lesions followed by a loss of endothelial cells of the sinusoids. In addition, electron microscopically, a rupture of the liver cells' membranes could be detected[2]. Thus allyl formate is not only a poison acting upon capillaries but is a hepatotoxic substance which leads to a blockade of energy metabolism in the hepatocytes.

Our findings are the results of giving single intraperitoneal injections of allyl formate to adult golden hamsters. In most cases we injected 0.0075 ml allyl formate/100 g body wt.; the animals were killed one, two and three hours after injection[3].

Allyl formate absorbed by the peritoneum is carried by the bloodstream through the portal vessels into the liver parenchyma. Necrosis starts periportally and progresses towards the microvasculatory periphery, the terminal hepatic venule. Histochemically using the PAS-reaction the necrotic hepatocytes can be characterised by their complete loss of glycogen whereas the still intact parenchyma is marked by a high glycogen content. Therefore the healthy and the damaged areas can easily be differentiated and it is possible to detect identical microvasculatory zones within the liver parenchyma.

From a small piece of liver in which nearly 80% of the parenchyma was destroyed, we made serial sections and built up a microreconstruction of the healthy parenchyma and the afferent portal branches at a magnification of 1:125[4].

At first sight the reconstruction shows parenchymal masses of irregular shape; these masses consist of the totality of the still intact hepatocytes in the vasculatory periphery (Figure 11.1). The portal vessels run inside the empty spaces, these spaces correspond to the degenerated zones 1 and 2 of the liver acinus following Rappaport's nomenclature[5]. On top of the reconstruction we can see two preterminal portal branches, each of which supply a part of the liver parenchyma which is called a *complex acinus*. From these preterminal branches there originate several terminal vessels, which are the axes of the *simple acini*. The *terminal hepatic venules* are always surrounded by the still intact parenchyma because they are situated at the most peripheral point of the microvascularisation. Therefore they are not 'central veins'. The irregular shape of the microvasculatory periphery is a result of the branching of the afferent vessels. What is important is, that the periportal and the perivenous zones of the liver parenchyma build up a continuum of equally supplied hepatocytes. This must be kept in mind when regarding a section of liver tissue: there are no insular remainders.

The fact, that the microvasculatory-dependent functional units can be destroyed step by step starting from the portal region up to the terminal hepatic venule suggested that allyl formate should be used for

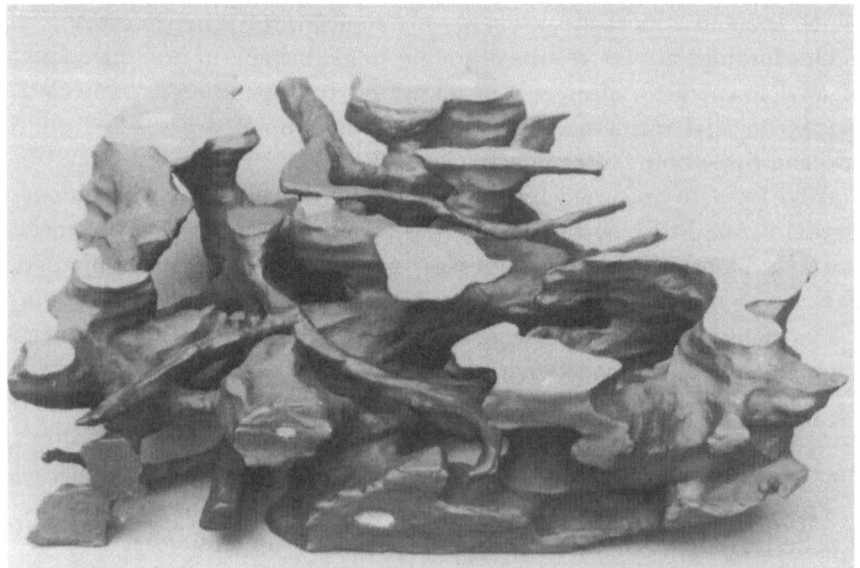

FIGURE 11.1   Microreconstruction of liver parenchyma after allyl formate poisoning. The peripheral zone 3 and the portal veins are reconstructed

the study of the enzymatic equipment of the parenchymal zones. However, there remains the question of what happens to those enzymes whose highest activities are normally situated in the periportal area, when this zone is damaged by allyl formate.

Using histochemical techniques the main activities of glycogen synthetase and phosphorylase can be demonstrated in the periportal zone. This contradicts Eger[6] who believed the essential steps of glycogen metabolism to be around the 'central vein'. Following the hypothesis that the functional units of the liver are rather steady ones, i.e. that the enzymatic equipment of the periportal hepatocytes differs from the equipment of the perivenous cells, then a clinical or experimental necrosis of the periportal field must necessarily lead to a complete breakdown of all metabolic functions which are bound to this area.

Under the experimental condition of allyl formate poisoning it is possible to demonstrate, however, that a necrosis of zone 1 does not lead to a loss of glycogen synthetase and phosphorylase activities but to a shifting of these activities towards the nearest healthy zone; at first to the outer border of zone 2, then to zone 3 (Figures 11.2 and 11.3). In

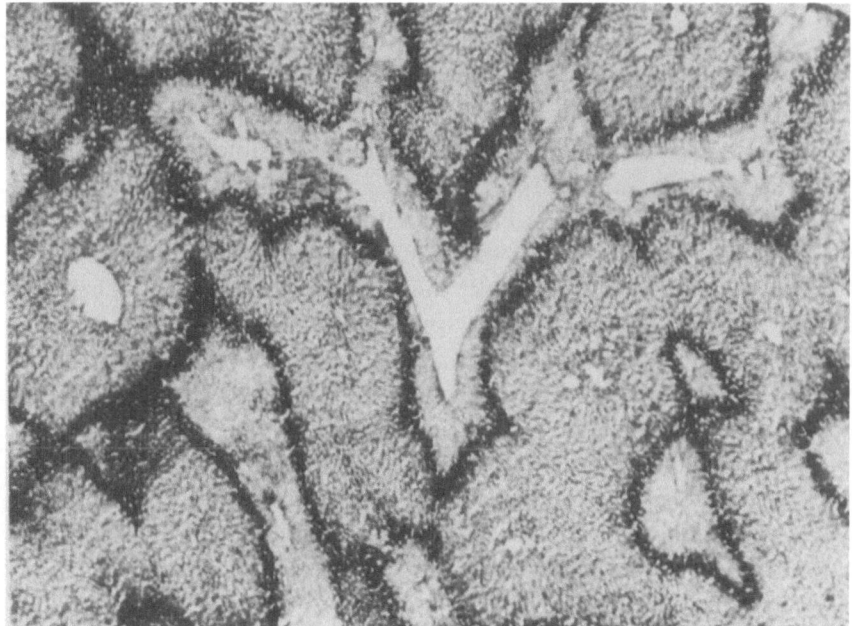

FIGURE 11.2   UDPGGT activity in the liver after allyl formate. Main enzyme activity is localised in zone 2 of the liver acinus

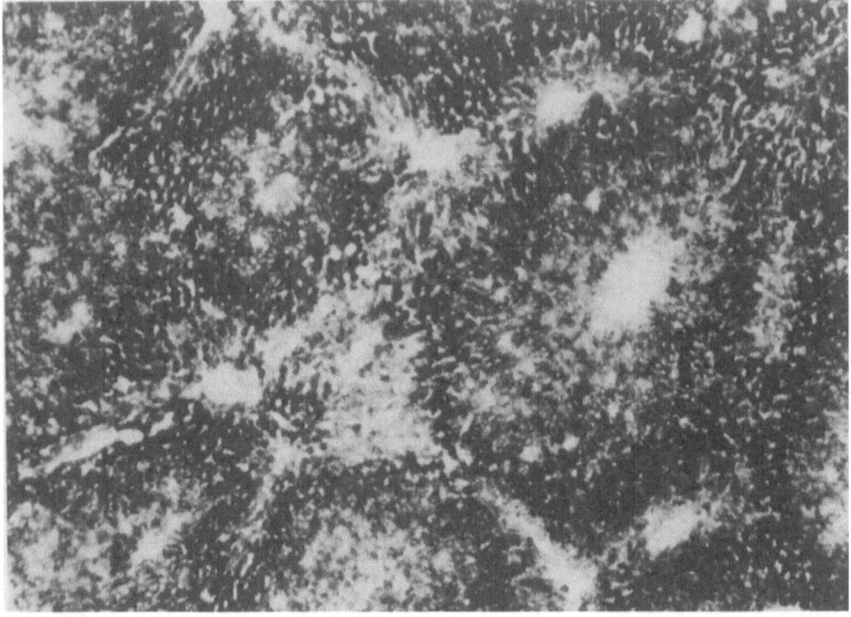

FIGURE 11.3   Phosphorylase activity in the liver after allyl formate. Most intense
reaction in zone 2 of the liver acinus

cases of more advanced necrosis the activity of glycogen synthetase is
shifted towards the extreme periphery around the terminal hepatic
venule (Figure 11.4). As yet it has not been possible to localise phosphorylase activity in this area.

The translocation of the enzyme activities of glycogen metabolism
could be interpreted in this way: glucose, transported by the afferent
vessels normally arrives at first at the periportal hepatocytes. Therefore
in this zone glycogen is built up by a high UDPGGT activity. In the
same field phosphorylase activity is necessary to compensate the synthetase activity and to enable the glucose to be transported towards the
terminal hepatic venule.

After poisoning the periportal zone by allyl formate the glycogen and
the glycogen-bound enzymes are discharged from these cells. Zone 1
now is metabolically mute. In this case the adjacent healthy zone 2 or 3
is the target field for the arriving glucose. By this the enzyme activities
are activated, or, perhaps, induced.

On the basis of the evidence provided, it can be concluded that by
using histochemical techniques it is possible to demonstrate a sub-

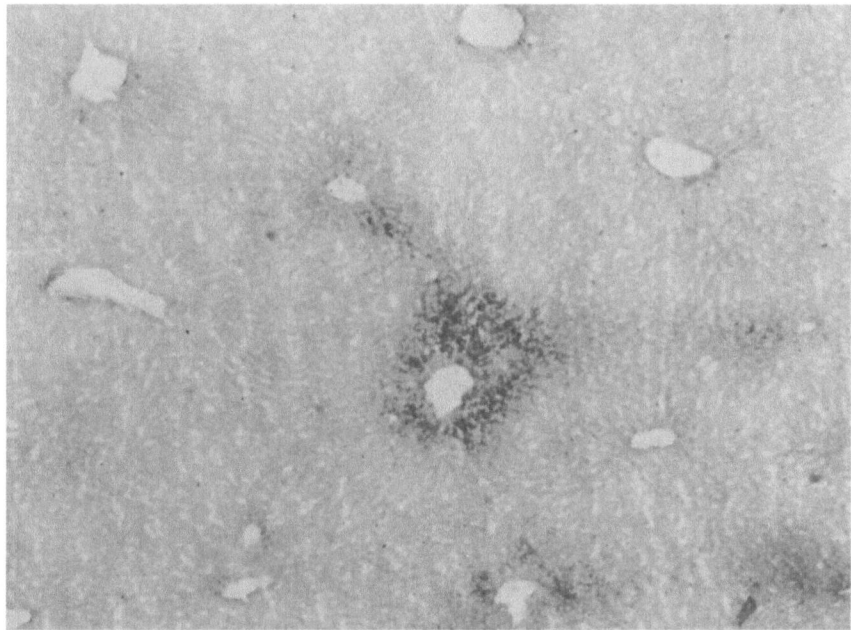

FIGURE 11.4 UDPGGT activity in the liver after allyl formate. Enzyme activity at the most peripheral point of the acinus, in zone 3 around the terminal hepatic venule

division of functions within the liver parenchyma. These functional units depend on vasculatory conditions and are therefore not steady but dynamic ones.

REFERENCES

1. Piazza, J. G. (1917). Zur Kenntnis der Wirkung von Allylverbindungen. *Z. Exp. Pathol. Ther.*, **17**, 318–341
2. Haenni, B. (1964). Les effects de l'intoxication aiguë au formiate d'allyl sur le foie du rat. Etude au microscope électronique. *Pathol. Microbiol.* (*Basel*), **27**, 974–1002
3. Sasse, D. and Köhler, J. (1969). Die Verlagerung von Funktionseinheiten des Glykogenstoffwechsels in der Leber durch Allylformiat. *Histochemie*, **18**, 325–336
4. Sasse, D. and Schenk, A. Die räumliche Darstellung der funktionellen Lebereinheit (Acinus). *Acta Anat.* (in press)
5. Rappaport, A. M. (1960). Betrachtungen zur Pathophysiologie der Leberstruktur (Übersicht). *Klin. Wschr.*, **38**, 561–577
6. Eger, W. (1954). Zur Pathologie des zentralen und peripheren Funktionsfeldes des Leberläppchens. *Zbl. Allg. Pathol. pathol. Anat.*, **91**, 255–267

The measurement of liver injury and protection, with special reference to paracetamol, dimethylnitrosamine and carbon tetrachloride

A. E. M. McLean

Paracetamol (N. acetyl *para*-amino phenol, acetaminophan 'Panadol', and many other trade names in USA, Germany and elsewhere) is a safe and effective analgesic, used like aspirin, but without aspirin's gastric irritant effect. It was well-described in 1894[1] and is practically without side-effects in normal use. However in gross overdose (12–50 g in man) it causes severe liver damage[2]. In 1973 there were about 5000 cases of self-poisoning with paracetamol in Britain, with 50 deaths (R. Goulding, Poisons Centre, Guy's Hospital, London, personal communication).

Acute overdosage in the rat (about 3 g/kg by mouth) causes liver necrosis in about 18 hours. The liver injury is unusual in its extreme variability. In a group of animals given the same dose, some will have no liver injury, some have massive necrosis of all lobes and some will have massive necrosis of one lobe, fading into centrilobular necrosis and with parts of lobes left uninjured (Figure 12.1). This makes histological assessment of the quantity of injury impossible and other means of measurement of liver injury have to be found. Plasma isocitrate dehydrogenase (ICD) activity correlates well with the proportion of liver involved in the injury, when the ICD is expressed as a logarithmic function and the weight of the affected part of the liver compared with that left unaffected.

It has been known for a long time that paracetamol is excreted largely as the glucuronide and sulphate conjugates[3]. Recent work by Mitchell and co-workers[4] has shown that phenobarbital pretreatment of mice makes them sensitive to paracetamol, that toxic effects are preceded by

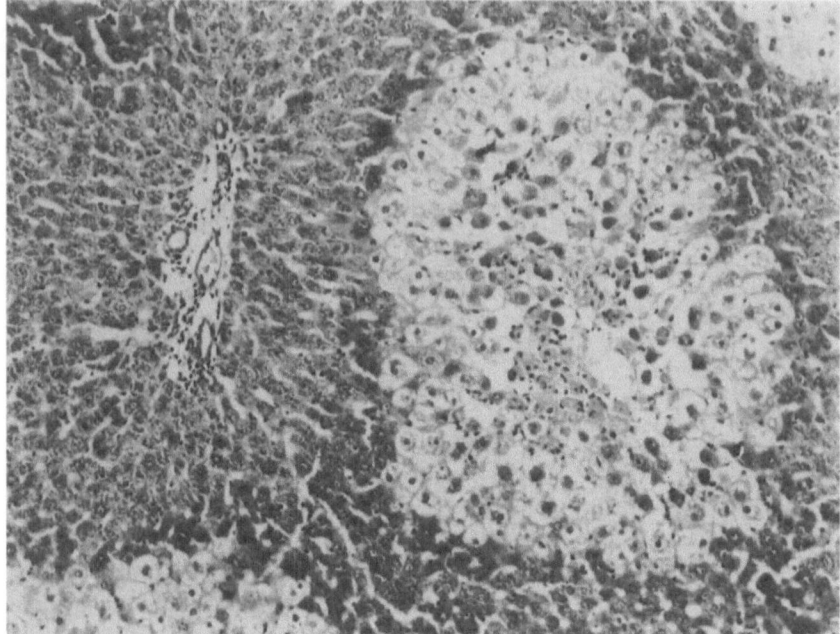

FIGURE 12.1   Centrilobular necrosis in part of a liver 24 hours after 1 g/kg oral dose of paracetamol phenobarbital pretreated rat[5] ($\times$ 85)

depletion of liver glutathione levels and that liver injury is accompanied by 'covalent binding' of paracetamol metabolites to liver proteins. They suggest that oxidative metabolism of paracetamol by the P_{450} system produces a reactive metabolite that attacks glutathione and when this is depleted, attack on liver cell organelles follows.

We have worked on the dietary factors that alter paracetamol toxicity[5]. Table 12.1 shows that feeding low protein diets lowers glutathione concentration in the liver and increases the sensitivity of the animals to paracetamol in spite of lower levels of cytochrome P_{450}.

The measurement of LD_{50} involves finding a dose–response relation. The doses required to achieve the predetermined response (in this case 50% mortality), vary as the diets and pretreatments of animals used are varied. The changes in LD_{50} give an indication not only that a change has occurred, but give a measure of how big the change is. The classical technique of experimental pathology is to give a single dose of toxin, and to measure the response at a single time with or without various pretreatments, or antidotes. This procedure can only tell us that some-

Table 12.1   THE EFFECT OF DIET AND PHENOBARBITONE ON THE LETHALITY OF PARACETAMOL AND ON CYTOCHROME P_{450} AND GLUTATHIONE CONTENT OF THE LIVER

Diet	Cytochrome P_{450} nmol/g liver	Gluta-thione μmol/g liver	Lethality of paracetamol LD_{50} g/kg	(95% limits)
Stock pellets (41B)	40 ± 9	6.9 ± 1.7	5.2	(4.6–6.0)
Stock pellets (41B) + phenobarbitone	142 ± 35	7.6 ± 1.0	2.0	(1.7–2.4)
3% casein, 5% olive oil diet	23 ± 5	2.2 ± 0.2	2.1	(2.0–2.3)
3% casein, 5% olive oil diet + phenobarbitone	81 ± 15	2.8 ± 0.3	0.9	(0.8–1.0)
25% yeast diet	37 ± 3	2.8 ± 0.5	0.4	(0.2–0.7)

LD_{50} values were determined on at least four groups of four rats and calculated by the method of Weil[5]. Other results are expressed as the mean of at least five determinations on different animals ± one standard deviation

thing has or has not happened at the particular dose. Since it may well be that our pretreatment has altered the shape of the dose response curve, no quantitative measure of change of toxicity can come from such a procedure.

For instance, the 'yeast diet' (Table 12.1) which is deficient in vitamin E, and methionine, not only makes the rats sensitive to paracetamol, but also changes the time of death from 24 hours after dosing to about four hours after dosing. This change in time course is associated with a new pathological picture. Instead of liver failure, we see a massive block of blood flow out of the liver. Table 12.2 shows that the rat's liver

Table 12.2   THE EFFECT OF PARACETAMOL 500 mg/kg I.P. *in vivo* ON RATS FED ON YEAST DIET PLUS PHENOBARBITONE IN DRINKING WATER

	Liver wt. g%	Haemoglobin in liver % of total body Hb	Plasma ICD nmol/ml/min	Pyramidon demethylation μM/g/hour by liver slice
Rat (1)	8.9	67%	107	1.2
Rat (2)	7.1	18%	1980	0.2
Rat (3-control) No paracetamol	5.2	7%	1	1.3

becomes grossly enlarged and a high proportion of the total body red cell mass is trapped in the liver. This effect is most easily explained as being caused by leakage of reactive metabolites from the hepatocytes. The metabolites can then damage vascular endothelium of centrilobular veins or else sinusoidal lining cells, and cause an outflow block to blood flow.

In measuring plasma enzymes another problem arises. Plasma enzyme activity of a group of animals (or persons) is not normally distributed, but log-normally distributed. If the statistical procedures appropriate to the normal distribution are applied to the arithmetic measurements, one gets results like 500 ± 400 for mean and standard deviation. This is ridiculous because some values must lie between one and two standard deviations below the mean and these would have to be negative enzyme activities! This meaningless application of a wrong statistic often produces spurious significance of results because it places undue weight on a few very high activities. If the logarithm of each enzyme activity is taken, then mean and standard deviations and tests of significance can be correctly calculated by the usual procedures. For ease of communication the antilog of the mean and the antilog of the mean +1SD and antilog mean −1SD can be used to show how the values are distributed in their ordinary biochemical units. Table 12.3 shows how phenobarbital pretreatment alters serum enzyme activity after paracetamol dosage.

Table 12.3 shows that the phenobarbital treated rat responds to 0.5 g

Table 12.3 DOSE RESPONSE RELATION BETWEEN PARACETAMOL AND PLASMA ISOCITRATE DEHYDROGENASE ACTIVITY

| | | ICD activity | |
| | | Geometric mean | ± 1 SD |
Paracetamol dose	Treatment		
2 g/kg	—	13	(2–86)
1 g/kg	—	11	(7–41)
2 g/kg	+ Phenobarbital	1360	(280–6630)
1 g/kg	+ Phenobarbital	115	(10–1470)
0.5 g/kg	+ Phenobarbital	33	(4–300)
0.25 g/kg	+ Phenobarbital	2	(1–3)
1 g/kg	+ Phenobarbital + Methionine 100 mg/kg	8	(1–48)

All rats were fed stock diet *ad libitum* with or without one week's pretreatment with phenobarbital in the drinking water. Methionine was given as a single oral dose at the same time as the oral dose of paracetamol

paracetamol with a more severe injury than the stock rat has in response to 2 g/kg. Although only a single point is shown it also indicates that 10% methionine brings the toxic effect down by a factor of at least more than two. Further quantitation would require a more complete dose response curve.

Figure 12.2 shows the effect of addition of 25% methionine to oral paracetamol doses. The lethal effects are largely abolished, so that an LD_{50} cannot be obtained in the presence of methionine. These techniques of *in vivo* measurement of toxicity have led us to suggest that paracetamol could be used more safely if a small amount of methionine or cystine were added to the formulation.

In vitro studies are often useful especially as screening techniques to find out if a particular molecule has an effect on some toxic process. Incubation of rat liver slices from the highly sensitive 'yeast phenobarbital' or 'Stock + phenobarbital' fed animals gives such a technique for paracetamol.

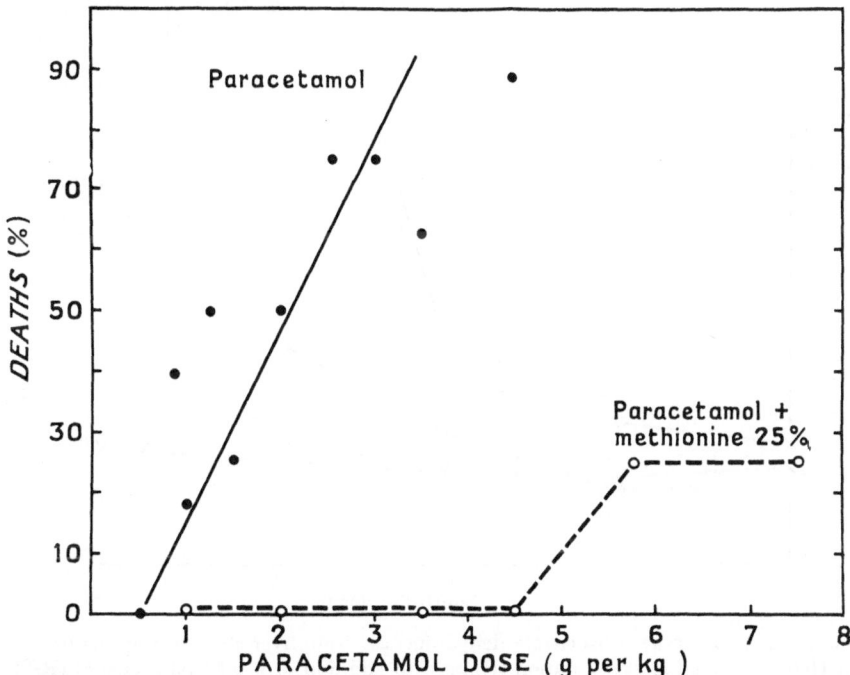

FIGURE 12.2 Effect on methionine on the lethal action of paracetamol in phenobarbital pretreated rats. Paracetamol or paracetamol–methionine mixtures (4–1) were given orally as a suspension and the rats observed for one week. At least four rats were treated at each dosage point

The system is not as complex as the whole animal, nor as far removed from life as microsomes, nor as laborious as the isolated perfused liver or liver cells. Liver slices incubated in Hepes Ringer, leak very little isocitrate dehydrogenase into the medium. If paracetamol is added large amounts leak out after a latent interval (Figure 12.3). The microsomal demethylation of pyramidon to 4-amino antipyrine by liver slices is also

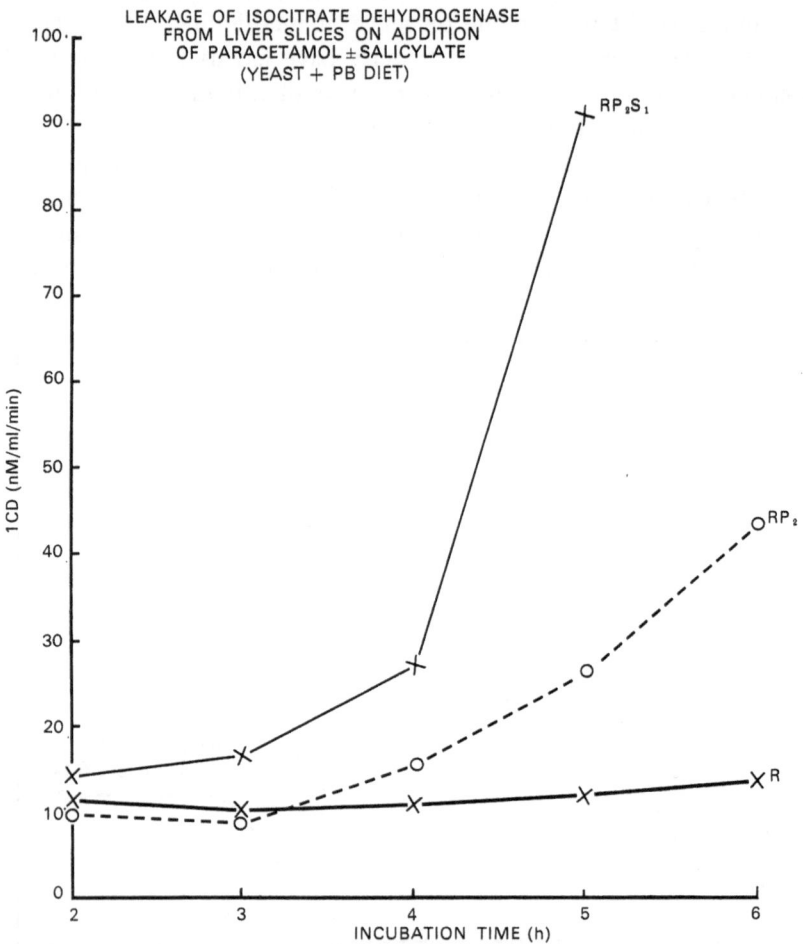

FIGURE 12.3   Leakage of isocitrate dehydrogenase from liver slice during incubation in Hepes buffered Ringer solution (R) or with addition of 2 mM paracetamol (RP_2) or addition of paracetamol + 1 mM salicylate (RP_2S_1). The salicylate blocks the metabolism of paracetamol to glucuronide or sulphate conjugates. The slices incubated in Ringer solution lost 4–6% of their total isocitrate dehydrogenase into the medium in six hours

blocked by preincubation with paracetamol. Slices are incubated for three hours with paracetamol at varying doses and then moved to a second fresh Ringer solution containing pyramidon. Pyramidon demethylation is seen to be powerfully inhibited by preincubation with paracetamol (Figure 12.4). This inhibition is prevented by addition of

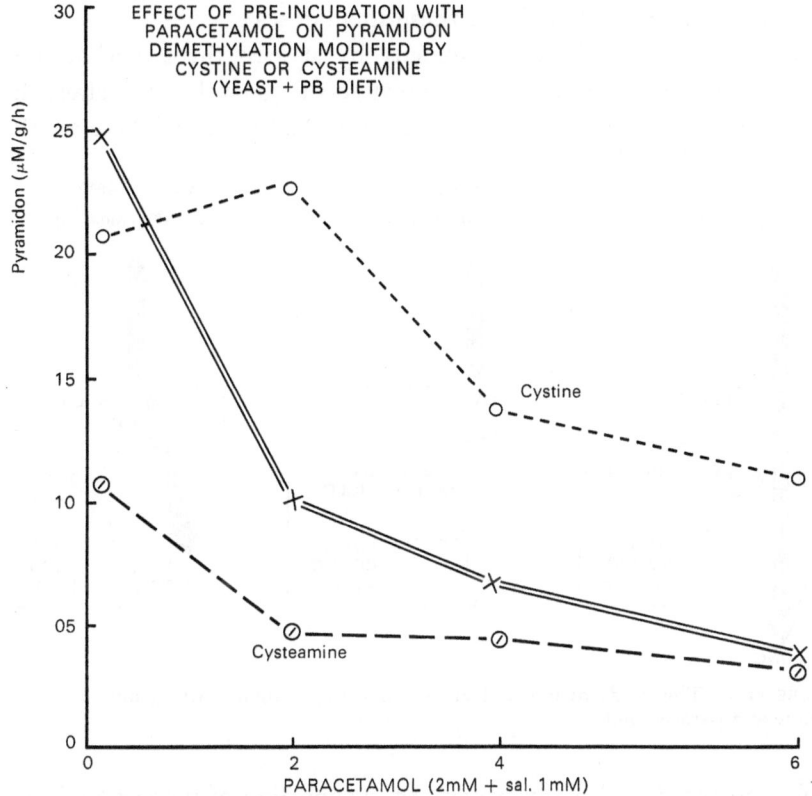

FIGURE 12.4   The effect of three hours' preincubation in Ringer solution containing paracetamol, on demethylation of pyramidon in a second incubation medium containing only Ringer plus pyramidon (2 mM)

cystine to the first incubation medium. Cysteamine which has been proposed as a treatment for paracetamol poisoning[4], irreversibly blocks pyramidon demethylation. It seems likely that the protective effect of cysteamine depends on its inhibiting effect on paracetamol metabolism through destruction of the microsomal system.

If we consider the metabolism of paracetamol, carbon tetrachloride

(CCl$_4$) and dimethyl nitrosamine (DMN) (Figure 12.5), we note that while CCl$_4$ can either be breathed out harmlessly or be metabolised to a toxic compound, no such alternative exists for DMN. DMN can only be metabolised slowly, or quickly. The amount of liver damage produced by a small (10–40 mg/kg) dose of DMN does not depend on the rate of DMN metabolism. Varying the diet varies the rate of DMN metabolism but does not alter the toxicity of these small doses[6].

For paracetamol, diet alters toxicity by at least three mechanisms. First, diet (including phenobarbitone) affects P$_{450}$ level and so alters the ratio between glucuronidation and oxidation pathways[5,6]. These are the

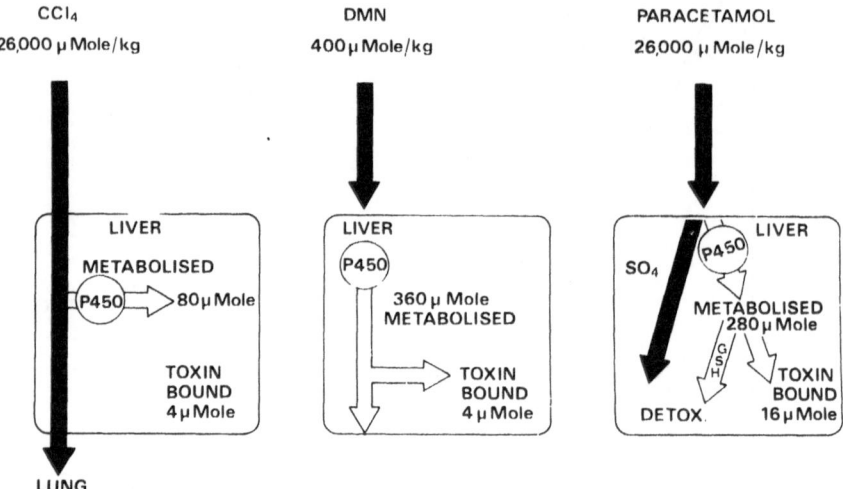

FIGURE 12.5   The mode of metabolism of three hepatotoxins, CCl$_4$, dimethylnitrosamine and paracetamol

'safe' and the 'toxic' pathways and the proportion of paracetamol dose that will be activated is varied in this way.

Secondly the diet can alter glutathione levels and so alter the amount of toxic metabolite that is rendered harmless by reaction with glutathione[5].

Thirdly an unknown factor, to which vitamin E deficiency may contribute a small part, makes the yeast fed rats highly sensitive. Which of these factors is important in man is yet unknown, but we can at least use our present knowledge to see if methionine is a safe and effective method of prevention or treatment of paracetamol self-poisoning.

REFERENCES

1. Hinsberg, O. and Treupel, G. (1894). Ueber die Physiologische Wirkung des *p*-Amido phenols und einiger Derivative Desselben. *Arch. Exp. Pathol.*, **33**, 216–250
2. Prescott, L. F., Wright, N., Roscol, P. and Brown, S. S. (1971). Plasma paracetamol half life and hepatic necrosis in patients with paracetamol overdosage. *Lancet*, **i**, 519–522
3. Williams, R. T. (1959). *Detoxication Mechanisms*, 328 (London: Chapman and Hall)
4. Mitchell, J. R., Thorgeiresson, S. S., Potter, W. Z., Jollow, D. J. and Keiser, H. (1974). Acetaminophen induced hepatic injury: Protective role of gluthathione in man and rationale for therapy. *Clin. Pharmacol. Ther.*, **16**, 676-684.
5. McLean, A. E. M. and Day, P. A. (1975). The effect of diet on the toxicity of paracetamol and the safety of paracetamol–methionine mixtures. *Biochem. Pharmacol.*, **25**, 37–42.
6. McLean, A. E. M. and Day, P. A. (1974). The use of new methods to measure the effect of diet and inducers of microsomal enzyme synthesis of cytochrome P_{450} in liver homogenates and a metabolism of dimethyl nitrosamine. *Biochem. Pharmacol.*, **23**, 1173–1180

CHAPTER 13

Hepatoprotective substances: a partial assessment

K. Aterman and G. Yüce

INTRODUCTION

The widespread use of carbon tetrachloride (CCl_4) has led to an equally widespread search for substances which would prevent or mitigate the effects of this toxin on the liver. The study of such 'hepatoprotective' agents has almost become a branch of the experimental pathology of the liver in its own right, for their number is large, and they include a curious assortment of unrelated substances such as honey given subcutaneously, or water from an Italian spa. Frequently no rational explanation can be given of some of these alleged protective effects, which have either not been re-examined at all by other workers or have been flatly contradicted. The scepticism engendered by this unsatisfactory state of affairs may lead to potentially valuable protective substances being overlooked or discarded. Yet the example of the 'antioxidants' has shown how important the continued search for such protective substances can be. Recknagel and Glende[1] have recently again pointed out what an effect the discovery of the protective action of antioxidants has had on current views of the mode of action of CCl_4. It was, therefore, thought desirable to offer a comparative basis for further study by reinvestigating some of the substances with real or alleged hepatoprotective properties, and to eliminate some of the variable factors which may have contributed to the ambiguous or contradictory results reported. The scope of this study has been limited to some of the better known or more interesting substances affecting the course of poisoning by CCl_4.

EXPERIMENTAL PROCEDURE

The procedure adopted was to follow in most instances the experimental details of the workers who had reported the hepatoprotective properties of a given substance, and then to test this substance under 'standard' conditions. These were intended to decrease the marked variability from animal to animal which is such a well-known feature of the liver damage produced by CCl_4, and included in the first place the use of littermates only. The experiments were based mainly on male rats of the Sprague–Dawley strain, although females were also used on occasion. Each experimental animal was only compared with its untreated littermate. The effect of cortisone on the protective action of N,N-diphenyl-p-phenylene-diamine or DPPD, for instance, was tested in four littermates in such a way that one rat was given only CCl_4, whereas the three brothers received in addition, respectively, cortisone, DPPD, and cortisone and DPPD together. In none of the experiments were fewer than eight animals used per group, with the corresponding number of controls. In many experiments the numbers were larger. Moreover, several important experiments were repeated after some time, in order to test their reproducibility. CCl_4 was mostly injected subcutaneously in a dose of 0.15 ml/100 g body wt. In some instances, however, CCl_4 was given by intraportal or intrasplenic injection, in order to eliminate a possible effect of the hepatoprotective substance on the absorption of CCl_4, which might have masqueraded as a protective effect on the liver itself.

The assessment of protective effects presents some difficulty. The importance of choosing appropriate criteria has been emphasised by Recknagel and Glende[1]. Some authors have used the survival time of animals after large doses of CCl_4 as an easily defined endpoint. While this may be a valid procedure, it may not be relevant for the assessment of hepatoprotective properties, since the effect of large doses of CCl_4 need not be limited to liver damage. This has recently been strongly emphasised by Slater[2] who criticised the use of large doses of CCl_4. Although the survival time of littermates was also tested in some instances of the present series, it was considered more appropriate to place the emphasis mainly on a combined histological and functional evaluation of liver damage. All livers were fixed in 10% neutral buffered formalin and the extent of necrosis, hydropic vacuolation and fatty change was determined in 7 μm sections. For liver function studies the serum levels of the glutamic-oxalacetic (SGOT) and the glutamic-pyruvic (SGPT) transaminases, as well as the degree of bromsulph-thalein retention (BSP), were ascertained. Since these tests were based on micromethods, they could be repeated in the same animal 24, 48, 72 and even 96 hours after the injection of CCl_4, so that the development of liver damage with and without hepatoprotective substances could be followed in relation to time. An attempt was, of course, made to corre-late the histological with the functional impairment of the liver. What correlation between these parameters of liver damage, however, could be found was only approximate. Although, in general, a severe func-tional disturbance was also accompanied by marked histological damage, a strict correlation could not always be found in the individual animals, if they were graded according to their serum enzyme levels and the histological appearance. Vorhaus and Vorhaus[3] had had a similar experience with regard to the BSP test. One reason may be found in the very nature of the histological changes. It is, perhaps, not widely known that the pathological changes following the administration of CCl_4 are not always uniformly distributed throughout the section—a fact seemingly ignored in those studies that rely only on histological appearances as an index of liver damage. Moreover, serious difficulties arise if one attempts to evaluate from a functional point of view the variable spectrum of changes—necrosis, hydropic change and fatty vacuolation—found histologically, since there are no indications avail-able as to how much each morphological component contributes to the functional impairment. This difficulty led to the emphasis being placed in the present experiments mainly on the functional changes observed, since their quantitative evaluation appeared to be less open to subjective judgments than the widely used method of the histological gradation of liver damage. In this context attention should be drawn to the fact that the functional evaluation did not rely only on the serum levels of the transaminases, but included also a test of the excretory capacity of the liver. No significant discrepancies between these functional parameters were observed.

RESULTS AND DISCUSSION

The first experiments undertaken were intended to study the effect of intrasplenic injections of CCl_4 on liver function. One such experiment is shown in Table 13.1. Under these conditions CCl_4 produces liver damage which appears to be proportional to the dose given. Larger doses were not studied from the functional point of view, because the animals tended to die rather rapidly with extensive liver necrosis. Smaller doses, however, can be used in studies of hepatoprotective substances. This was done, for instance, when the favourable effects of zinc chloride given subcutaneously, or of DPPD given intraperitoneally, were evaluated and clearly demonstrated. The intraportal or the more convenient intrasplenic injection of CCl_4, therefore, offers a convincing

Table 13.1   THE EFFECT OF GRADED INTRASPLENIC INJECTIONS OF CCl_4 ON THE LIVER FUNCTION OF MALE AND FEMALE RATS

Dose (µl)	SGOT	SGPT	BSP
2 ♀	714	399	28.5
4 ♀	961	509	32.8
5 ♂	2460	1640	58.7
6 ♀	2268	1272	53.6
7.5♂	3731	2706	65.5
10 ♂	10,010	8296	93.3

means of evaluating hepatoprotective substances; it should always be used when such claims are to be confirmed.

One of the first substances for which hepatoprotective properties have been claimed was *xanthine* given subcutaneously or intramuscularly[4]. It will perhaps be recalled that the alleged ameliorating effects of some liver extracts were also attributed to xanthine, but its effect could then be explained as little as it can be now; it was finally viewed as 'non-specific'—as if this label added one iota to our understanding—, because it was later maintained that the injection of other inert substances inducing localised inflammatory changes also could produce hepatoprotective effects[5,6]. Table 13.2 shows that under the conditions of the present experiment the administration of xanthine has no demonstrable effect on the liver damage caused by CCl_4. The functional impairment is the same in the rats given xanthine as in their brothers not receiving it. It is ironical that experiments which served as a potent stimulus for further studies should years later not be confirmed. There is, apparently, no need to invoke an ill-defined 'non-specific' effect. This applies also to the next series of experiments presented here in which the claims of Stenger *et al.*[7] were tested. These workers had at first maintained that 'blockade' of the reticuloendothelial system favourably affected the degree of liver damage produced by CCl_4[8], but

Table 13.2 THE FAILURE OF TWO SUBCUTANEOUS DOSES OF XANTHINE (50 mg/100 g BODY WT.) TO AFFECT THE LIVER DAMAGE BY A SUBCUTANEOUS DOSE OF CCl_4 (0.15 ml/100 g BODY WT.)

Time	Treatment	SGOT*	SGPT*	BSP*
24 h	CCl_4	1841.13 ± 185.71	1309.60 ± 171.07	48.48 ± 5.60
	CCl_4 + Xanthine	1874.66 ± 237.17	1257.93 ± 196.00	48.87 ± 6.36
48 h	CCl_4	1970.08 ± 226.40	1398.84 ± 161.40	50.95 ± 5.68
	CCl_4 + Xanthine	2018.14 ± 166.81	1409.64 ± 194.08	51.62 ± 5.53

* Mean ± S.D.

were later led to postulate an unexplained, perhaps mechanical, effect of substances that stimulated the phagocytic cells of the liver. They supported their contention by treating rats with *India ink* before the injection of CCl_4. India ink was one of the substances that had also been tested, with rather questionable results, by earlier workers when the alleged effects of xanthine became more widely known. In the series of Stenger *et al.*[7,8] pretreatment with India ink was stated to mitigate the effect of CCl_4 on the liver even if this poison was given as long as one month after the intravenous injections of India ink. It should be noted that the claims of Stenger's group were based on morphologic, including electron microscopic, but not on liver function studies. Re-examination of these claims under the standard conditions of the present experimental series, however, did not bear them out. Table 13.3 shows the results of one of several such experiments: no significant differences in liver impairment by CCl_4 were found after pretreatment with India ink.

Table 13.3 THE FAILURE OF THE SEX OF THE ANIMAL AND OF THREE INTRA-VENOUS INJECTIONS (0.7 ml) OF INDIA INK (I.I.), TO INFLUENCE THE SEVERITY OF LIVER DAMAGE ASSESSED 24 HOURS AFTER THE SUBCUTANEOUS INJECTION OF A SINGLE DOSE OF CCl_4 (0.1 ml/100 g BODY WT.)

	SGOT	SGPT	BSP	
CCl_4	1216.10 ± 368.45	593.30 ± 392.20	58.21 ± 7.09	
CCl_4 + I.I. ♂	1179.90 ± 354.96	549.50 ± 410.09	55.58 ± 7.91	< 0.05
CCl_4	1154.90 ± 342.90	494.60 ± 345.97	50.38 ± 7.36	
CCl_4 + I.I. ♀	1139.20 ± 351.25	544.50 ± 410.82	52.29 ± 6.22	

Nor were such differences seen if instead of India ink *trypan blue*, another substance stimulating the RES, was used. According to Petrelli and Stenger[9] pretreatment with trypan blue also reduced the liver damage produced by CCl_4. Table 13.4 shows that this claim could

Table 13.4 THE LACK OF EFFECT OF AN INTRAVENOUS INJECTION OF TRYPAN BLUE (3 ml OF A 2.5% SUSPENSION/250 g BODY WT.) ON THE LIVER DAMAGE PRODUCED IN FEMALE RATS BY AN INTRAPERITONEAL DOSE OF CCl_4 (0.5 ml)

		SGOT	SGPT
24 hours	CCl_4	2492.75 ± 376.62	1302.88 ± 107.85
	CCl_4 + T.B.	2476.00 ± 189.06	1293.50 ± 194.80
48 hours	CCl_4	2652.40 ± 114.28	1257.40 ± 294.98
	CCl_4 + T.B.	2341.40 ± 440.64	1477.40 ± 70.91

not be confirmed. It is hoped to publish these experiments in detail elsewhere. Here it may be sufficient merely to state that a modifying effect of the RES activated by India ink or by trypan blue, which would in any case be difficult to explain in the light of current views of the mode of action of CCl_4, has by no means been proved.

It has already been pointed out that in most of the experiments of the present series only male rats have been used. This choice was based on the repeatedly stated assertion that male rats were more susceptible to damage by CCl_4 than were female animals[10]. It was, therefore, conceivable that the protective effects against CCl_4 might also be determined or influenced by the sex of the experimental animal: India ink, for instance, ineffective in male rats, might still protect female animals. From Table 12.3, based on littermate male and female rats, it can be seen that this is not the case. This table, however, also shows that by the criteria chosen here the functional impairment after CCl_4 alone also is not significantly influenced by the sex of the experimental animals. Only with the BSP retention test could a somewhat greater impairment—of questionable statistical significance—be noted in male than in female rats. That the sex of the experimental animal does not appear to be of striking importance in the response of the liver to CCl_4 seems to be borne out also by the data presented in Table 13.1. Neither could there be found conspicuous differences when the protective effects of α-tocopherol were studied in male and in female rats, as will be shown. This lack of an effect of the sex of the animals is in contrast to the findings or assumptions of other workers and should, therefore, be further tested.

A considerable body of data has been assembled concerning the protective effects of 'antioxidants'. The stimulus for this line of investigation was given when the effects of α-tocopherol on the course of poisoning by CCl_4 were studied[11]. The published data concerning α-tocopherol, however, were by no means conclusive. Some of the discrepancies have been reviewed by Recknagel and Glende; to some extent these may be accounted for by the criteria chosen to assess the protective effects. It would be difficult, for instance, to claim any significant effect of pretreatment by α-tocopherol, given intraperitoneally 40 hours before a massive oral dose of CCl_4, on the survival time of littermate rats (Table 13.5). This contrasts with the results summarised by Recknagel and Glende[1]. In experiments on the survival time of the animals of the present series it was found that a clear-cut separation of

Table 13.5 THE NUMBER OF MALE RATS SURVIVING A SINGLE TOXIC ORAL DOSE OF CCl_4 (4 ml/kg BODY WT.) WITH AND WITHOUT α-TOCOPHEROL (95 INTERNATIONAL UNITS/150 g BODY WT. INTRAPERITONEALLY)

	CCl_4 (4 ml/kg)	$CCl_4 + \alpha$ — tocopherol (95 I.U./150 g)
Short term (< 3 days)	14	9
Long term (> 7 days)	0	3

the results could be obtained, if the survival times were arbitrarily divided into a 'short-term', i.e. fewer than three days, and a 'long-term', i.e. more than seven days, survival period. One such experiment is shown in Table 13.5, but, although the actual figures may differ, the conclusions drawn from other experiments were essentially the same. Following an oral dose of CCl_4 of 4 ml/kg body wt., for instance, six rats survived fewer than three, and eight rats more than seven days. The corresponding survival times of their littermates—although pairs only were compared, in these instances the conclusions are the same if the group as a whole is considered—given an intraperitoneal injection of 95 international units of α-tocopherol 40 hours earlier, were seven rats for the short, and nine rats for the longer term—obviously no significant difference. Similarly, a third group of littermates, given intraperitoneally 50 mg of *nicotinic acid*[12] three times in two daily divided doses, showed survival times which did not differ significantly from those of their brothers in the other two groups just mentioned (six rats short-, six rats long-term). Of interest in this context is the unexplained variability of the survival times of the control rats given CCl_4 only in experiments undertaken at different times. This is another reason why in such experiments littermates should be used. Another possible fallacy is that not only the dose of the protective agent but, above all, also the toxic dose of CCl_4 given may have to be more carefully adjusted and evaluated than was the case in some of the published experiments, if possible protective effects are not to the overshadowed by too high a dose of the toxin. This is illustrated in Table 13.6 which shows that pretreatment with *sodium selenite*—a trace metal that can prevent dietary liver necrosis in rats deficient also in vitamin E—may have protective effects, if the

Table 13.6 THE NUMBER OF FEMALE RATS SURVIVING VARIABLE ORAL TOXIC DOSES OF CCl_4 WITH AND WITHOUT FOUR INTRAPERITONEAL DOSES (0.25 mg/ 150 g BODY WT.) OF SODIUM SELENITE

	CCl_4 (2.7 ml/kg)	CCl_4 + Sod. selenite (0.25 mg/150 g × 4)
Short term (< 3 days)	6	3
Long term (> 7 days)	4	7
	CCl_4 (4 ml/kg)	CCl_4 + Sod. selenite (0.25 mg/150 g × 4)
Short term	14	9
Long term	1	4

toxic dose of CCl_4 given is reduced from 4 to 2.7 ml/kg body wt. In the higher dose, chosen because of some published findings, sodium selenite was here considered to be ineffective. It could, however, be argued that it should be precisely the high doses of CCl_4 with whose help significant protective effects should be demonstrated. That this is, indeed, possible is shown in Table 13.7, from which it is quite apparent that, even with

Table 13.7 THE NUMBER OF FEMALE RATS SURVIVING AN ORAL TOXIC DOSE OF CCl_4 (4 ml/kg BODY WT.) WITH AND WITHOUT THREE INTRAPERITONEAL DOSES OF DPPD (100 mg/150 g BODY WT.)

	CCl_4 (4ml/kg)	CCl_4 + DPPD (100 mg/150 g)
Short term (< 3 days)	34	12
Long term (> 7 days)	0	19

the high dose of CCl_4 given, *N,N-diphenyl-p-phenylenediamine (DPPD)*, a strong antioxidant, has a marked protective effect. For reasons already stated, however, experiments involving survival times were performed only if reports taken from the published findings of other workers demanded it, and only as a preliminary screening procedure to be followed in some instances by an evaluation of liver function. The results of some of these experiments are shown in Tables 13.8, 13.9 and 13.10. From Table 13.8 it can be seen that in the doses given here α-tocopherol exerted only a mild favourable effect, if a standard dose of

Table 13.8 THE EFFECT OF INTRAPERITONEAL α-TOCOPHEROL (95 I.U./150 g BODY WT.) ON THE LIVER FUNCTION OF RATS GIVEN A SUBCUTANEOUS DOSE OF CCl_4 (0.15 ml/100 g BODY WT.) (*p* VALUES BETWEEN LINES)

		SGOT	SGTP	BSP
24 hours	CCl_4	2134 ± 437.4	1410 ± 200.1	63.5 ± 7.9
		< 0.02	< 0.01	< 0.02
	α-Toc + CCl_4	1702 ± 384.2	1155 ± 204.6	54.9 ± 7.8
48 hours	CCl_4	2273 ± 506.5	1501 ± 215.2	67.9 ± 6.56
		< 0.05	< 0.05	< 0.01
	α-Toc + CCl_4	1822 ± 391.0	1298 ± 250.4	58.0 ± 6.55
96 hours	CCl_4	582 ± 140.5	385 ± 133.5	33.3 ± 4.06
	α-Toc + CCl_4	436 ± 114.3	272 ± 64.8	22.0 ± 8.78

30♀

0.15 ml/100 g body wt. of CCl_4 was given subcutaneously. It is interesting to note that this effect was more clearly seen with the more specific SGP-transaminase, and that it appeared mainly in the early phases of the experiment. Attention should be drawn here to the fact that no fundamental differences were observed if male, instead of the female rats shown in Table 13.8, were used. This observation does not agree with other published reports[1]. This mild effect found here is in marked contrast to the pronounced and protracted effect produced by DPPD (Tables 13.9 and 13.13), apparently one of the strongest protective agents against CCl_4. A significant protective effect was also seen if the antihistaminic *Phenergan* was given intraperitoneally in a dose of 12.5

Table 13.9 THE PROTECTIVE EFFECT OF THREE INTRAPERITONEAL DOSES OF DPPD (100 mg/150 g BODY WT.) ON THE LIVER FUNCTION OF MALE RATS SUBSEQUENTLY GIVEN AN INTRAPERITONEAL INJECTION OF CCl_4 (0.5 ml/100 g BODY WT.)

	Treatment	SGOT	SGPT	BSP
24 hours	CCl_4	1479.13 ± 415.94	1039.60 ± 190.87	44.24 ± 7.42
	CCl_4 + DPPD	469.92 ± 156.92	292.57 ± 96.47	20.96 ± 5.27
48 hours	CCl_4	1605.15 ± 432.18	1149.92 ± 201.04	47.29 ± 9.47
	CCl_4 + DPPD	505.93 ± 182.23	330.07 ± 170.62	22.25 ± 6.28
72 hours	CCl_4	873.70 ± 236.71	630.10 ± 181.11	36.62 ± 6.45
	CCl_4 + DPPD	244.23 ± 80.71	163.08 + 57.70	13.88 ± 3.73
96 hours	CCl_4	499.50 ± 162.51	207.60 ± 94.89	27.51 ± 5.97
	CCl_4 + DPPD	138.08 ± 44.35	78.46 ± 29.94	9.48 ± 2.95

All $P < 0.001$

mg/kg 30, 24 and six hours before, and at the time of, the administration of an oral dose of CCl_4 of 1.25 ml/kg (Table 13.10).

One of the variable factors in many experiments concerned with toxic effects appears to be the nutritional state of the animal. It has been known for a considerable time that a *protein-free diet* could protect rats against CCl_4 poisoning. This had been shown histologically[13], but the quantitative evaluation of the extent of this protective effect is

Table 13.10 THE PROTECTIVE EFFECT OF FOUR INTRAPERITONEAL DOSES OF 'PHENERGAN' (12.5 mg/kg BODY WT.) ON THE LIVER FUNCTION OF FEMALE RATS GIVEN A SINGLE ORAL DOSE OF CCl_4 (1.25 ml/kg BODY WT.)

	SGOT	SGPT	BSP
CCl_4	3091.38 ± 466.92	1624.75 ± 288.57	69.91 ± 7.29
	< 0.001	< 0.005	< 0.05
CCl_4 ± Phenergan	2040.67 ± 461.39	1111.56 ± 310.17	56.24 + 12.03

presented here in Table 13.11. It is again of interest to see that the
determination of the SGPT appears to be the most sensitive indicator of
liver damage by CCl_4 under these conditions, followed by the BSP-
retention test. The effect of the protein-free diet was compared with
that of a somewhat *protracted fast* of the animals of three days. It should
be stated here that in all the experiments of the present series all animals
were fasted for about 16–18 hours before liver function tests were done.
This includes the untreated controls supplying the base-line values.

Table 13.11 THE PROTECTIVE EFFECT OF A PROTEIN-FREE DIET GIVEN TO
MALE RATS FOR SEVEN DAYS BEFORE INJECTING SUBCUTANEOUSLY A SINGLE DOSE
OF CCl_4 (0.15 ml/100 g BODY WT.)

		SGOT	*SGPT*	*BSP*
	PFD	110.5 ± 28.83	45.0 ± 11.29	8.2 ± 3.64
24 hours	PFD + CCl_4	1292.9 ± 681.70	875.4 ± 447.63	38.1 ± 13.30
		< 0.05	< 0.01	< 0.02
	CCl_4	1781.7 ± 231.38	1349.5 ± 166.04	50.7 ± 5.97
	PFD	105.2 ± 24.73	41.2 ± 9.16	7.0 ± 2.90
48 hours	PFD + CCl_4	1446.7 ± 724.4	993.0 ± 508.89	43.2 ± 15.66
		< 0.05	< 0.01	< 0.02
	CCl_4	2040.1 ± 257.02	1537.2 ± 245.77	58.2 ± 7.36

The fast of three days produced in otherwise untreated rats a minor, but
nevertheless significant, impairment of liver function as judged by the
SGPT and the BSP-tests (Table 13.12). The most striking feature,
however, was the severe liver damage which resulted when such fasted
animals were given the standard dose of CCl_4 (Table 13.12). Presumably
the enzyme systems metabolising CCl_4 are activated in the process of
adjusting to the state of starvation. The exact mechanism is at the
moment not clear, but it is interesting to note that a similar striking
deterioration of liver function by CCl_4 can also be produced in normally

Table 13.12 THE DELETERIOUS EFFECT OF STARVATION FOR THREE DAYS ON THE LIVER FUNCTION OF MALE RATS 24 HOURS AFTER A SINGLE SUBCUTANEOUS DOSE OF CCl_4 (0.15 ml/100 g BODY WT.)

	SGOT	*SGPT*	*BSP*
Normal diet	90.50 ± 11.18	36.60 ± 3.47	4.79 ± 0.96
		< 0.005	< 0.01
Starvation	113.22 ± 35.50	57.00 ± 16.44	7.20 ± 2.45
Normal diet + CCl_4	2381.22 ± 766.82	1533.33 ± 369.62	55.93 ± 7.33
	< 0.01	< 0.001	< 0.001
Starvation + CCl_4	5331.10 ± 1512.53	3382.20 ± 1005.96	78.18 ± 10.38

fed animals that had been treated with high doses of *cortisone* for a few days before the administration of CCl_4 (Table 13.13). Earlier experiments[14] had demonstrated this effect, but they had not been done under 'standard' conditions, and the number of animals was rather small because of the limited amounts of cortisone then available. Moreover, the results obtained were not in keeping with the conclusions of some other workers[3]. It was, therefore thought desirable to elaborate these findings, and to use them to underline the fact that the effect of cortisone on the liver may vary with the type of liver damage produced. The favourable effect of cortisone on the course of dietary liver necrosis[15], for instance, has to be contrasted with its deleterious effect in poisoning by CCl_4 demonstrated here. This effect of cortisone also raises the question whether the effect of starvation, demonstrated in the preceding experiment, may not have been mediated by an adrenal cortex activated by the longish fast—a severe 'stress' for a small rodent. This possibility needs to be investigated further. Of interest is also the fact that the more severe liver damage induced by CCl_4 in rats treated with cortisone can be ameliorated by DPPD, but not to the same extent as in rats not given cortisone (Table 13.13). The example of this experiment shows that an approximate quantitative assessment can be easily arrived at by the appropriate experimental design.

Finally, two interesting hepatoprotective substances should be briefly discussed. Their mode of action is unknown, and much more work will be required to elucidate it. *5-hydroxytryptamine* has been shown to prevent the development of liver fibrosis[16] and while this effect could be

Table 13.13 THE EFFECTS OF CORTISONE ACETATE (EIGHT INTRAMUSCULAR DOSES OF 1.5 mg/100 g BODY WT.), DPPD (THREE INTRAPERITONEAL DOSES OF 100 mg/150 g BODY WT.), AND OF CORTISONE PLUS DPPD ON THE LIVER FUNCTION OF MALE RATS GIVEN A SINGLE SUBCUTANEOUS DOSE OF CCl_4 (0.15 ml/100g BODY WT.)

Treatment	Time (h)	SGOT	SGPT	BSP
	24	1616 ± 396.0	966 ± 110.93	42.0 ± 5.18
CCl_4	48	1891 ± 197.3	1164.2 ± 68.58	48.2 ± 6.11
	96	319 ± 139.5	185 ± 30.58	14.0 ± 3.91
	24	2726 ± 372.7	1590 ± 300.90	57.4 ± 3.45
CCl_4 + Cortisone	48	3001 ± 405.6	1870.4 ± 380.42	66.9 ± 6.83
	96	730 ± 90.1	320 ± 32.63	26.6 ± 1.80
	24	675 ± 119.2	492 ± 107.58	22.2 ± 1.88
CCl_4 + DPPD	48	831 ± 107.0	635 ± 184.95	24.9 ± 1.90
	96	116 ± 22.8	76.2 ± 22.8	10.1 ± 1.85
	24	1170 ± 211.4	733.8 ± 191.66	32.7 ± 2.62
CCl_4 + Cortisone + DPPD	48	1381 ± 187.2	943.8 ± 255.94	38.2 ± 0.70
	96	192 ± 23.8	103.8 ± 23.27	12.6 ± 2.95

Table 13.14 A COMPARATIVE STUDY OF THE PROTECTIVE EFFECTS OF ZINC CHLORIDE (ELEVEN SUBCUTANEOUS DOSES OF 4 mg/100 g BODY WT.) AND OF 5-HYDROXYTRYPTAMINE (SIX DOSES OF 100 mg/kg BODY WT.) ON THE LIVER DAMAGE PRODUCED IN MALE RATS BY SIX SUBCUTANEOUS DOSES OF CCl_4 (0.15 ml/100 g BODY WT.)

	Treatment	SGOT	SGPT	BSP
	CCl_4	2077.2 ± 813.9	1516.10 ± 447.58	52.33 ± 8.20
		< 0.001	< 0.001	< 0.001
24 hours	CCl_4 + $ZnCl_4$	717.37 ± 184.28	347.37 ± 183.10	28.54 ± 8.20
		< 0.005 < 0.005	< 0.01 < 0.001	< 0.001
	CCl_4 + Serotonin	1073.11 ± 428.33	646.0 ± 218.13	28.54 ± 8.20
	CCl_4	2156.40 ± 854.42	1594.10 ± 503.55	53.36 ± 10.21
		< 0.001	< 0.001	< 0.001
48 hours	CCl_4 + $ZnCl_4$	815.75 ± 168.76	490.87 ± 189.85	24.13 ± 2.34
		< 0.001	< 0.001	< 0.001
	CCl_4 + Serotonin	996.33 ± 345.79	591.11 ± 325.06	28.63 ± 8.91

attributed to an inhibition of the proliferation of the connective tissue, Table 13.14 shows that this cannot be the whole story, since treatment with serotonin also significantly decreases the impairment of liver function. This agrees with the conclusions of Fiore-Donati and Chieco-Bianchi[16]. A similar, but even more marked, effect is also seen if *zinc chloride* is injected subcutaneously for several days. This confirms the findings of Voigt and Saldeen[17] and Saldeen and Brunk[18]. The effect of zinc chloride is quite remarkable, and should be further defined. Since, as has already been stated, zinc chloride also appears to be effective against CCl_4 given intrasplenically, an effect of this compound on the absorption of CCl_4 can be excluded. A comparison of the data in Table 13.14 shows that the protective effect of zinc chloride surpasses that of serotonin, but comparisons should perhaps end here.

CONCLUSIONS

A summary of all the findings presented is given in Table 13.15. It is hoped that the data presented here will serve as a basis for future studies. It is apparent that some order can be brought into the chaos of the many conflicting reports published, if a systematic study under standard conditions is undertaken in one laboratory. Perhaps the most obvious conclusion to be drawn is that due attention must be paid to the criteria by which hepatoprotective substances are to be evaluated. An assessment of liver function appears to be the most convenient tool for comparative studies. While no attempt has been made to survey the whole field, or to interpret the results obtained with a view of fitting them into the framework of current opinion on the mode of action of CCl_4, the effects of hepatoprotective substances and their mechanisms clearly will have to be brought in line with these views. It was for this reason that the partial survey presented here has been undertaken, so that some of the seeming discrepancies, or ill-understood findings, could be properly evaluated.

ACKNOWLEDGMENT

The investigation presented here was supported by a grant from the Medical Research Council of Canada, to whom our thanks are due.

Table 13.15 A SUMMARY OF THE EFFECTS OF THE VARIOUS AGENTS TESTED ON THE LIVER DAMAGE PRODUCED BY CCl_4

Favourable	No Effect	Unfavourable
Protein-free diet	Sex	Starvation
DPPD	Xanthine	Cortisone (high dose)
Phenergan	Liver extract* ("Ripason")	
Serotonin	India ink	
Zinc chloride	Trypan blue	
? α-Tocopherol	Sodium selenite	
	Vitamin B_{12}*	

* Older findings

REFERENCES

1. Recknagel, R. O. and Glende, E. A. J. (1973). Carbon tetrachloride hepatotoxicity: An example of lethal cleavage. *CRC. Crit. Rev. Toxicol.*, **2**, 263–297
2. Slater, T. F. (1972). *Free Radical Mechanisms in Tissue Injury* (London: Pion Limited)
3. Vorhaus, E. F. and Vorhaus L. J. (1954). Protective effects of pretreatment with cortisone, aureomycin and folic acid in carbon tetrachloride induced hepatic injury in rats. *Gastroenterology.*, **26**, 887–894
4. Forbes, J. C. and Outhouse, E. L. (1940). Studies on the mechanism of the protective action of xanthine against carbon tetrachloride poisoning. *J. Pharmacol. Exp. Ther.*, **68**, 185–193
5. Ravdin, I., Vars, H. M. and Goldschmidt, S. (1939). The non-specificity of suspensions of sodium xanthine in protecting the liver against injury by chloroform and the probable cause of its action. *J. Clin. Invest.*, **18**, 633–640
6. Calder, R. M. (1942). The protective action of xanthine and other insoluble substances on the liver. *J. Pathol. Bacteriol*, **54**, 369–373
7. Stenger, R. J., Petrelli, M., Segel, A., Williamson, J. N. and Johnson, E. A. (1969). Modification of carbon tetrachloride hepatotoxicity by prior loading of the reticuloendothelial system with carbon particles. *Amer. J. Pathol.*, **57**, 689–706

8. Stenger, R. J., Williamson, J. N. and Johnson, E. A. (1968). The effect of reticuloendothelial blockade upon carbon tetrachloride hepatotoxicity. A light and electron microscopic study. Abstracts of 65th Annual Meeting of the Amer. Assoc. Pathol. Bacteriol., *Amer. J. Pathol.*, **52**, 11a

9. Petrelli, M. and Stenger, R. J. (1969). The effect of trypan blue on the hepatotoxicity of carbon tetrachloride in the rat. *Exp. Molec. Pathol.*, **10**, 115–128

10. György, P., Seifter, J., Tomarelli, R. M. and Goldblatt, H. (1946). Influence of dietary factors and sex on the toxicity of carbon tetrachloride in rats. *J. Exp. Med.*, **83**, 449–462

11. Hove, E. L. (1948). Interrelation between α-tocopherol and protein metabolism. III. The protective effect of vitamin E and certain nitrogenous compounds against CCl_4 poisoning in rats. *Arch. Biochem.*, **17**, 467–474

12. Gallagher, C. H. (1960). The effects of nicotinic acid in experimental carbon tetrachloride poisoning of sheep. *Austr. J. Agric. Res.*, **11**, 1009–1016

13. Aterman, K. and Darlington, D. (1959). A re-examination of the effect of vitamin B_{12} concentrate on the hepatic injury produced by carbon tetrachloride. *Brit. J. Nutr.*, **13**, 168–177

14. Aterman, K. and Ahmad, N. D. (1953). Cortisone and liver function. *Lancet*, **i**, 71–73

15. Aterman, K. (1972). The role of the adrenal cortex in experimental dietary liver necrosis. *Beitr. Pathol.*, **146**, 162–179

16. Fiore-Donati, L. and Chieco-Bianchi, L. (1960). Effect of 5-hydroxytryptamine on the development of the carbon tetrachloride-induced cirrhosis in rats. *Lab. Invest.*, **9**, 625–638

17. Voigt, G. E. and Saldeen, T. (1965). Über den Schutzeffekt des Zinks gegenüber Mangansulfat- oder Kohlenstofftetrachlorid-induzierten Leber-schäden. *Frankf. Ztschr. Pathol.*, **74**, 572–578

18. Saldeen, T. and Brunk, U. (1967). Enzyme histochemical investigations of the inhibitory effect of zinc on the injurious action of carbon tetrachloride on the liver. *Frankf. Ztschr. Pathol.*, **76**, 419–426

Liver morphology and enzyme release: further studies in the isolated perfused rat liver

E. Schmidt, F. W. Schmidt, J. Möhr, P. Otto,
I. Vido, K. Wrogemann and Ch. Herfarth

Based on studies with the isolated, haemoglobin-free perfused rat liver, three topics concerning enzyme release as an indication of liver cell damage, and extracellular enzyme patterns as a mean to its description will be discussed.

MATERIAL AND METHODS

Male Wistar rats; body wt. 236 ± 18 g; liver wt. 11.1 ± 1.2 g; fed *ad libitum* on Altromin R (1320®).

STANDARD CONDITIONS[1,2]

Perfusion temperature 23 °C; flow 2.6–3.6 ml/min/g liver; duration four hours; closed system[1].

Perfusion medium[2,5] (200 ml): Bovine Albumin (Behring) 25 g/l; NaCl 137 mM; KCl 2.7 mM; $CaCl_2$ 1.8 mM; $MgCl_2$ 0.49 mM; $NaHCO_3$ 12 mM; NaH_2PO_4 0.68 mM; glucose 5.1 mM; pyruvate 0.095 mM; lactate 1.3 mM; pH 7.3; Oxygenation by 95% O_2 + 5% CO_2. Enzyme activities, metabolite concentrations and oxygen consumption have been determined as described previously[3-6]. The *in vitro* effects on the enzyme activities during the circulation have been accounted for by way of calculation[4].

THE SIGNIFICANCE OF THE PHENOMENON AS COMPARED TO OTHER BIOCHEMICAL PARAMETERS AND TO MORPHOLOGICAL FINDINGS

The isolated haemoglobin-free perfused rat liver loses intracellular enzymes into the perfusion medium. Under standard conditions, as described, the rate of release of a given enzyme depends in the first place on its concentration gradient between intracellular and extracellular space, on its molecular weight and on its intracellular localisation[6]. Table 14.1 shows that less than 1% of the amount of enzymes in the

Table 14.1 TOTAL ENZYME RELEASE INTO THE MEDIUM AFTER FOUR HOURS OF PERFUSION UNDER STANDARD CONDITIONS (MEAN VALUES)

	U/200 ml	*U/liver*	*% released*
MDH	39	4185	0.93
LDH	29	3830	0.76
ICDH	1.3	213	0.62
GPT	1.4	318	0.44
GOT	3.6	1200	0.30
GLDH	0.05	488	0.01

liver is lost after four hours of perfusion under standard conditions, and that the relative release rates differ by an order of magnitude between MDH and GLDH, as could be expected from the foregoing. Nevertheless, the course of enzyme elevation in the medium can be reliably determined. Besides some enlargement of the sinusoids due to the perfusion technique, the histology before and after four hours of perfusion is normal.

For the investigation of the effects of anoxia, we equilibrated the perfusion system with oxygenated medium for one hour; then oxygen was replaced by argon for the second hour and afterwards oxygenation restored for another two hours. Figure 14.1 shows that during the second hour the rise of enzyme activities in the medium becomes steeper, mostly pronounced with GLDH. After the restitution of oxygen supply this accelerated increase continues, with the exception of GLDH, for the last two hours. This is somewhat surprising, with respect to the complete restoration of the oxygen consumption and of

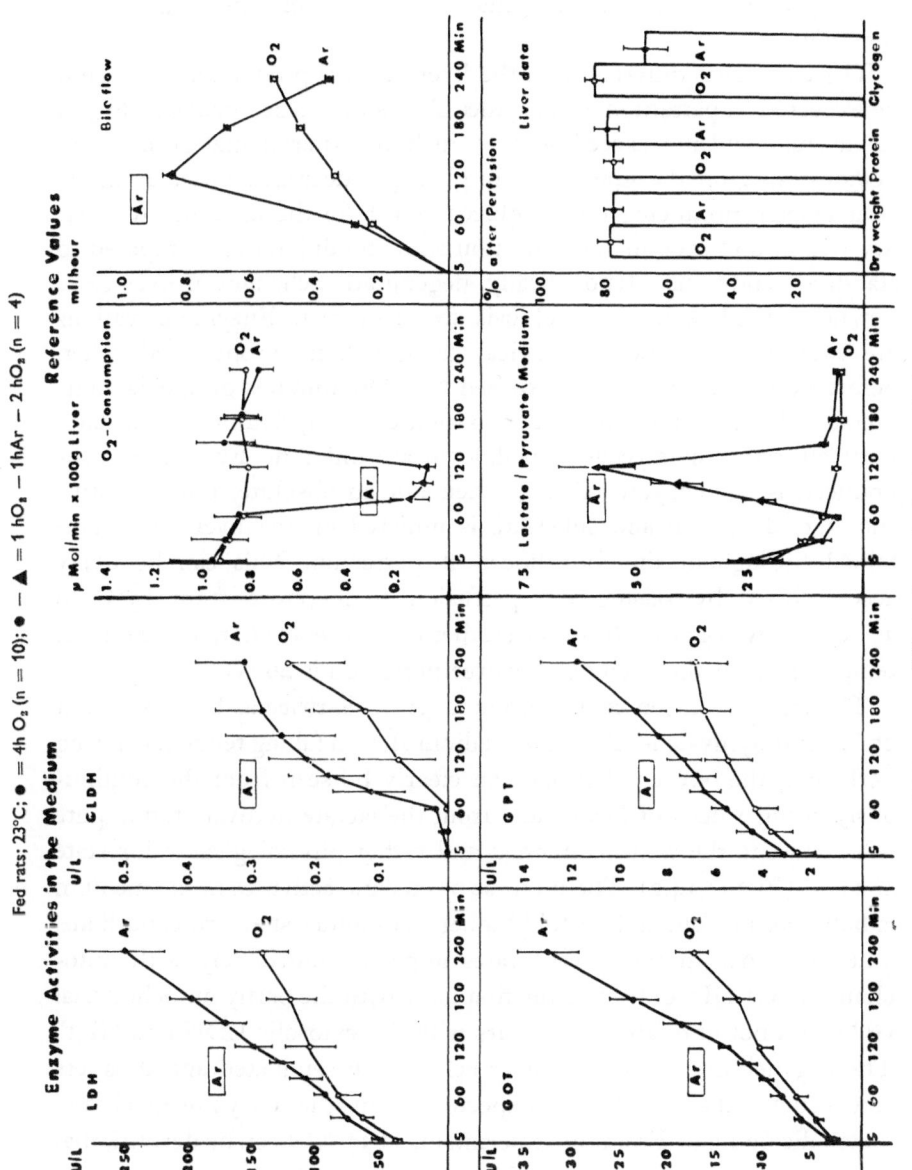

FIGURE 14.1   Effect of anoxia during perfusion

the cytosolic redox state as reflected by the lactate/pyruvate ratio. The reaction of bile flow to acute anoxia is conspicuous. It denotes that bile production is not always a suitable indicator of unimpaired liver function.

The enzymatic differences in the liver are less pronounced, as could be expected: a pattern of 12 enzymes shows only small changes, 6% in the average and not exceeding 20% in both experimental groups (not demonstrated on the graph). Only glycogen decreases twice as much after anoxia, producing higher glucose levels in the medium, whereas dry weight and protein concentration show no differences compared to standard conditions. Histologically, degenerative changes of liver cells, but no marked signs of necrobiosis are to be seen. Enzyme elevations are twice as high and histological changes more pronounced, when before perfusion the liver is exposed to a few minutes of anoxia combined with stasis, though neither oxygen consumption nor the lactate/pyruvate ratio nor glycogen breakdown are different. Even more pronounced is the enzyme release, when not an absolute, but a relative shortage of oxygen and substrate is inflicted on the liver and maintained throughout the four hours of perfusion. This can be easily accomplished by raising the perfusion temperature from 23°C to 37 °C. It is well-known from the studies of Kessler *et al.*[7] that the critical temperature for the haemoglobin-free perfusion is 26 °C.

Though the oxygen consumption at 37 °C is twice as high as that at 23 °C, and pyruvate levels in the medium show a falling tendency during perfusion, the oxygen shortage can clearly be seen from the continuously rising values of lactate and from the lactate/pyruvate ratio, quite in contrast to the well-maintained and rather physiological redox state at 23 °C (Figure 14.2). The increase of enzyme activities in the medium is between ninefold and 19-fold higher than under standard conditions. The difference in the release rates appears immediately with mitochondrial GLDH, only after the first hour with the partly mitochondrial GOT and not until after two hours with the cytosolic LDH and GPT. The degenerative changes of liver cells are disseminated and thus less conspicuous than could be expected from the enzymological and metabolic findings. From the experiments at 37 °C it can be derived, that concomitant relative shortage of both oxygen and substrates seem not only to add up, but to multiply in their respective effects on enzyme release.

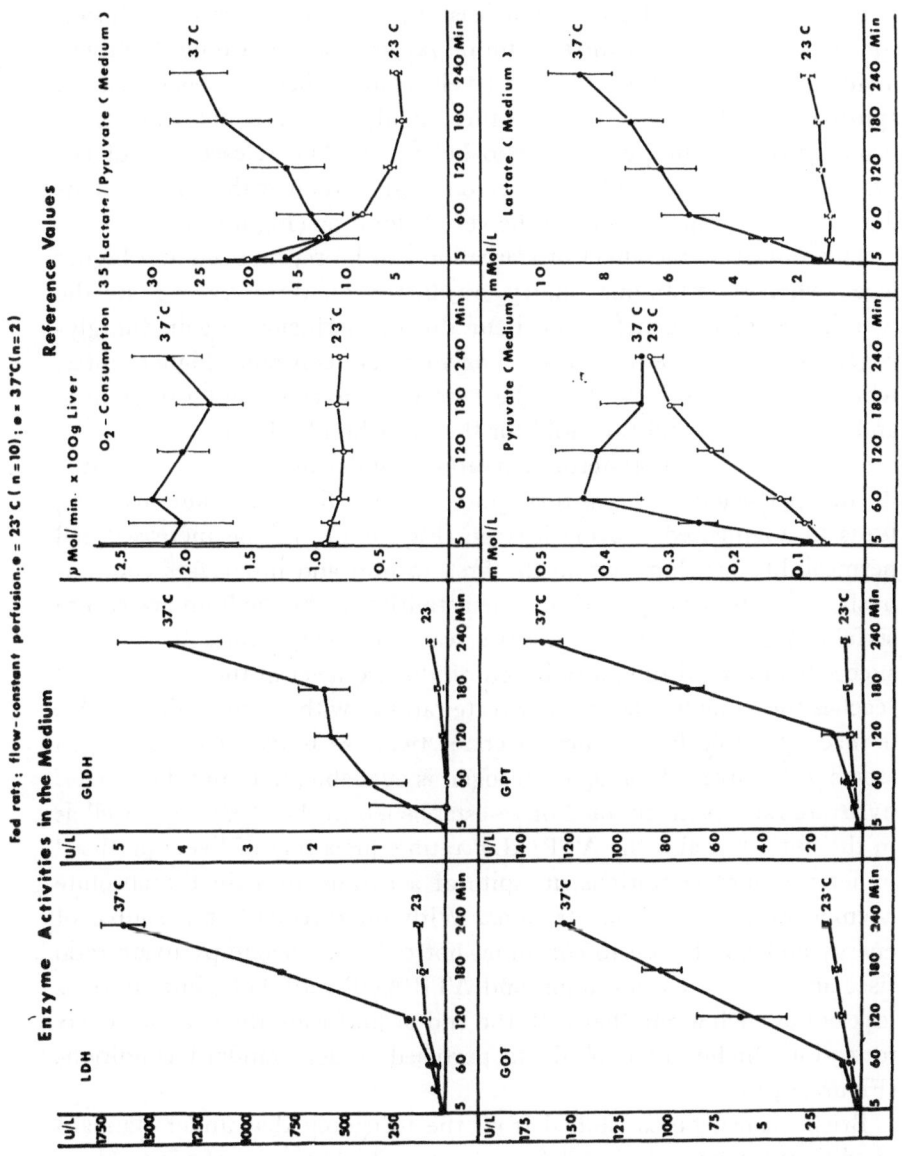

FIGURE 14.2 Effect of temperature

The net effect of starvation on enzyme release was studied by two methods:

The livers of rats fasted for at least 15 hours previous to perfusion consume virtually the same amount of oxygen and differ only slightly in maintaining extracellular glucose levels though their glycogen content approximates to zero. On the other hand, they are not capable of bringing the lactate/pyruvate ratio below 10. The release rate of enzymes, is between 2.5-fold and fivefold higher than with fed rats. This difference is conspicuous from the very beginning (Figure 14.3).

This unfavourable effect of starvation can be reproduced at a higher level, when an additional injury is inflicted on the liver, e.g. by the withdrawal of oxygen for one hour during perfusion. Again the glycogen-depleted livers release enzymes at constant higher rates, which are four to fivefold for the cytosolic enzymes and isoenzymes, and between two and threefold for the mitochondrial ones.

Like previous short-term starvation, undernutrition of the liver during perfusion, by omitting glucose from the perfusion medium, leads to augmented enzyme leakage (Figure 14.4). The increased cell permeability develops within the first 30 min and progresses continuously. After four hours the enzyme activities in the medium are two to sixfold higher, when no glucose was supplied, although the liver succeeds in establishing a satisfactory glucose level in the medium and reaches the same low lactate/pyruvate ratio as with glucose added. This is made possible by consuming about twice as much of the glycogen stores of the liver. As long as glycogen is available, not only the lactate/pyruvate ratio is maintained or re-established in the medium as well as in the liver, but also the ATP/ADP ratio equals that of livers perfused under standard conditions, in spite of a certain drop in the absolute adenine nucleotide concentrations. With no glycogen as a source of energy and no glucose to consume, not only the lactate/pyruvate ratio rises and oxygen consumption and ATP/ADP ratio falls, but enzymes leak out at such a rate that with the end of perfusion their levels are six to 15-fold higher than in livers perfused under standard conditions (Figure 14.5).

Briefly it can be concluded from the foregoing that under standard conditions enzymes leak out from livers, which after perfusion appear normal from the histological point of view. Increased release of enzymes can occur though oxygen consumption is satisfactory, and the ratios of lactate/pyruvate and ATP/ADP are in the favourable range of between

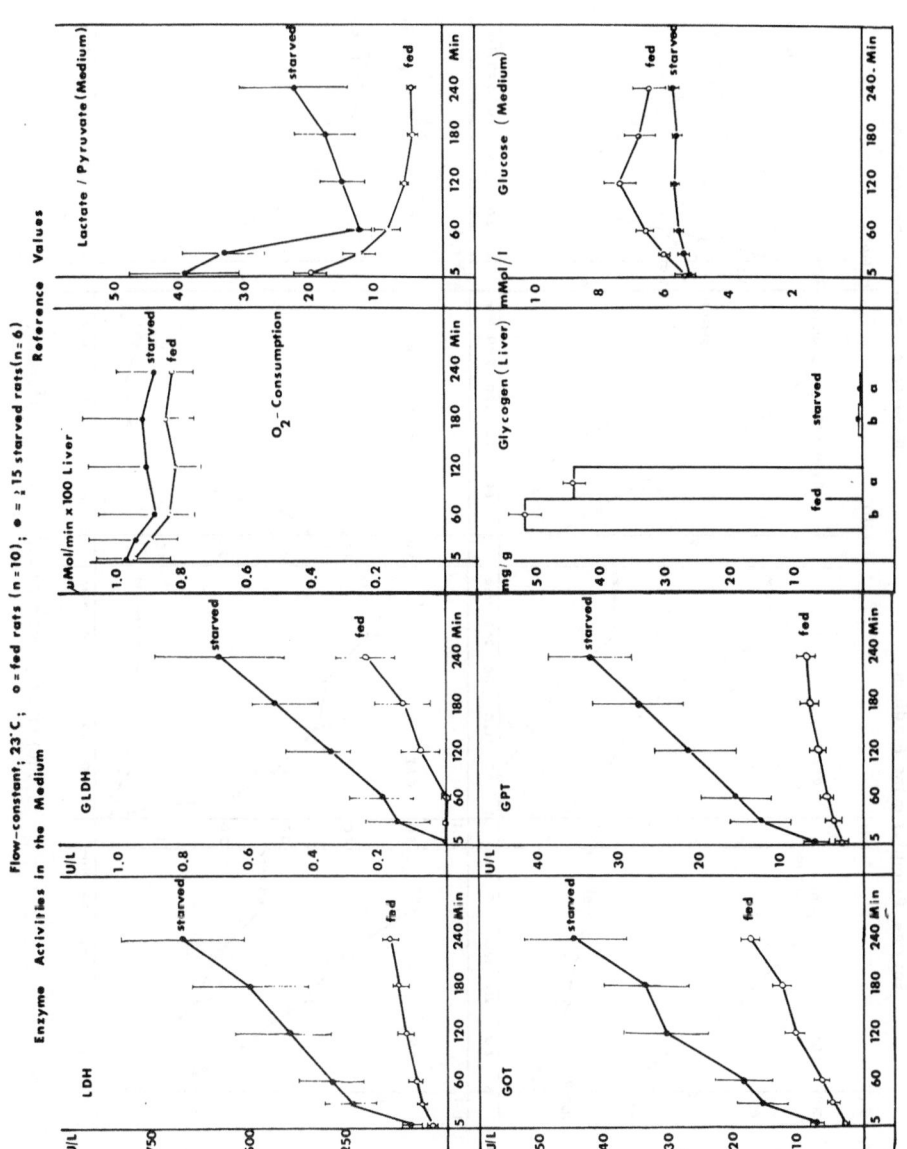

FIGURE 14-3   Effect of the nutritional state

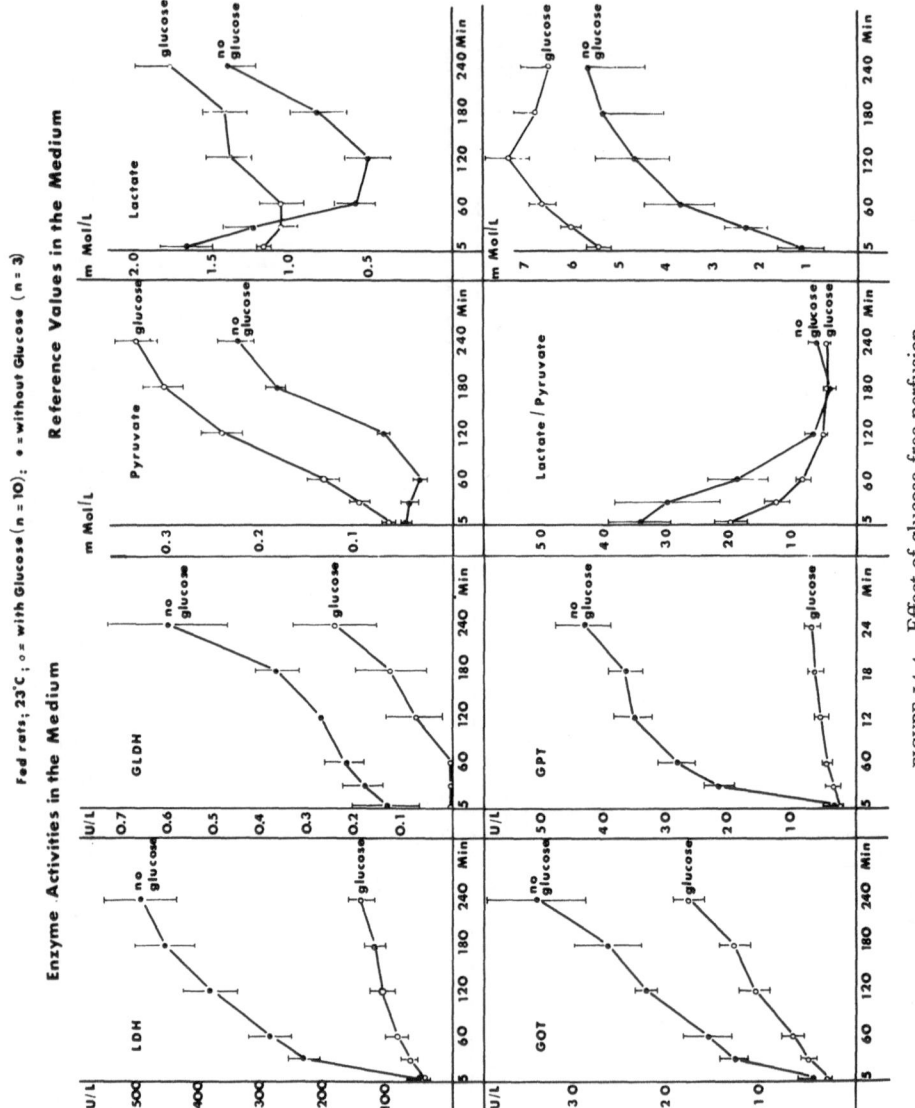

FIGURE 14.4   Effect of glucose-free perfusion

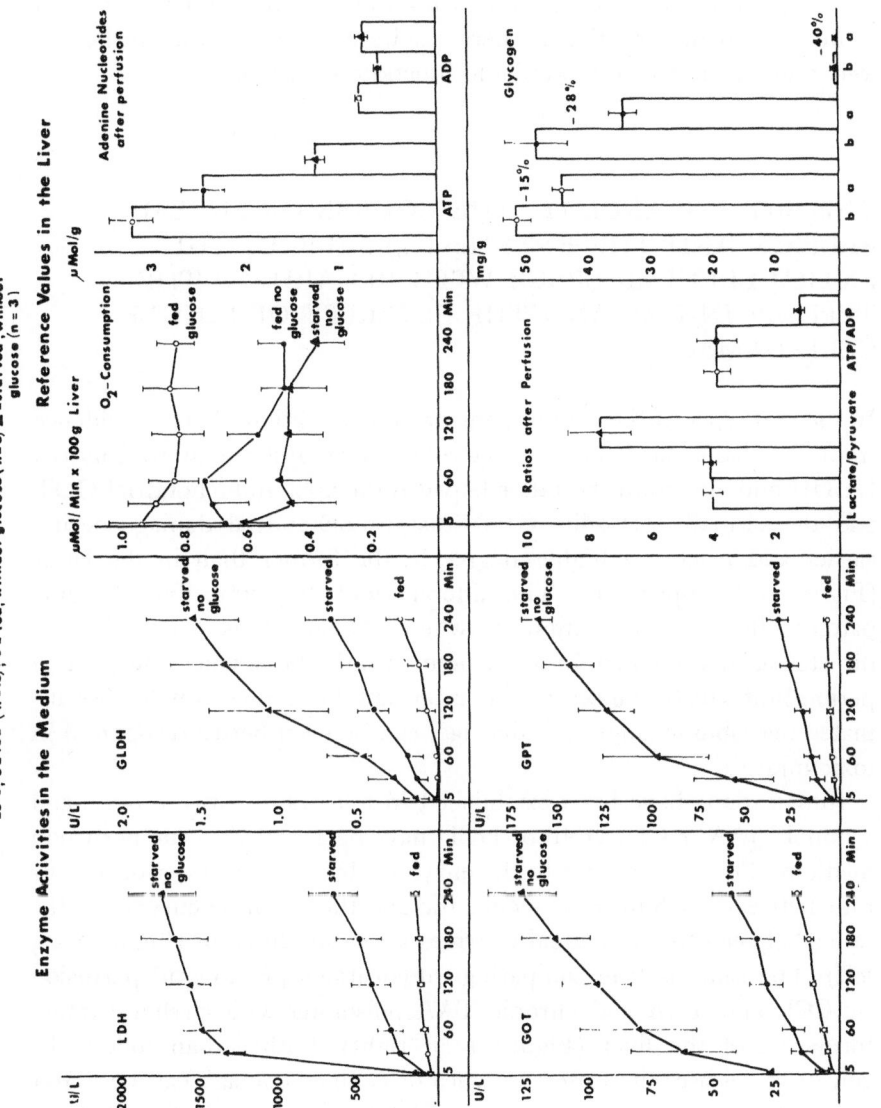

FIGURE 14.5   Effect of the nutritional state and glucose-free perfusion

3 and 5. Impaired oxygen supply, as long as it is not combined with stasis, and especially, as long as the liver can fall back to energy production from glycolysis by consuming its own glycogen reserve or exogenously conveyed glucose, is less injurious to the tightness of cell membranes than conditions, where respiration may be undisturbed or well-restored, but readily available substrate is lacking.

THE SIGNIFICANCE OF THE COURSE OF ENZYME RELEASE AND THE ENZYME PATTERN IN THE EXTRACELLULAR SPACE WITH REGARD TO THE TYPE OF INJURY AND THE SEVERITY OF SINGLE CELL DAMAGE

In the two types of liver injury, anoxia and starvation, there is evidence from the ratios between the cytosolic LDH and the mitochondrial GLDH and also from the ratios between the 60% mitochondrial GOT and the virtually cytosolic GPT, that mitochondrial damage occurs earlier and reaches a higher degree in the former than in the latter (Figure 14.6, upper part). The differences of the extracellular enzyme patterns between such injuries, where the attack is predominantly directed against the membrane structures and others, where the general permeability disturbances are unimportant in comparison to disseminated necrobiotic single cell damage, can be even better recognised in toxic injuries.

Intoxications have been established in two ways: On the one hand 1 mmol/l JAA, KCN, DNP or DCH have been added to the perfusion medium. The release rates of the enzymes differ by an order of magnitude between the four toxic agents, but also the elevation curves and the ratios between the individual enzymes are quite different (Figure 14.7, left). The same is true comparing intoxications previous to perfusion by CCl_4 and TAA and chronic TAA poisoning with cirrhotic transformation of the liver (Figure 14.7, right). Rather than follow the course of release, the different types of cellular damage can be better demonstrated by the average ratios of LDH/GLDH and of c-GOT/m-GOT in the medium (Figure 14.6, lower part). The more severe single cell damage in KCN poisoning than after application of DCH is evident, in spite of the tenfold higher average elevation of the enzyme activities

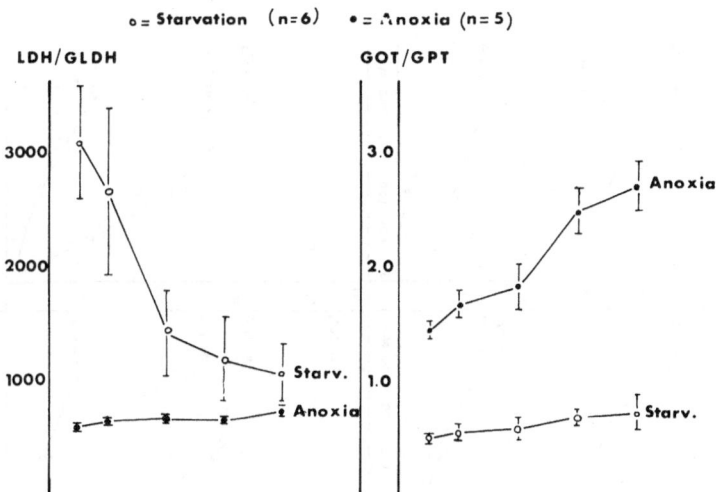

Enzyme Ratios in the Medium (23°C)

o = Starvation (n=6)   • = Anoxia (n=5)

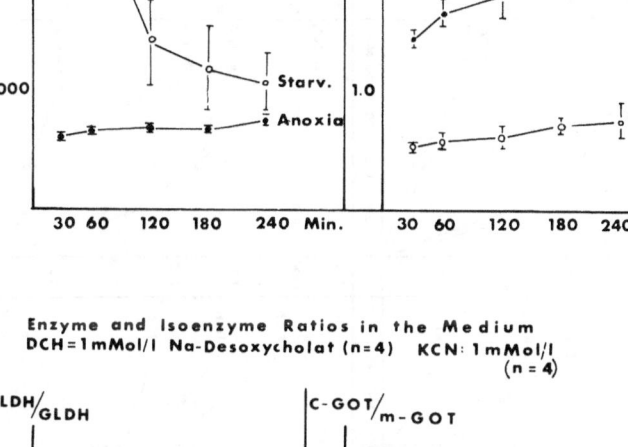

Enzyme and Isoenzyme Ratios in the Medium
DCH = 1 mMol/l Na-Desoxycholat (n=4)   KCN: 1 mMol/l
(n = 4)

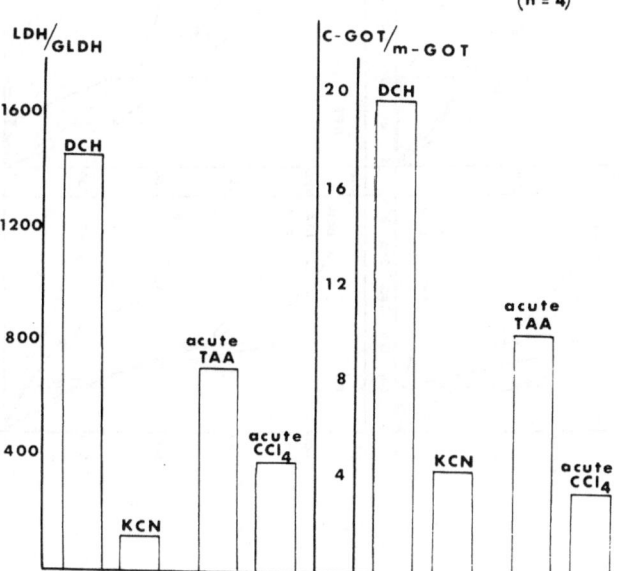

FIGURE 14.6   Upper panel; Slight *v.* severe single cell damage. Lower panel; 'Membrane lesion' *v.* 'necrobiosis'

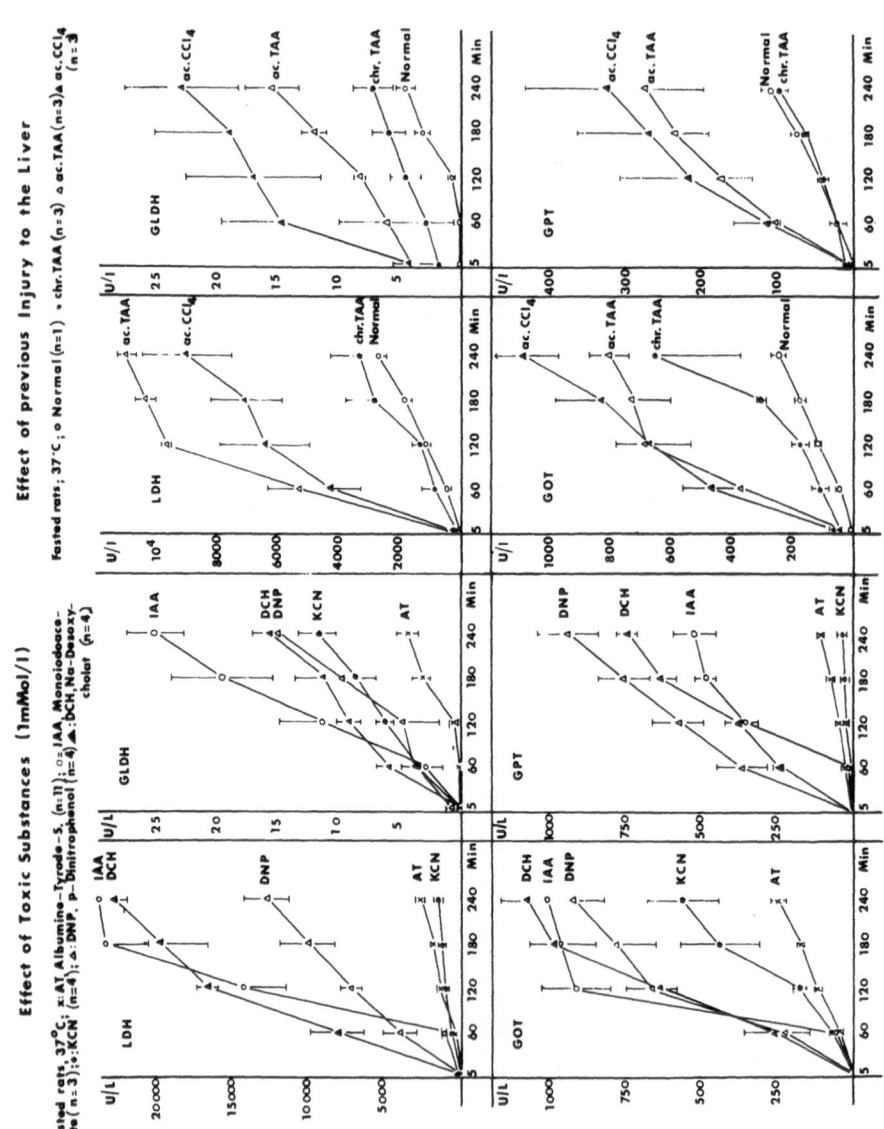

FIGURE 14.7 Enzyme activities in the medium: Effect of toxic substances and effect of previous injury on the liver

in the latter. Histologically the difference is not so striking; in fact, it is scarcely recognisable.

In acute CCl_4 and TAA intoxication the elevation of enzymes in the medium is very similar in degree, but the enzyme pattern in CCl_4 poisoning shows much lower ratios between cytosolic and mitochondrial enzymes and isoenzymes than that in acute TAA poisoning. In this case, the difference is also reflected in the well-known histological pictures.

It can be concluded, that in very early stages of liver cell damage, the type of injury is better recognisable by the extracellular enzyme pattern than by the histological picture, due to the time needed by the morphological symptoms to develop their characteristic features.

As a whole, the ratio GOT/GPT is less suitable for this purpose due to its very complex nature, even when the different half-lives are not taken into consideration as in the perfusion studies; the second complicating factor lies namely in the distribution of the individual enzymes within the hepatic lobule. This leads to the last topic.

THE SIGNIFICANCE OF THE EXTRACELLULAR ENZYME PATTERNS WITH RESPECT TO THE LOCALISATION OF THE CELLULAR DAMAGE

As GPT activity is about three times higher in the periportal than in the central part of the liver lobule and ICDH and ADH have only two-thirds of their activity in the periphery of the lobule than in its central field[8-11], it can be expected, that for example the ratio ICDH/GPT, both cytosolic of origin, gives an indication where the actual injury is predominantly localised. This is in fact possible, as it can be seen from Figure 14.8. The cell damage in KCN poisoning is not only focal but also more marked around the central veins, whereas JAA produces a diffuse cell damage which is most pronounced in the vicinity of the portal tracts. Of course the main lesion in acute CCl_4 poisoning is a central one, whereas in chronic TAA intoxication piece meal necroses in the periportal fields prevail. The last example refers again to the differences between lack of oxygen and lack of substrate, the former leading in marked cases to the well-known central necrobiotic processes, the latter predominating in the peripheral areas. Understandably, the manifestation of the site of the cellular damage in the enzyme pattern is

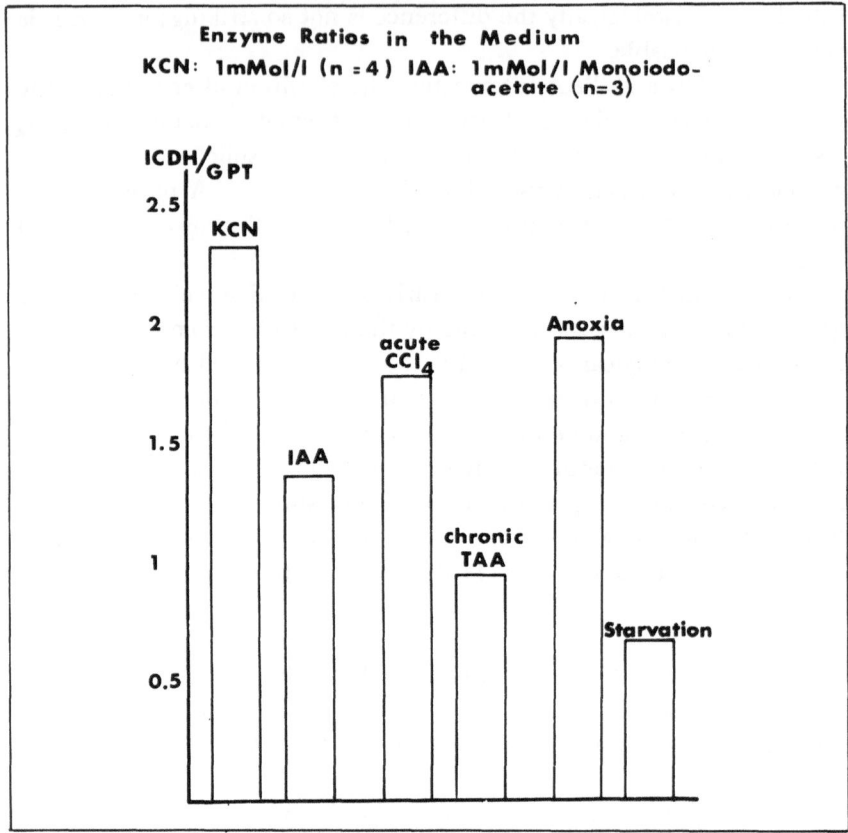

FIGURE 14.8   Central *v.* peripheral or diffuse damage

most conspicuous during the early stages. Later on, the more the lesion expands and becomes diffuse, the more the characteristic ratios between centrally predominating and peripherally prevailing enzyme activities become blurred.

SUMMARY

The release of intracellular enzymes in liver cell injury occurs early when the process is still reversible. It is a more sensitive indicator of cellular damage than are most other biochemical parameters and most morphological findings. The courses of release and especially the enzyme patterns in the extracellular space, analysed with respect to the intracellular and the intralobular localisation of the hepatic enzymes, reflect the variability of the severity and the sites of the injurious processes.

ABBREVIATIONS

DCH : Na-desoxycholate
DNP : 2,4-dinitrophenol
GLDH: Glutamic dehydrogenase (EC 1.4.1.3)
GOT : Glutamic oxalacetic transaminase (EC 2.6.1.1)
GPT : Glutamic pyruvic transaminase (EC 2.6.1.2)
JAA : Monoiodoacetate
ICDH : Isocitric dehydrogenase (EC 1.1.1.42)
LDH : Lactic dehydrogenase (EC 1.1.1.27)
MDH : Malic dehydrogenase (EC 1.1.1.37)
TAA : Thioacetamide

REFERENCES

1. Scholz, R. (1968). Untersuchungen zur Redoxkompartimentierung bei der hämoglobinfrei perfundierten Rattenleber. In: *Stoffwechsel der isoliert perfundierten Leber*, 25–47 (W. Staib and R. Scholz, editors) (Berlin, Heidelberg, New York: Springer-Verlag)
2. Schimassek, H. (1962). Perfusion of isolated rat liver with a semi-synthetic medium and control of liver function. *Life Sci.*, **11**, 629–634
3. Schmidt, E. and Schmidt, F. W. (1962). Untersuchungen über optimale Reaktionsbedingungen für Enzym-Aktivitäts-Bestimmungen in Leber-extrakten, und Extrakten anderer Organe und im Serum. *Enzym. Biol. Clin.*, **2**, 201–222
4. Schmidt, E., Schmidt, F. W. and Herfarth, C. (1966). Studien zum Austritt von Zell-Enzymen am Modell der isolierten perfundierten Ratten-leber; I. Mitt.: Schmidt, E., Schmidt, F. W. and Dettmar, K. H. Zur Stabilität von Zell-Enzymen in verschiedenen zur Organ-Durchströmung geeigneten Lösungen. *Enzym. Biol. Clin.*, **7**, 53–72
5. Schmidt, E., Schmidt, F. W., Herfarth, C., Dettmar, K. H. and Fabel, H. (1966). Studien zum Austritt von Zell-Enzymen am Modell der isolierten, perfundierten Ratten-Leber. II. Mitt.: Untersuchungs-Methoden und Studien über Wahl des Perfusions-Mediums und Vergleichbarkeit der Enzym-Muster verschiedener Leber-Lappen. *Enzym. Biol. Clin.*, **7**, 167–184
6. Schmidt, E., Schmidt, F. W., Herfarth, C., Opitz, K. and Vogell, W. (1966). Studien zum Austritt von Zell-Enzymen am Modell der isolierten,

perfundierten Ratten-Leber. III. Mitt.: Analyse des bei Perfusion unter Hypoxie entstehenden extracellulären Enzym-Musters. *Enzym. Biol. Clin.*, **7**, 185–202

7. Kessler, M. and Schubotz, R. (1968). Die O_2-Versorgung der hämoglobinfrei perfundierten Rattenleber. In: *Stoffwechsel der isoliert perfundierten Leber*, 12–20 (W. Staib and R. Scholz, editors) (Heidelberg, Berlin, New York: Springer-Verlag)

8. Shank, R. E., Morrison, G., Cheng, C. H., Karl, I. and Schwartz, R. (1959). Cell heterogeneity within the hepatic lobule (quantitative histochemistry). *J. Histochem. Cytochem.*, **7**, 237–239

9. Morrison, G. and Brock, F. E. (1967). Quantitative measurement of alcohol dehydrogenase in the lobule of normal livers. *J. Lab. Clin. Invest.*, **70**, 116–120

10. Pette, D. and Brandau, H. (1966). Enzym-Histogramme und Enzym-Aktivitäts-Muster der Rattenleber. *Enzym. Biol. Clin.*, **6**, 79–122

11. Reith, A., Schüler, B. and Vogell, W. (1968). Quantitative und qualitative elektronenmikroskopische Untersuchungen zur Struktur des Leberläppchens normaler Ratten. *Z. Zellforsch.*, **89**, 225–240

CHAPTER 15

Phalloidin, a membrane specific toxin

M. Frimmer

For some years two fundamental misinterpretations have been disseminated in the field of phalloidin research: (a) The endoplasmic
reticulum has been regarded as the site of action of phalloidin[1]; (b) A
toxication of phalloidin by microsomal enzymes has been postulated[2-6].
Both speculations were based on presumptive evidences and have been
disproved by experimental facts[1,7]. Today it is undoubted that phalloidin acts as a genuine chemically unchanged compound[1] and that
alterations of the endoplasmic reticulum (ER) are secondary effects[8].
Based on experimental findings[9] in perfused livers in 1967 we suspected
that the primary effect of phalloidin is located in the plasma membranes
of liver cells. Initially we had argued that phalloidin might possess
valinomycin-like properties, because perfused livers release considerable amounts of potassium. However phalloidin is not a complexing
agent for potassium nor it is an ouabain-like drug[10], since it fails to
inhibit transport ATPases in isolated plasma membranes.

Our understanding of phalloidin action was improved by using a
generous gift from T. Wieland of labelled desmethylphalloin. Thus, we
were able to perform binding studies with purified subcellular fractions
obtained from non-poisoned livers[7].

In Figure 15.1 the binding of tritium labelled desmethylphalloin to
plasma membranes is compared with its binding to microsomes or
mitochondria. At low concentrations of the toxin, plasma membranes
bind much greater amounts of desmethylphalloin than other subcellular
particles. From Scatchard plots two dissociation constants (2.2×10^{-8}
and 1.2×10^{-6}M) could be calculated[7]. However the second binding
site might be non-specific. Our results were confirmed by T. Wieland's
group. Additional electron microscopical observations of the same
group suggested that phalloidin interacts with filamentous structures of
the membrane (see Chapter 16). In our hands, isolated hepatocytes

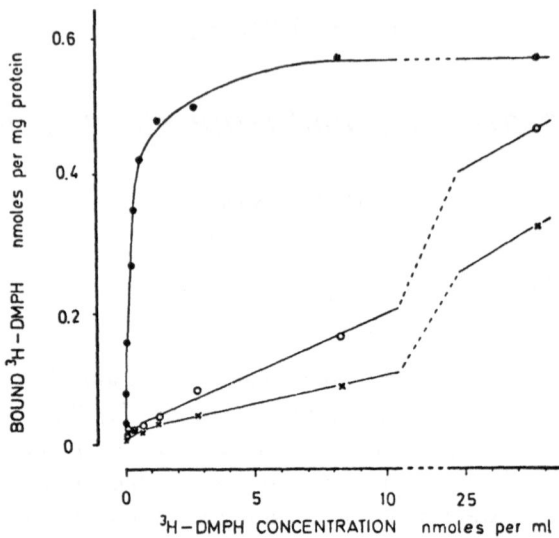

FIGURE 15.1   Binding of ^{3}H-desmethylphalloin by subcellular fractions of rat liver. Points represent mean values of three experiments. ●——● plasma membranes; o——o microsomes; x——x mitochondria (From Lutz *et al.* (1972). 'Binding of ^{3}H-desmethylphalloin to isolated plasma membranes from rat liver.' *Naunyn-Schmiedeberg's Arch. Pharmacol.*, **273**, 341–351, by courtesy of Springer-Verlag)

proved to be a useful tool for the study of the next step of phalloidin poisoning[12,21] since this method allowed us to keep the conditions constant and to avoid the influence of microcirculatory disturbances in the liver. R. Kroker prepared completely intact cells neither releasing potassium nor remarkable amounts of other components.

Figure 15.2 presents a scanning electron micrograph from untreated freshly prepared rat hepatocytes. The whole surface of isolated hepatocytes is covered with microvilli. If we exposed such cells *in vitro* to phalloidin the appearance of the surface was completely changed within 5–10 min. Figure 15.3 shows a scanning electron micrograph from cells 10 min after treatment with 65 μg phalloidin/ml of cell suspension. Amoeboid coral-like protrusions were formed[12].

The morphological effect of phalloidin can be explained by a labilisation of the membrane structure. The softening of the plasma membrane is not ubiquitous. It is localised in distinct areas of the cell surface as shown by many electron micrographs. We feel that this morphological effect could be caused by the interaction of phalloidin with contractile proteins as observed in the laboratory of B. Agostini. The consequences

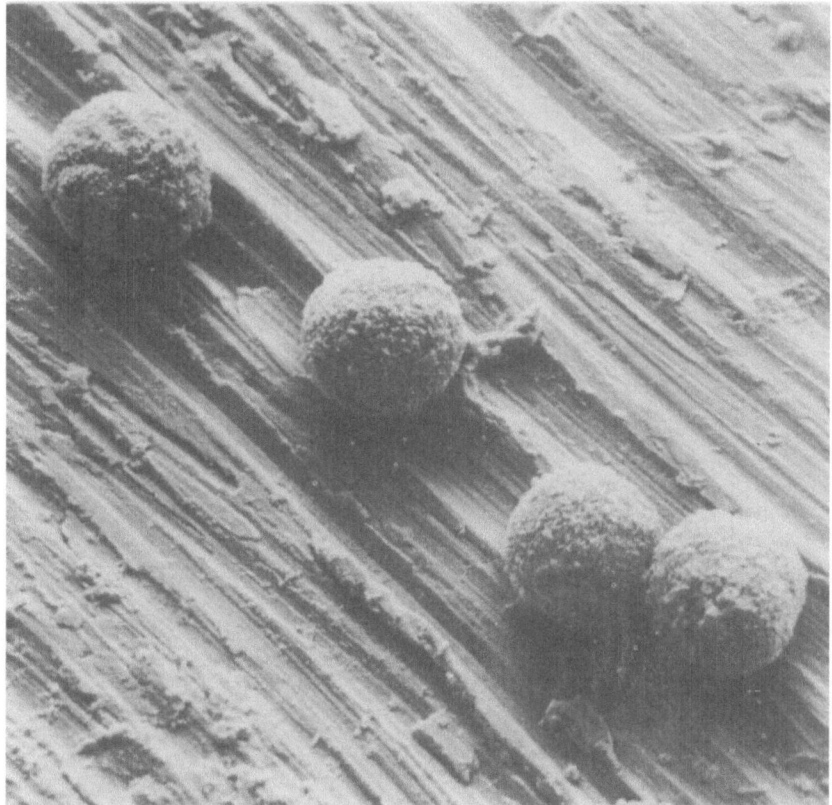

FIGURE 15.2 Scanning electron micrograph of untreated rat hepatocytes. (Photograph taken by E. Petzinger, Giessen)

of membrane softening by phalloidin will be discussed later. Before then I would like to report on some spectroscopical investigation$ by D. Hegner and R. Kroker[10] partially done in the MPI for spectroscopy (Göttingen) in the laboratory of A. Stier. The typical u.v. spectrum of phalloidin is changed, when this cyclopeptide interacts with plasma membranes. The spectrum of phalloidin is shifted towards a longer wavelength and transformed into a single peak spectrum. These optical changes were prevented by trypsination of the isolated plasma membranes. The solubilised material contained the substance interacting with phalloidin as shown with the optical method. Obviously this optical test lacks satisfactory theoretical interpretation. Nevertheless some

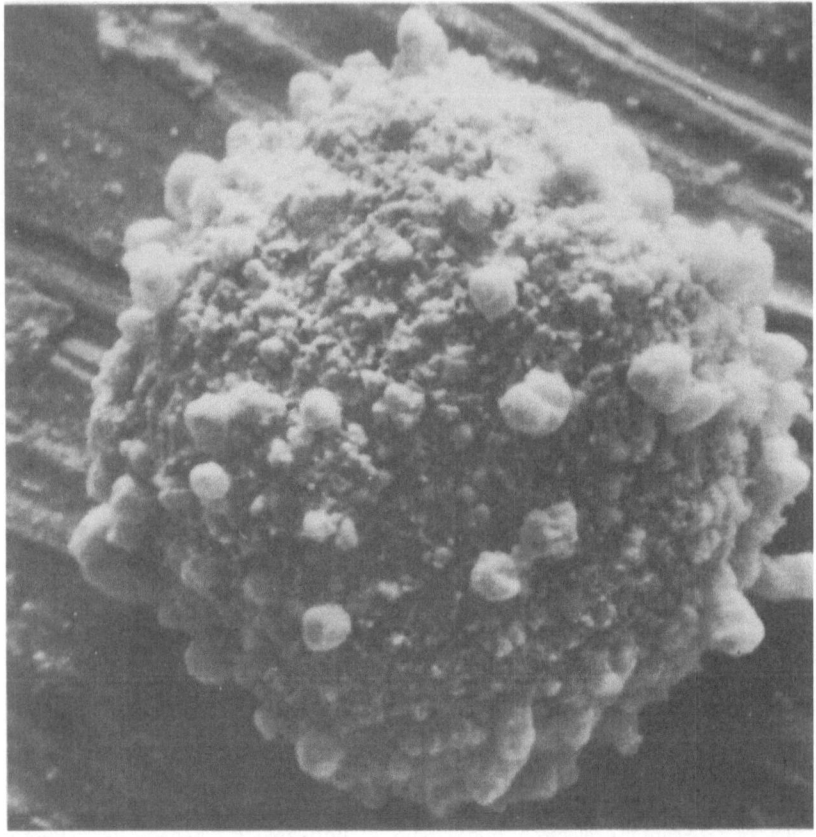

FIGURE 15.3   Isolated hepatocyte 10 min after treatment with 65 μg phalloidin/ml cell suspension. (Scanning electron micrograph taken by E. Petzinger, Giessen). (× 6000)

biological data can be correlated with the results of the spectroscopical studies, which indicates the validity of the optical method.

In Table 15.1 some data from experiments with isolated hepatocytes are summarised. Figure 15.4 demonstrates the toxic effect of phalloidin in isolated hepatocytes observed with phase microscopy. If the cell suspension were quickly trypsinated before the treatment no protrusions could be observed. Thus a good correlation exists between the spectroscopical data and the sensitivity of hepatocytes *in vitro*. It should be mentioned that the optical test used by our group is not specific for phalloidin. Non-toxic derivatives like secophalloidin show the same behaviour as phalloidin itself. As yet we have not postulated a site of

Table 15.1 CHANGES OF THE U.V. SPECTRUM OF PHALLOIDIN DUE TO INTER-ACTION WITH DIFFERENTLY PRETREATED HEPATOCYTES, AS COMPARED WITH ITS CELLULAR EFFECTS

Coincidence of spectral changes and sensitivity		
Treatment	*Spectral changes*	*Cellular alterations*
None	+	Up to 80% of cells form protrusions in presence of phalloidin. The number of the damaged cells depends on the concentration of phalloidin[14]
Trypsination *in vitro*	o	Up to 20% of cells form protrusions in presence of phalloidin[14]
Cells prepared from rats previously poisoned with CCl_4 *in vivo*	Decreased[15]	Rats poisoned with CCl_4 are less sensitive to phalloidin[5]
Cells prepared from baby rats (16–20 days)	Mostly decreased[16]	Baby rats are less sensitive to phalloidin [3, 17]
Cells pretreated *in vitro* with silybin	Decreased independence on the concentration of the drug[18]	Cells form no protrusions in presence of phalloidin. Silybin protects animals against phalloidin when given simultaneously with the toxin[19]

action for phalloidin from these findings. Our present view is that the reacting structure might represent the binding site for phalloidin responsible for its specificity. We tried to isolate this phalloidin binding material which can be solubilised by trypsination. Preliminary data suggest sialoglycoproteins[20]. Possibly one of these proteins is a component or a subunit of the receptor. Further studies should elucidate this problem.

What is the significance of the softening of membrane areas by phalloidin? How can we explain the death of hepatocytes by this mechanism? Table 15.2 furnishes some experimental data useful for an approach. Figure 15.5 presents our interpretation of the various findings in isolated cells and in perfused livers respectively. In both cases softening of the sensitive areas is a precondition of two different types of deformation. In isolated hepatocytes the osmotic pressure gradient is

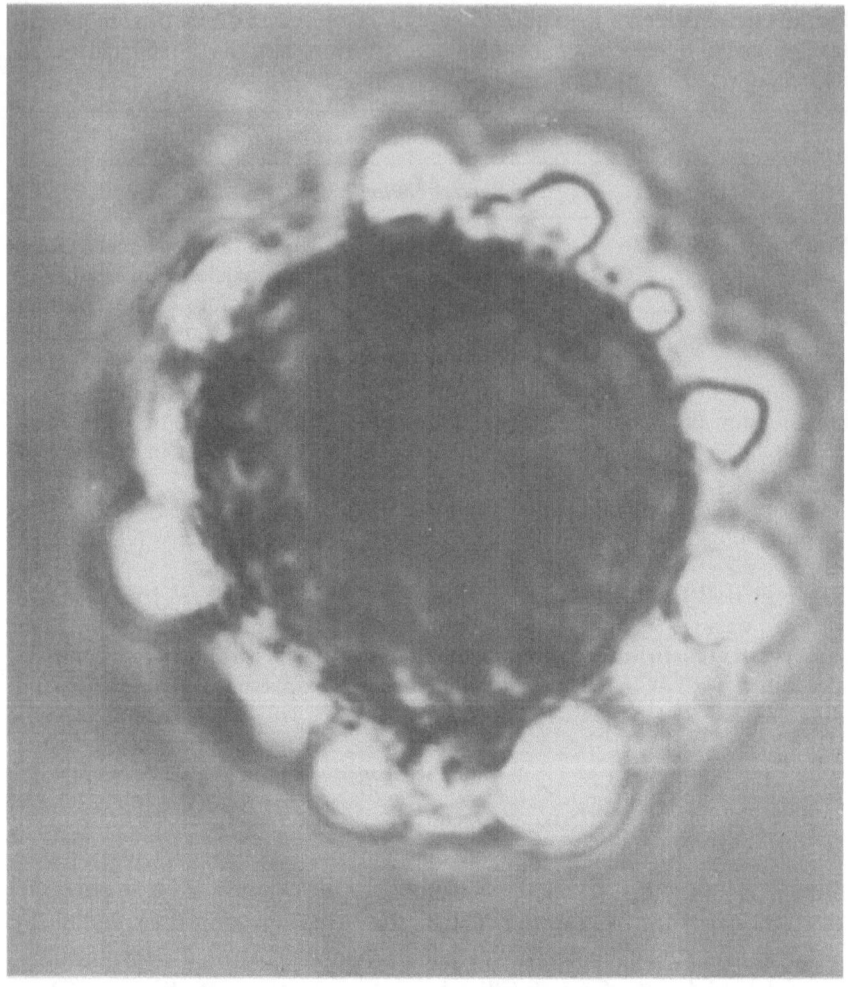

FIGURE 15.4a   Effect of phalloidin on isolated hepatocytes without pretreatment. 95μg phalloidin/ml cell suspension, 10 min at 37°C. (Phase contrast photograph taken by E. Petzinger). (× 4000)

directed from inside out. The colloid osmotic pressure difference was high in all experiments with isolated cells, because the medium contained no protein. Consequently protrusions are formed. In the perfused tissue a hydrostatic pressure difference might exist from outside in. Invaginations of the softened areas result from the actual intrasinusoidal pressure. Large vacuoles are shaped from these invaginations. In contrast phalloidin does not stimulate active phagocytosis in isolated hepatocytes[21].

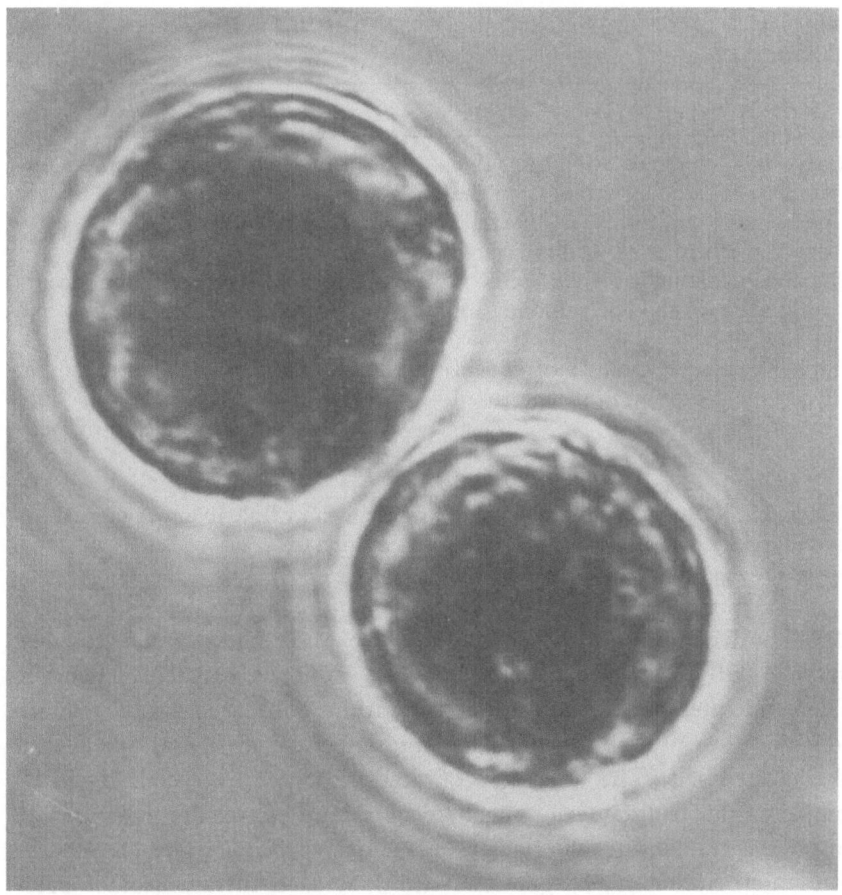

FIGURE 15.4b   Hepatocytes pretreated for 5 min with trypsin and subsequently exposed to 95 μg phalliodin/ml cell suspension. (× 2500)

A similar approach can be made to the dilatation of the ER. In this case the extracellular fluid might enter the channels of the ER followed by a dilatation of these structures. The latter hypothesis can be supported by several biochemical data produced by our laboratory[8]. Obviously the ER is not injured by phalloidin itself, because isolated microsomes are completely insensitive to phalloidin *in vitro*. The enzymatic behaviour of microsomes from poisoned livers is completely identical with those from livers damaged by a partial outflow block[8,22]. The yield of microsomal protein and the kinetic data (K_m, V_{max}) of glucose-6-phosphatase and esterase activities (E.C.3.1.1.1) were analysed.

Table 15.2   PHALLOIDIN EFFECTS *in vivo*, IN PERFUSED LIVERS AND IN ISOLATED
HEPATOCYTES

Livers in vivo, *and perfused livers*	*Isolated hepatocytes*
Rapid and marked swelling. The amount of swelling depends on the perfusion pressure[22]. Maximal effect at PR of > 3.5 ml/min/g	The total cell volume remains unchanged in absence of a hydrostatic gradient[22]
The vacuolisation of liver cells is correlated with the amount of swelling[21]	No additional vacuolisation occurs in presence of phalloidin. No stimulation of phagocytosis[21]
Marked release of potassium and of lysosomal enzymes in perfused livers[9, 22]	The K^+-loss is smaller than in perfused livers. Phalloidin does not stimulate the release of lysosomal enzymes[11]

Conclusion: The microcirculatory conditions in the whole liver are crucial for
secondary effects following the 'softening' of surface areas

Under both conditions the V_{max} of glucose-6-phosphatase and of esterase
was markedly increased, whereas the K_m values remained unchanged.
This indicates that microsomal alterations observed in phalloidin
poisoning are probably caused by micromechanical stress, but not by
phalloidin itself. The alteration of the surface of liver cells by phalloidin might facilitate the mechanical dilatation of the ER. In the
absence of phalloidin a similar process is only possible during a remarkable microcirculatory stagnation with increased intrasinusoidal pressure. The possible role of lysosomes in the mechanism of phalloidin
poisoning was overestimated for some years. Isolated lysosomes are
insensitive to phalloidin *in vitro*[9]. The marked release of lysosomal
enzymes, observed in perfused livers poisoned with phalloidin[9], might
be a secondary effect caused by swelling and change of the intracellular
pH.

My comprehensive thesis of phalloidin action on liver tissue is as
follows: Phalloidin reacts with distinct areas of the cell surface. The
primary effect consists of a softening of membrane structures which
again is a precondition for both the vacuolisation and the increased
permeability of liver cells.

Isolated hepatocytes

Protuberances

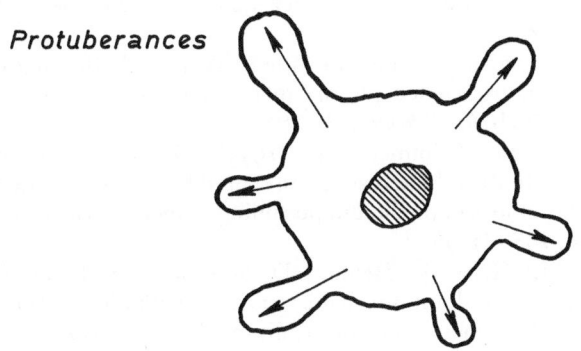

Liver cells in situ

Invaginations   Vacuolization
                       of the ER

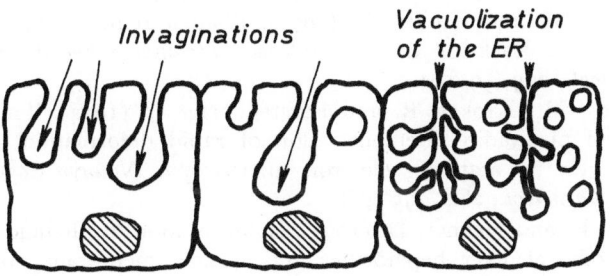

FIGURE 15.5   (see text)

REFERENCES

1. Puchinger, H. and Wieland, T. (1969). Suche nach einem Metaboliten bei Vergiftung mit Desmethylphalloin (DMP). *Eur. J. Biochem.*, **11**, 1–6
2. von der Decken, A., Löw, H. and Hultin, T. (1960). Über die primären Wirkungen von Phalloidin in Leberzellen. *Biochem. Z.*, **332**, 503–518
3. Fiume, L. (1965). Mechanism of action of phalloidin. *Lancet*, **i**, 1284–1285
4. Rehbinder, D., Löffler, G., Wieland, O. and Wieland, T. (1963). Studien über den Mechanismus der Giftwirkung des phalloidins mit radioaktiv markierten Giftstoffen. *Z. Physiol. Chem.*, **331**, 132–142
5. Floersheim, G. L. (1966). Schutzwirkung hepatotoxischer Substanzen

gegen letale Dosen eines Toxins aus *Amanita phalloides* (phalloidin). *Biochem. Pharmacol.*, **15**, 1589–1593

6. Floersheim, G. L. (1966). Protektion gegen Amanitatoxine. *Helv. Physiol. Pharmacol. Acta*, **24**, 219–228

7. Lutz, F., Glossmann, H. and Frimmer, M. (1972). Binding of ³H-des-methylphalloin to isolated plasma membranes from rat liver. *Naunyn-Schmiedeberg's Arch. Pharmarcol.*, **273**, 341–351

8. Homann, J. and Frimmer, M. (1975). Glucose-6-phosphatase and arylesterase activities of microsomes prepared from perfused rat livers after partial outflow block or phalloidin poisoning. *Naunyn-Schmiedeberg's Arch. Pharmacol.*, **288**, 87–96

9. Frimmer, M., Gries, J., Hegner, D. and Schnorr, B. (1967). Unter-suchungen zum Wirkungsmechanismus des Phalloidins: Freisetzung von lysosomalen Enzymen und von Kalium. *Naunyn-Schmiedeberg's Arch. Pharmacol.*, **258**, 197–214

10. Hegner, D., Lutz, F., Eckermann, V., Gries, J. and Schnorr, B. (1970). Effect of phalloidin in Mg²-ATPase, (K⁺-Na⁺) ATPase and K⁺ depen-dent *p*-nitrophenylphosphatase activity of plasma membranes isolated from rat liver. *Biochem. Pharmacol.*, **19**, 487–493

11. Frimmer, M. and Kroker, R. (1973). Phalloidin poisoning of isolated hepatocytes: Lack of enzyme release. *Naunyn-Schmiedeberg's Arch. Pharmacol.*, **279**, 99–104

12. Frimmer, M., Kroker, R. and Porstendörfer, J. (1974). The mode of action of phalloidin: Demonstration of rapid deformation of isolated hepatocytes by scanning electron microscopy. *Naunyn-Schmiedeberg's Arch. Pharmacol.*, **284**, 395–398

13. Kroker, R. and Hegner, D. (1973). Solubilisation of phalloidin binding sites from rat liver hepatocytes and plasma membranes by trypsin. *Naunyn-Schmiedeberg's Arch. Pharmacol.*, **279**, 339–346

14. Petzinger, E. and Frimmer, M. (unpublished data)

15. Kroker, R. and Frimmer, M. (1974). Decrease of binding sites for phalloidin on the surface of liver cells during carbon tetrachloride intoxication. *Naunyn-Schmiedeberg's Arch. Pharmacol.*, **282**, 109–111

16. Kroker, R. and Frimmer, M. (1974). The mechanism of phalloidin tolerance in baby rats and in animals poisoned with carbon tectrachloride. *Naunyn-Schmiedeberg's Arch. Pharmacol.*, **Suppl. 284**, R 51

17. Wieland, O. and Szabados, A. (1966). On the nature of phalloidin toler-ance in newborn rats. *6th Int. Congr. Clin. Chem. Munich*; **vol. 4**, *Advances in Clinico-Biochemical Research*, 59–66 (Basle, New York: Karger; 1968)

18. Frimmer, M. and Kroker, R. (1975). Phalloidinantagonisten: 1. Mitteilung. Wirkung von Silybinderivaten an der isoliert perfundierten Rattenleber. *Arzneim. Forschg. (Drug Res.)*, **25**, 394–396

19. Petzinger, E., Homan, J. and Frimmer, M. (1975). Phalloidinantago-nisten: 2. Mitteilung. Protektive Wirkung von Disilybin bei Vergiftung

isolierter Hepatozyten mit Phalloidin. *Arzneim. Forschg.* (*Drug Res.*), **25**, 571–576.

20. Abdel Raheem, M. (1975) (University of Giessen: Thesis)
21. Weiss, E., Sterz, I., Frimmer, M. and Kroker, R. (1973). Electron microscopy of isolated rat hepatocytes before and after treatment with phalloidin. *Beitr. Pathol.*, **150**, 345–356
22. Frimmer, M. (1972). The influence of physical conditions on swelling and K^+-release in perfused rat livers poisoned with phalloidin. *Naunyn-Schmiedeberg's Arch. Pharmacol.*, **275**, 393–403

CHAPTER 16

Morphological changes induced by phalloidin in the rat liver

B. Agostini, V. M. Govindan and W. Hofmann

INTRODUCTION

The phallotoxins, components of the poisonous mushroom *Amanita phalloides* (for review see Ref. 1), lead to death of experimental animals within a few hours by a characteristic haemorrhagic dystrophy of the liver. On histological examination, this final stage is preceded by a formation of numerous non-fatty vacuoles, which begin at the periphery of the lobule and then extend to the central zone. The pathogenesis of this alteration has been disputed. Lutz et al.[2], found that [3][H]desmethylphalloin is strongly bound to plasma membranes of hepatocytes rather than to microsomal or mitochondrial fractions. Some time ago, it was demonstrated in this laboratory, by electron microscopy of isolated membrane preparations, that phalloidin affects the plasma membranes of hepatocytes *in vivo* and *in vitro*[3]. Furthermore, it was shown that [3][H]desmethylphalloin binds mainly to the protein filaments which appear with increased frequency in poisoned plasma membrane fractions[4].

In this report, substantiating observations on sectioned liver and immunofluorescence investigations will be presented. It will be shown that the interaction of phalloidin with the plasma membrane is an early link in the chain of events leading to the known dramatic alteration of the liver. Furthermore it will be confirmed that phalloidin causes a characteristically striking increase of actin filaments in the hepatocytes.

MATERIALS AND METHODS

Male Wistar rats, weighing about 200 g, were fasted overnight before injection of the toxin. Phalloidin[1] and [3][H]desmethylphalloin[5], with specific activity of 32.5 μCi/mg, were used as poisons and O-carbomethyl-[6]Tyr-antamanide[6] was used as an antidote.

Rats were injected intravenously with 1–5 μg phallotoxin/g body wt. and killed by decapitation 10–60 min after poisoning. The liver was prepared for isolation of plasma membranes, for immunological investigations and for studies by light and electron microscopy. The liver of a non-poisoned animal served as a control.

MEMBRANE PREPARATION

Plasma membranes of liver cells were isolated by homogenising liver in a medium containing 1.0 mM $NaHCO_3$ and 0.5 mM $CaCl_2$ (pH 7.5) according to Ray[7]. In several experiments, Ray's fraction was fractionated by a modified Evans[8] procedure on a linear sucrose gradient (45–30%) in a Spinco Rotor SW-25-1 at 20 000 rpm for 15 hours[4]. Protein was estimated according to Lowry *et al.*[9], 5-nucleotidase by the method of Emmelot *et al.*[10], and glucose-6-phosphatase according to Swanson[11].

In vitro EXPERIMENTS

Membrane suspensions in 1.0 mM $NaHCO_3$ and 0.5 mM $CaCl_2$ (pH 7.5), were incubated with 10 μg phalloidin per 0.1 mg protein for 10 min at 37 °C with or without preincubation[3] and for 20 min with 10 or 50 μg of the phallotoxin antidote antamanide.

IMMUNOFLUORESCENCE

Liver sections from control- and phalloidin-poisoned rats were cut at 5 μ in a cryostat microtome, moistened with a drop of Coons buffer, containing 0.01 M Na-barbiturate and 0.144 NaCl (pH adjusted to 7.2 with HCl) and covered with a drop of rabbit antiserum against actomyosin of chicken stomach, labelled with fluorescein isothiocyanate. This was prepared by Professor U. Gröschel-Stewart; for review on methods see Ref. 12. The sections were kept for 30 min in a moist chamber at room temperature and carefully rinsed and washed several times for 90 min with Coons buffer. Thereafter sections were embedded with a mixture of 30% 0.1 M glycine buffer (pH 8.6) and 70% glycerol, observed in a Leitz Ortholux epifluorescence microscope, using filter combinations BG 480 and K 510 and lamp: Hg 200 W and photographed with an Ilford film HP 4 (27–29 DIN).

Smear preparations of plasma membrane of control and *in vivo* poisoned animals prepared according to Ray[7] were also processed for immunological investigation. Ray's fraction challenged with the labelled antibody for 30 min at 37 °C was purified by the above modified Evans procedure and processed for detection of the immunological reaction or used for a specificity test.

Specificity test: Cryostat sections and membrane fractions from control and poisoned animals were covered with a drop of a mixture of labelled antibody, and membrane fraction from poisoned rats observed with higher fluorescence in the fluorescence microscope after careful washing.

LIGHT MICROSCOPY

Fresh liver tissue was fixed with Bouin's solution, Baker's formaldehyde-calcium, absolute alcohol or neutral formalin and embedded in paraffin. Sections (4–6 μ) were stained with haematoxylin and eosin, the PAS technique, Masson's trichrome and Van Gieson's technique.

ELECTRON MICROSCOPY

Droplet material: Various membrane preparations, including those incubated with antibodies, were examined by negative staining technique, according to standard procedures. Usually 1% phosphotungstic acid (PTA), adjusted to pH 7.1–7.2 with KOH, or 1% uranyl acetate at pH 4.5 were applied. In a few cases 2% ammonium molybdate or a mixture of v/v 1% PTA—2% ammonium molybdate, both at pH 7.1–7.2 were used.

Sectioned material: Suspensions of membrane fractions from control and poisoned animals were fixed with glutaraldehyde for 45 min, adding the fixative to the test tube to a final concentration of 5%. Specimens were postfixed for one hour with 1% OsO_4 solution in Na-Veronal and Na-acetate buffer, which also contained 12.5 mM $CaCl_2$ at pH 6.1–6.2 adjusted with HCl according to Kellenberger *et al.*[13].

Small portions of liver tissue were rapidly excised from the left and the right lobes of the liver and placed in the fixative at 4 °C where they were further minced. Samples were usually fixed for two hours with 2.5% glutaraldehyde and 2.5% formaldehyde in 0.1 M phosphate buffer (pH 7.2) and postfixed for one hour with 1% OsO_4 in Veronal-acetate buffer, pH 7.2[14], with added sucrose[15]. In a few cases, samples were fixed directly with 1% OsO_4 in 0.1 M phosphate buffer (pH 7.2), or only with the glutaraldehyde–formaldehyde solution as above.

After washing and in most experiments, counterstaining for one hour with 0.5% uranyl acetate, material was dehydrated in alcohol and embedded in Epon 812. Sections cut on an LKB ultratome were picked up on formvar coated grids and observed directly or after staining with uranyl acetate[16] and/or lead citrate[17]. A Siemens Elmiskop 101 electron microscope, equipped with a double condenser illumination, 300 μ Pt condenser and 30 μ Pt objective aperture, accelerating voltage of 80 kV and an emission current of 20 μA, was used.

RESULTS AND DISCUSSION

Figure 16.1a, taken by light microscopy of a paraffin section of a poisoned rat liver, shows a characteristic advanced stage of vacuolisation of the hepatocytes. Most vacuoli appear to be located close to the plasma membrane. In some places erythrocytes appear to be contained in vacuolar formations. Vacuoli of hepatocytes from a rat poisoned with phalloidin have been reported to display a positive immunofluorescence reaction, when challenged with labelled antirat whole serum[18]. As reported also by Tuchweber *et al.*[19], the electron microscope shows that vacuoli observed by light microscopy may simply represent a cross-section of invaginations of the cytoplasmic membrane of the hepatocytes (Figures 16.1b and 16.2). Electron microscopy also confirms that some vacuoli contain erythrocytes. In the final stage of haemorrhagic dystrophy, hepatocytes and endothelial cells display various degrees of alteration of the cytoplasmic structures, and the sinusoidal lumen and the space of Disse are filled with erythrocytes. Vacuolisation of hepatocytes by endocytosis has been observed recently in this laboratory[20] also in the isolated rat liver perfused with phalloidin.

Significant support to such a mechanism of cytoplasmic vacuolisation has been provided by correlated biochemical and ultrastructural studies

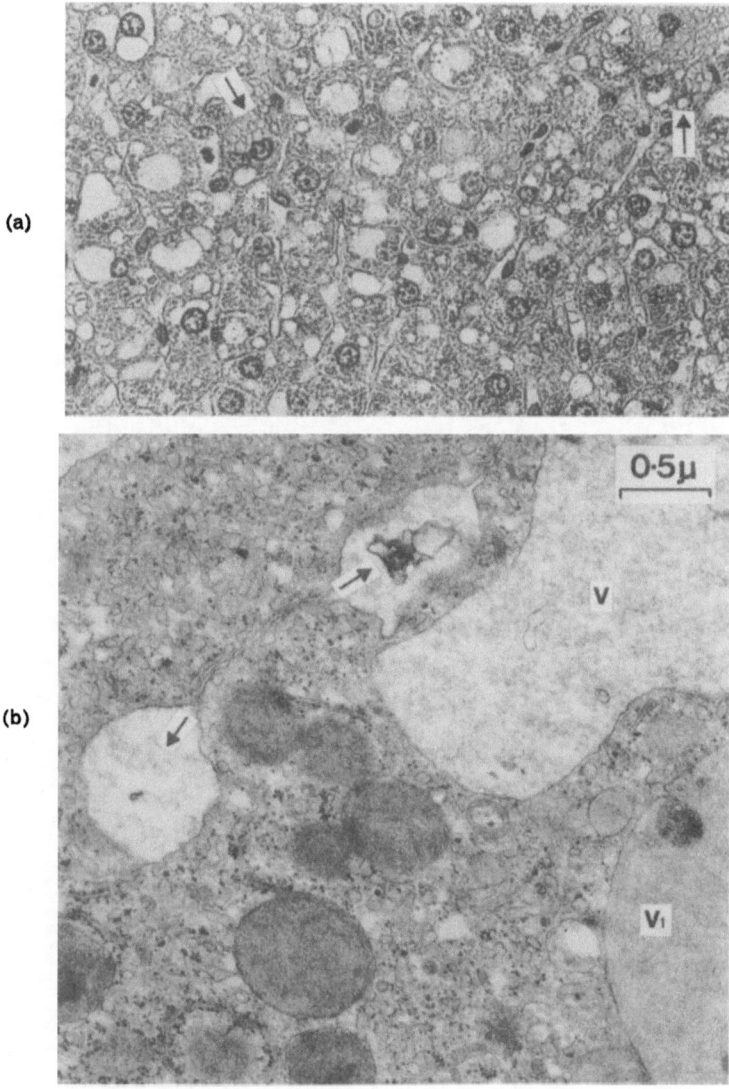

FIGURE 16.1 (a) Midzone of hepatic lobule of a rat, killed 30 min after phalloidin injection. Strong vacuolisation of hepatocytes. Vacuoli may contain erythrocytes (arrows). Haematoxylin–eosin (× 760)
(b) Electron micrograph of an epon section through two hepatocytes from the same liver as in (a). Arrows indicate widening of the intercellular space resulting in vacuole-like formations. The upper arrow points to a cavity which may correspond to an altered bile canaliculus. v and v_1 indicate vacuoli with content of various electron density (× 24 000)

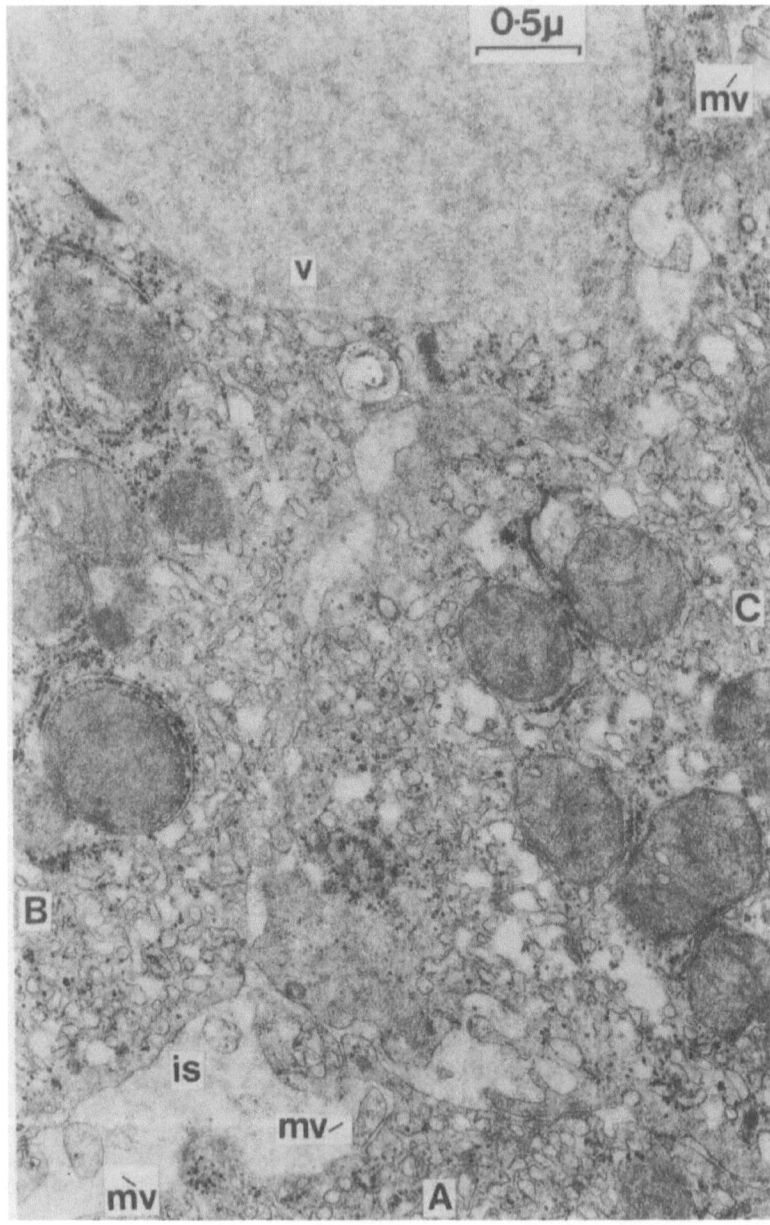

FIGURE 16.2   Section through three hepatocytes (A, B and C) 60 min after phalloidin poisoning, displaying advanced alteration of cytoplasmic structure. Top, near the cell border, vacuole (v) filled with material similar to plasma; bottom, enlarged intercellular space (is); mv: microvilli ($\times$ 25 200)

on plasma membrane preparations of hepatocytes of *in vivo* poisoned rats and on plasma membrane preparations poisoned *in vitro*[3,4,21].

Negative staining has proved a very suitable technique for investigating the surface structure and alteration of various membranes. Negatively stained plasma membrane preparations from control liver of rat (Figure 16.3a) appear in the electron microscope to consist of many elongated, collapsed, or distended sacs, the edges of which are characteristically coated with fine particles 60 Å in diameter[22]. Plasma membrane preparations of *in vivo* poisoned rats as well as plasma membrane preparations poisoned *in vitro* differ significantly from the control ones in the presence of a greatly increased frequency of filamentous structures[3]. Figure 16.3b—a preparation poisoned *in vitro*—shows a membrane sac, the edges of which do not display the fine surface particles characteristic of the control (Figure 16.3a), and numerous beaded filamentous structures, about 60 Å in width and up to 0.1 μ in length, scattered throughout the picture, which appear identical with actin filaments from muscle fibres. However, filaments of poisoned membrane preparations are stable in the presence of 0.6 M KI and also during homogenisation in 5 mM ATP, while native filamentous actin (F-actin) from muscle fibres depolimerises to the monomer under these conditions. Figure 16.3a shows that filaments are isolated from, and yet intimately associated with the membrane sacs. It could be shown[4] that [3][H]desmethylphalloin binds mainly to the fraction enriched with these filaments in a sucrose gradient. Such filamentous structures are only occasionally present in plasma membrane preparations obtained under the same conditions from control liver. The filament producing effect of phalloidin is prevented by antamanide[3], which is known to antagonise the lethal action of the phallotoxins[6].

Observation in the electron microscope of epon sections through pellets of plasma membrane preparations (Figures 16.4a and b) confirms the tremendous increase of filamentous structures on poisoned samples and provides important information on the topographic relation between filaments and the plasma membrane. Filaments can be observed on the cytoplasmic site of the plasma membrane close to the inner leaflet of the unit membrane, which *per se* is not altered. While in the control (Figure 16.4a) only a few filamentous structures (arrows) can be observed, which are limited to the level of special structures recognisable as the junctional complexes of Farquhar and Palade[23], on poisoned samples (Figure 16.4b), numerous free filaments can also be found

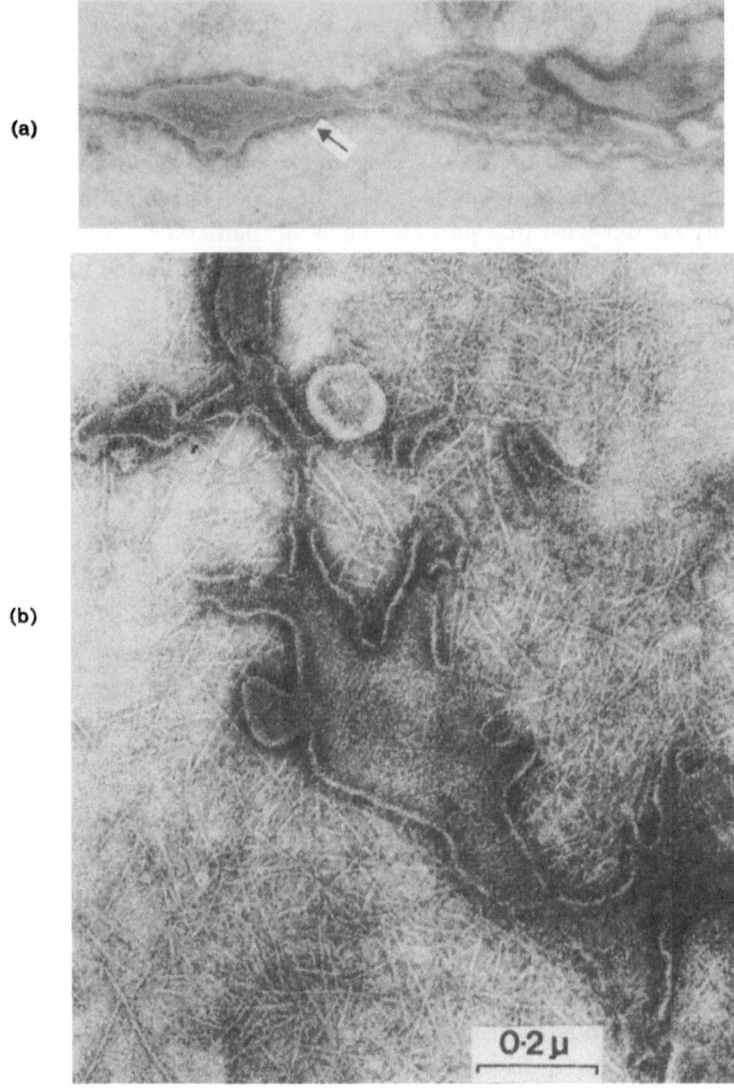

FIGURE 16.3   Electron micrographs of isolated plasma membranes of rat hepatocytes
negatively stained with PTA.
(a)   Control
(b)   After incubation *in vitro* at 37 °C with 10 μg phalloidin/mg protein for 10 min.
Arrow in (a) indicates the characteristic 60 Å surface particles. In (b) numerous beaded
filaments variously interlaced with each other, separated or intimately associated
with the membrane fragments, from which they appear to protrude, can be observed
(× 76 000)

(a)

(b)

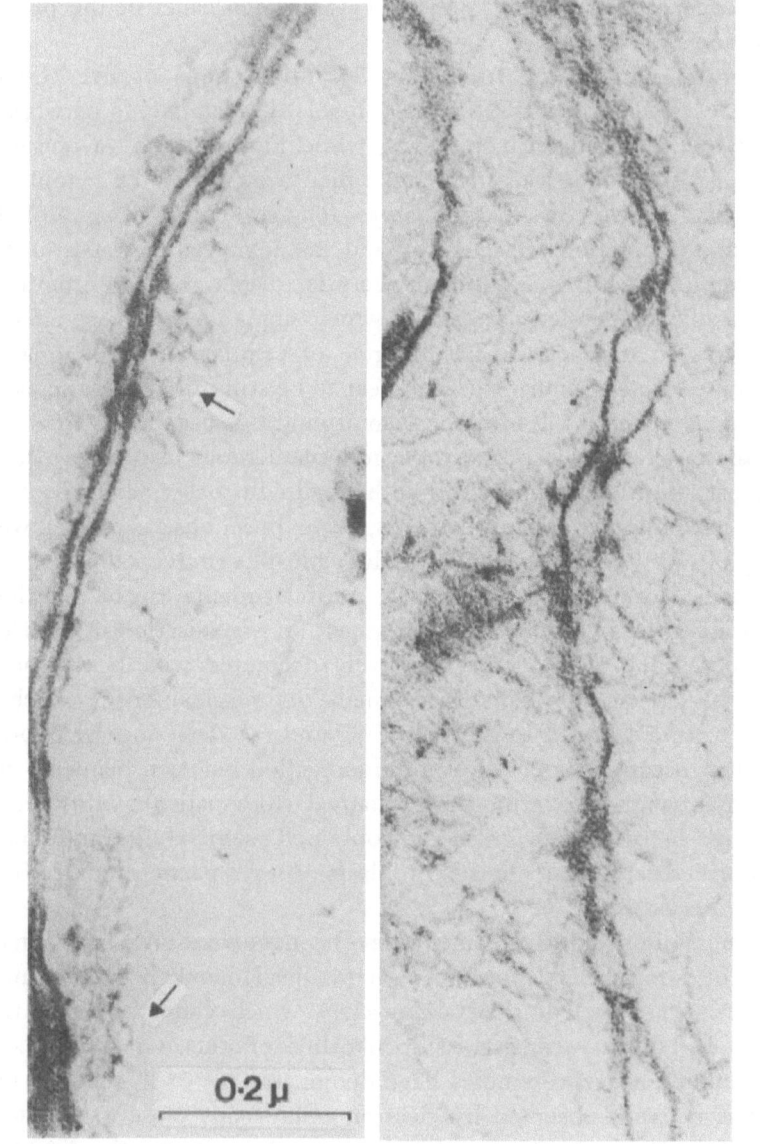

FIGURE 16.4 Epon sections through pellets of plasma membrane preparations of liver cells from control (a) and phalloidin-poisoned rat (b). While in (a) only a few filamentous structures, limited to the level of the junctional complexes (arrows) can be observed, in (b) filaments are more numerous and scattered throughout the picture (× 125 000)

which appear to break off from the cytoplasmic leaflet of the plasma membrane[21].

A similar pattern can be observed with sections of liver tissue. Figure 16.5a illustrates that in the control the filamentous network is limited to the junctional complexes, while Figure 16.5b—a poisoned liver—displays bundles of filaments which are free in the cytoplasm. Figure 16.6 shows two contiguous hepatocytes, which, in spite of the unsuitable orientation of sectioning and the advanced alteration of the cytoplasmic structures with areal necrosis, display a very prominent network of filamentous material, in which single filaments are difficult to resolve. In spite of the high degree of cellular alteration, plasma membranes of neighbouring cells appear to be still preserved. Increased filamentous material can often be seen around bile canaliculi.

In the last few years intracytoplasmic filamentous structures which, like those induced by poisoning with phalloidin described here, have similar structure to actin filaments, have been observed in a wide variety of non-muscular cells. Actually, actin-like proteins appear to be ubiquitous (for review see Ref. 24). Actin filaments can be identified and localised by two different techniques: (1) visualisation in the electron microscope of filaments selectively decorated with heavy meromyosin—a specific proteolytic fragment of muscle myosin which is known to interact with muscle actin[25,26] and (2) detection by fluorescence microscopy of a positive immunoreaction between filaments and labelled antiactin autoantibodies[27] obtained from patients with chronic aggressive hepatitis[28], or antibodies obtained from rabbits immunised with purified actin from mouse fibroblasts[29], or with actin prepared from human uterus[30].

The phalloidin-induced filaments have been shown to bind heavy meromyosin of rabbit skeletal muscle in an arrow-head manner like the filamentous actin (F-actin) of skeletal muscle[31], which confirms our earlier conception[21] that they consist of actin, like those of other non-muscle cells.

Immunofluorescence studies have demonstrated[27,30,32], that the filamentous network observed by electron microscopy close to the inner leaflet of the plasma membrane of hepatocytes do contain actin. A regular polygonal pattern of staining of the borders of the hepatocytes can characteristically be observed when antiactin antibodies are applied to liver cryostat sections.

Figure 16.7 depicts liver cryostat sections and smears of plasma membrane suspensions challenged with fluorescence antiserum against

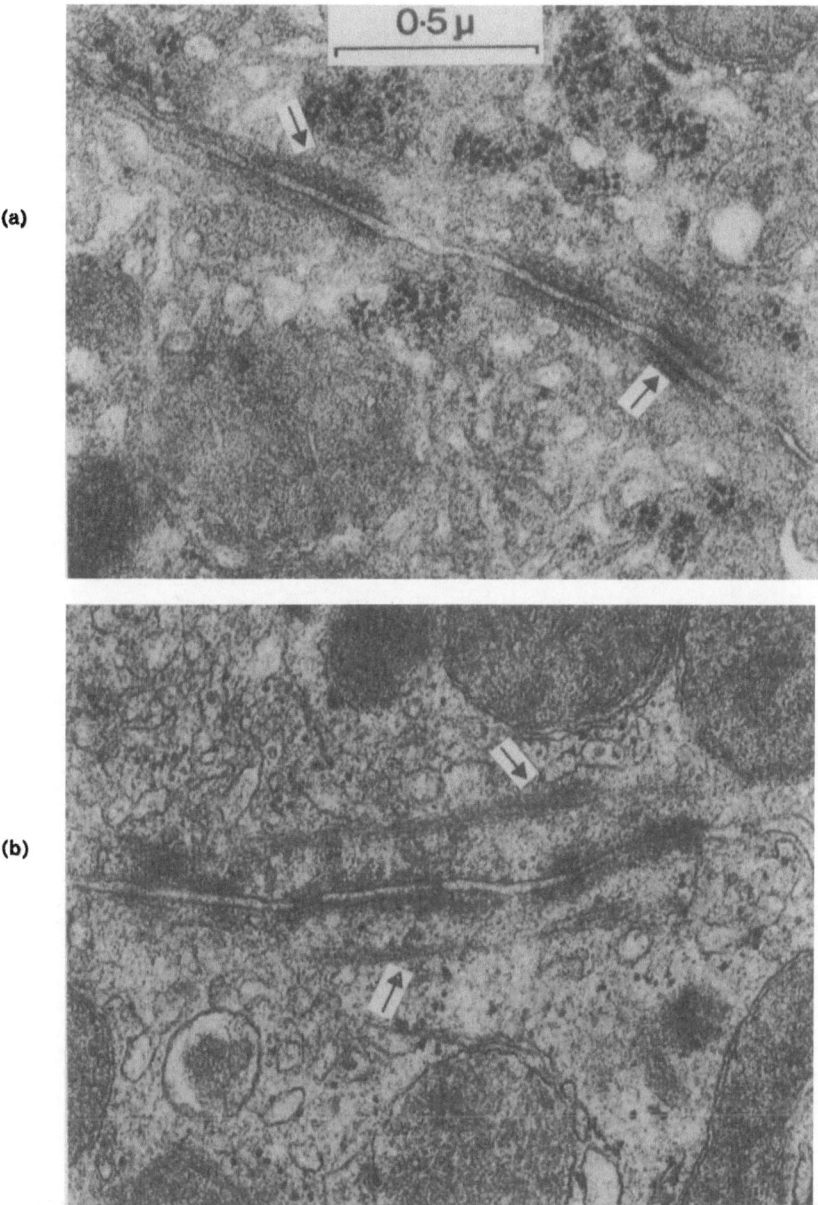

FIGURE 16.5 Sections through junctional complexes of contiguous hepatocytes of a control rat (a) and 20 min after phalloidin injection, (b). In the control (a), the filamentous network is limited to the junctional complexes (arrows), while on poisoned cells (b) bundles of free filaments (arrows) can also be observed (× 54 000)

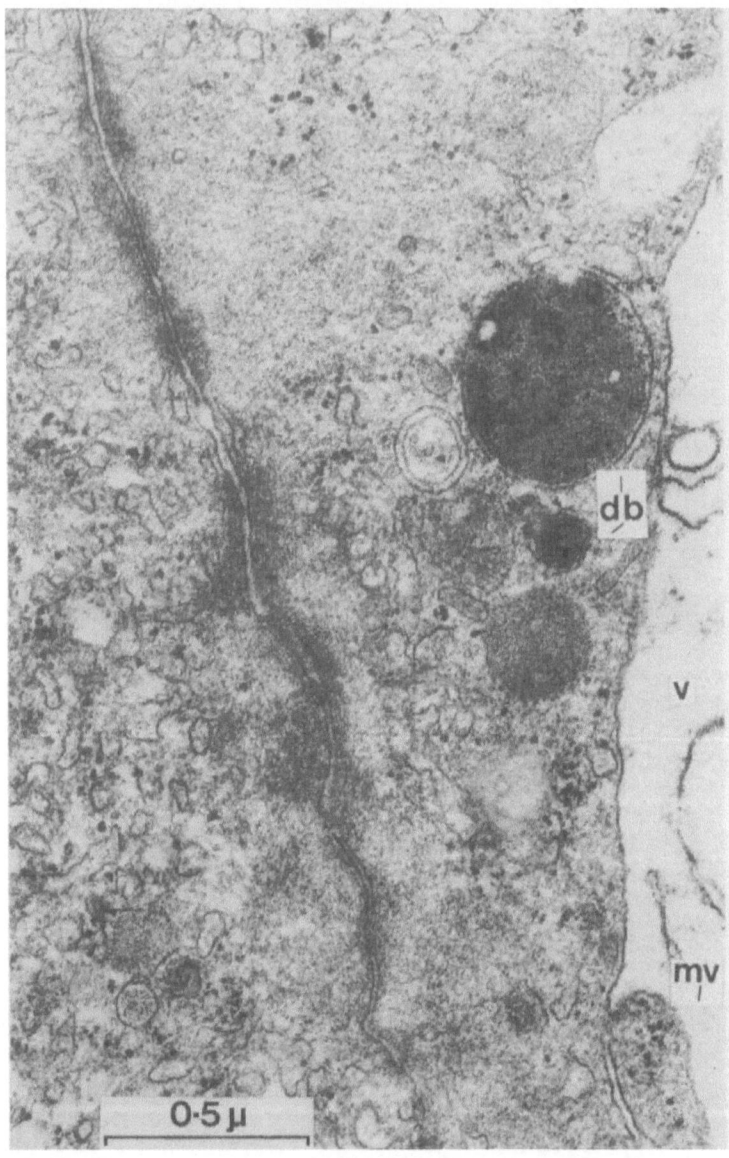

FIGURE 16.6 Section of two contiguous hepatocytes, 60 min after poisoning, displaying a prominent network of filamentous material near the plasma membrane and an advanced alteration of cytoplasmic structures with areal necrosis. On the right side of the figure, part of a vacuole (v) or invagination of plasma membrane, containing membranous structures and a microvillus (mv), can be seen. db: dense bodies ($\times$ 54 000)

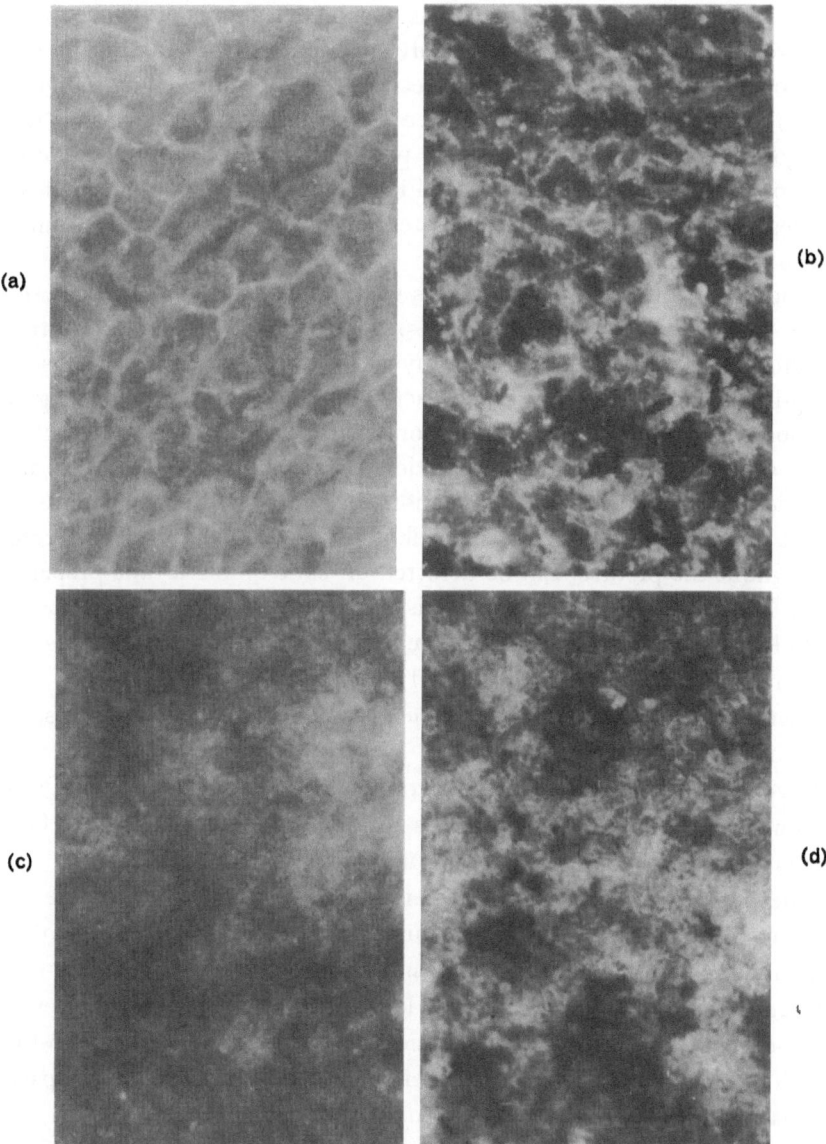

FIGURE 16.7   (a) and (b) Cryostat sections of a normal and a poisoned rat liver challenged with fluorescent anti-actomyosin antibodies. The polygonal pattern of staining
of hepatocyte borders characteristic of the control (a), is almost absent in the poisoned
liver (b), in which cytoplasmic fluorescence is strongly increased.
(c) and (d) Smear preparations of control and poisoned membranes incubated as in (a)
and in (b). The degree of fluorescence of poisoned membranes (d) is higher than in
the control (c) ($\times$ 915)

actomyosin from chicken stomach. As expected, sections of control liver (Figure 16.7a) display a regular polygonal pattern of staining of the hepatocyte borders; whereas on sections of poisoned liver (Figure 16.7b) the cytoplasmic fluorescence is strongly increased and the polygonal pattern is almost absent, probably due to alteration of the hepatocyte borders. Comparison of Figure 16.7c with 16.7d shows that the degree of fluorescence in smear preparations of poisoned membranes is also higher than in the control.

Binding of antibodies to filaments was confirmed by electron microscopy of negatively stained samples. Figure 16.8a depicts the ultrastructural aspect of the anti-actomyosin antibodies which we used. Irregular polygonal aggregates, characteristic of negatively stained I g G antibodies[33], can be observed. For comparison, a few filaments isolated from a plasma membrane preparation poisoned with phalloidin are represented at the same magnification in Figure 16.8b. Figure 16.8c shows that no definite binding of antibody particles, which are scattered throughout the picture, can be detected on control membrane preparations. When such a control sample is well washed, almost no antibody particles appear to be attached to the membrane. In contrast to this, in preparations of phalloidin-poisoned membranes (Figure 16.8d) the filamentous structures appear to be covered with antibody particles, in spite of repeated washings.

Cryostat sections and smear preparations covered for a specificity test with a mixture of labelled antibodies and membrane enriched with filaments never showed a positive immunoreaction.

The results of immunofluorescence investigations, like those of previous biochemical and ultrastructural studies[2,3,21], indicate that phalloidin affects primarily the plasma membrane of hepatocytes and interacts with the actin-like protein located close to the inner leaflet of the membrane resulting in a dramatic increase in actin filaments in the cell. This initiates the toxicological effect and provides, at least in part, the basis for endocytotic vacuolisation of the hepatocytes.

Similar relations between endocytotic vacuoli and microfilaments have been observed in cultures of Chang liver cells with added labelled sucrose[34]. Addition of cytochalasin to the medium alters microfilaments and reduces vacuolisation.

In vitro phalloidin has been demonstrated to be capable of polymerising globular actin (G-actin) from rabbit skeletal muscle to F-actin[22].

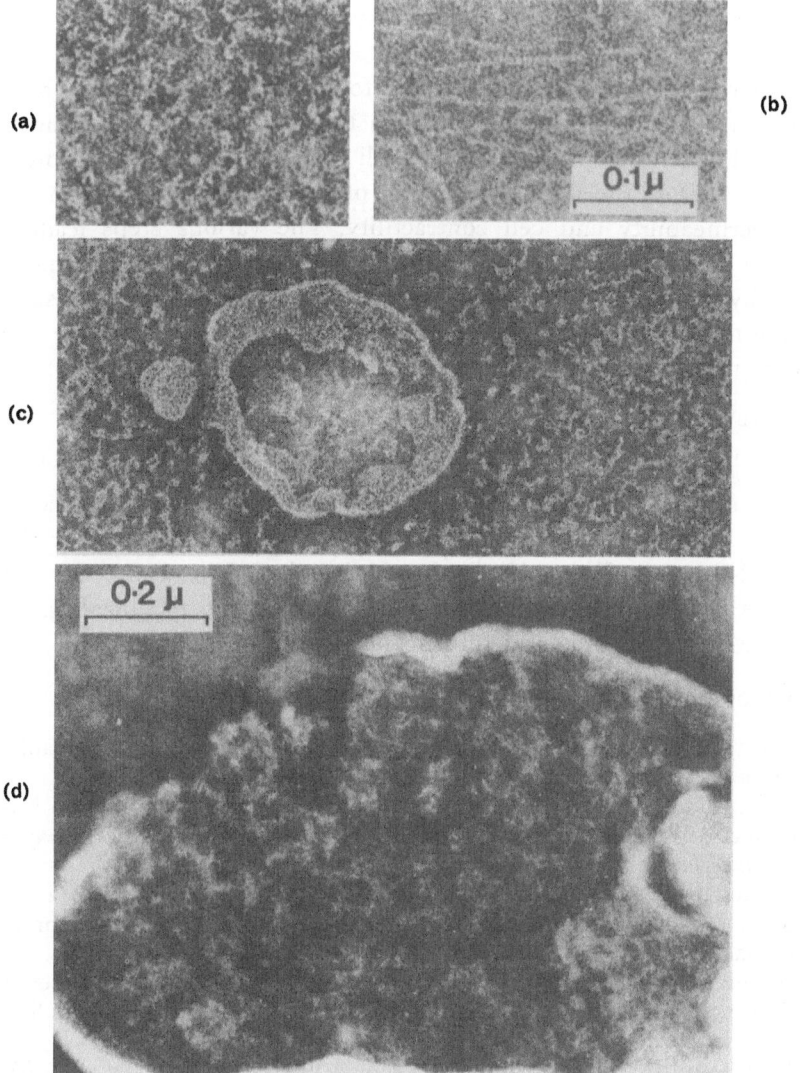

FIGURE 16.8   Electron micrographs of negatively stained preparations:
(a) Fluorescein-conjugated anti-actomyosin antibodies
(b) Filaments isolated from poisoned membrane preparation
(c) A control membrane incubated with antibody
(d) A poisoned membrane incubated with the antibody
Filaments of poisoned membrane (d) are clearly covered with antibody particles, which in the control (c) are scattered throughout the picture. (a) and (b): × 160 000; (c) and (d): × 80 000

This, in contrast to native F-actin from skeletal muscle, and like the phalloidin-induced filaments from rat liver is not depolymerised with 0.6 M KI.

Further investigations are necessary to clarify the means by which phalloidin penetrates into the liver cell to interact with the sensitive protein. The possible role of microtubuli has to be investigated, which would also allow the better evaluation of the relation between membrane permeability and cell contractility. The various steps leading from the endocytotic vacuolisation of hepatocytes to the haemorrhagic dystrophy of the liver also need further investigation. These results indicate that phalloidin is a very useful substance for studying the role of actin filaments in cell pathophysiology.

ACKNOWLEDGMENTS

We are grateful to Professor W. Hasselbach and to Professor Th. Wieland for important advice and suggestion in part of the experiments and for helpful discussion of the results. We thank Professor U. Gröschel-Stewart, Frauenklinik der Universität, Würzburg, for her generous donation of labelled antibodies. The skilled technical assistance of Mr K. Jelinek is gratefully acknowledged.

REFERENCES

1. Wieland, Th. and Wieland, O. (1972). The toxic peptides of Amanita species. *Microbial Toxins*, **8**, 249–280
2. Lutz, F., Glossman, H. and Frimmer, M. (1972). Binding of ^{3}H-desmethylphalloin to isolated plasma membranes from rat liver. *Naunyn-Schmiedeberg's Arch. Pharmacol.*, **273**, 341–351
3. Govindan, V. M., Faulstich, H., Wieland, Th., Agostini, B. and Hasselbach, W. (1972). *In vitro* effect of phalloidin on a plasma membrane preparation from rat liver. *Naturwissenschaften*, **59**, 521–522
4. Govindan, V. M., Rohr, G., Wieland, Th. and Agostini, B. (1973). Binding of a phallotoxin to protein filaments of plasma membrane of liver cell. *Hoppe-Seyler's Z. Physiol. Chem.*, **354**, 1159–1160
5. Puchinger, H. and Wieland, Th. (1969). ^{3}H-desmethylphalloin. *Liebigs Ann. Chem.*, **725**, 238–240
6. Wieland, Th., Rietzel, C. and Seeliger, A. (1972). Einige Derivate der phenolischen Seitenkette des Tyrosin^5- und Tyrosin^6-Antamanids. *Liebigs Ann. Chem.*, **759**, 63–70
7. Ray, T. K. (1970). A modified method for the isolation of the plasma membrane from rat liver. *Biochim. Biophys. Acta*, **196**, 1–9
8. Evans, W. H. (1970). Fractionation of liver plasma membranes prepared by zonal centrifugation. *Biochem. J.*, **166**, 833–842

9. Lowry, O. U., Rosenbrough, N. J., Farr, A. L. and Randall, R. J. (1951). Protein measurement with the folin phenol reagent. *J. Biol. Chem.*, **143**, 265–275

10. Emmelot, P., Bos, C. J. and Benedetti, E. L. (1964). Chemical composition and enzyme content of plasma membranes isolated from rat liver. *Biochim. Biophys. Acta*, **90**, 126–145

11. Swanson, M. A. (1955). Glucose-6-phosphatase from liver. *Meth. Enzym.*, **2**, 541–543

12. Groschel-Stewart, U. (1971). Comparative studies of human smooth and striated muscle myosins. *Biochim. Biophys. Acta*, **229**, 322–324.

13. Kellenberger, E., Ryter, A. and Sechaud, J. (1958). Electron microscopy study of DNA-containing plasms. II. Vegetative and mature phage DNS as compared with normal bacterial nucleids in different physiological states. *J. Biophys. Biochem. Cytol.*, **4**, 671–678

14. Palade, G. E. (1952). A study of fixation for electron microscopy. *J. Exp. Med.*, **95**, 285–297

15. Caulfield, J. B. (1957). Effects of varying the vehicle for OsO_4 in tissue fixation. *J. Biophys. Biochem. Cytol.*, **3**, 877–830

16. Watson, M. L. (1958). Staining of tissue sections for electron microscopy with heavy metals. I. *J. Biophys. Biochem. Cytol.*, **4**, 475–478

17. Reynolds, E. S. (1973). The use of lead citrate at high pH as an electron-opaque stain in electron microscopy. *J. Cell Biol.*, **17**, 208–212

18. Baccino, F. M. (1971). Biochemical evaluation of the lysosomal damage: investigations with an experimental model. *Quad. Sclavo Diagn.*, **7**, 907–936

19. Tuchweber, B., Kovacs, K., Khandekar, J. D. and Garg, B. D. (1973). Peliosis-like changes induced by phalloidin in the rat liver. *J. Med.*, **4**, 327–340

20. Lengsfeld, A. and Jahn, W. (1974). Endocytose an der isoliert perfundierten Rattenleber nach Phalloidinvergiftung. *Cytobiologie*, **9**, 391–400

21. Agostini, B. and Govindan, V. M. (1973). Elektronenmikroskopische Üntersuchungen an der Zellmembran der Leber bei Phalloidin-Vergiftung. *Verh. Dtsch. Ges. Pathol.*, **57**, 436

22. Benedetti, E. L. and Emmelot, P. (1965). Electron microscopic observations on negatively stained plasma membranes isolated from rat liver. *J. Cell Biol.*, **26**, 299–305

23. Farquhar, M. G. and Palade, G. E. (1963). Junctional complexes in various epithelia. *J. Cell Biol.*, **17**, 375–412

24. Bray, D. (1972). Cytoplasmic actin: a comparative study. *Cold Spring Harbor Symp. Quant. Biol.*, **37**, 567–571

25. Huxley, H. E. (1963). Electron microscope studies on the structure of natural and synthetic protein filaments from striated muscle. *J. Mol. Biol.*, **7**, 281–308

26. Ishikawa, H., Bischoff, R. and Holtzer, H. (1969). Formation of arrowhead complexes with heavy meromyosin in a variety of cell types. *J. Cell Biol.*, **43**, 312–328

27. Gabbiani, G., Ryan, G. B., Lamelin, J. P., Vassalli, P., Majno, G., Bouvier, C. A., Cruchaud, A. and Lüschner, E. F. (1973). Human smooth muscle autoantibody. Its identification as antiactin antibody and a study of its bindings to 'non-muscular' cells. *Amer. J. Pathol.*, **72**, 473–488
28. Johnson, G. D., Holborow, E. J. and Glynn, L. E. (1965). Antibody to smooth muscle in patients with liver disease. *Lancet*, **ii**, 878
29. Lazarides, E. and Weber, K. (1974). Actin antibody: the specific visualisation of actin filaments in non-muscle cells. *Proc. Nat. Acad. Sci. (USA)*, **71**, 2268–2272
30. Trenchev, P., Sneyd, P. and Holborow, E. J. (1974). Immunofluorescent tracing of smooth muscle contractile protein antigens in tissue other than smooth muscle. *Clin. Exp. Immunol.*, **16**, 125–136
31. Lengsfeld, A., Löw, I., Wieland, Th., Dancker, P. and Hasselbach, W. (1974). Interaction of phalloidin with actin. *Proc. Nat. Acad. Sci. (USA)*, **71**, 2803–2807
32. Farrow, L. J., Holborow, E. J. and Brighton, W. D. (1971). Reaction of smooth muscle antibody with liver cells. *Nature (London)*, **232**, 186–187
33. Valentine, R. C. and Green, N. M. (1967). Electron microscopy of an antibody-hapten complex. *J. Molec. Biol.*, **27**, 615–617
34. Wagner, R., Rosenberg, M. and Estensen, R. (1971). Endocytosis in Chang liver cell. Quantitation by sucrose-^{3}H uptake and inhibition by cytochalasin B. *J. Cell Biol.*, **50**, 804–817

CHAPTER 17

Interaction of phalloidin with actin

Th. Wieland, A. Schäfer, V. M. Govindan and H. Faulstich

In 1972, in search of the biological receptor molecule of the phallotoxins, microfilamentous structures were detected in liver membrane preparations of poisoned rats. These microfilaments were scattered over or loosely attached to the plasma membrane fragments[1]. The chemical nature of the microfilaments was suspected to be actin; the filaments, however, could not be dissolved in 0.6 M KI, conditions which normally depolymerise filamentous actin and hence are a reliable test for this protein. It took more than a year for the microfilaments to be identified as actin by other methods, and it was then realised that the experiment with KI had failed because the toxic action of phalloidin causes irreversible polymerisation of actin.

As a consequence of the blocked depolymerisation of actin, structural changes in the plasma membrane occur, causing for example the efflux of K^+ ions off the perfused liver and the bulges and protrusions in isolated hepatocytes as shown in the electron microscopic pictures by Frimmer[2]. In our experiments we obtained these protrusions with concentrations as low as 2×10^{-6} M. The effect was antagonised by antamanide, a cyclic decapeptide also isolated from *Amanita* mushrooms[3]. Since antamanide also suppresses the formation of microfilaments by phalloidin in plasma membrane preparations[1], the sensitivity to antamanide of the phalloidin effect on hepatocytes suggests that the protrusions in these cells are a consequence of the formation of the microfilaments by the toxin.

Concerning the identification of the filaments as actin by methods other than the iodide treatment, the first evidence of and consequence was provided by Wieland and co-workers[4] who studied the interaction of actin with cytochalasin B. Cytochalasin B reduced the formation of microfilaments by phalloidin. In a second experiment the phalloidin-induced microfilaments were decorated with heavy meromyosin[4].

When compared to decorated microfilaments of muscle actin, the pictures looked very similar with respect to the characteristic arrow-headed structures on both microfilaments. This gave further evidence that the chemical nature of the microfilaments in hepatocytes is not far from that of muscle actin.

In a third experiment Löw and Wieland[5] studied the action of phalloidin on muscle actin itself. They found that phalloidin also accelerates the polymerisation of the monomeric form of actin obtained from muscles (G-actin), and that also these filaments are resistant to KI-treatment. Interaction of phalloidin with actin in this case was studied by viscosimetry: A solution of G-actin had an outflow time of 32 sec; on addition of KCl polymerisation occurred raising the outflow time to 65 sec.

The effect was reversed on addition of KI (28 sec). The solution of G-actin treated with phalloidin likewise gave an outflow time of 65 sec. On addition of KI, however, the value was only slightly decreased to 58 sec, indicating the blocked depolymerisation. With the non-toxic phalloidin-sulphoxide[6] G-actin was likewise polymerised the outflow time being 60 sec; on addition of KI, however, the time of outflow decreased to 30 sec, indicating that polymerisation in this case was reversed by treatment with KI.

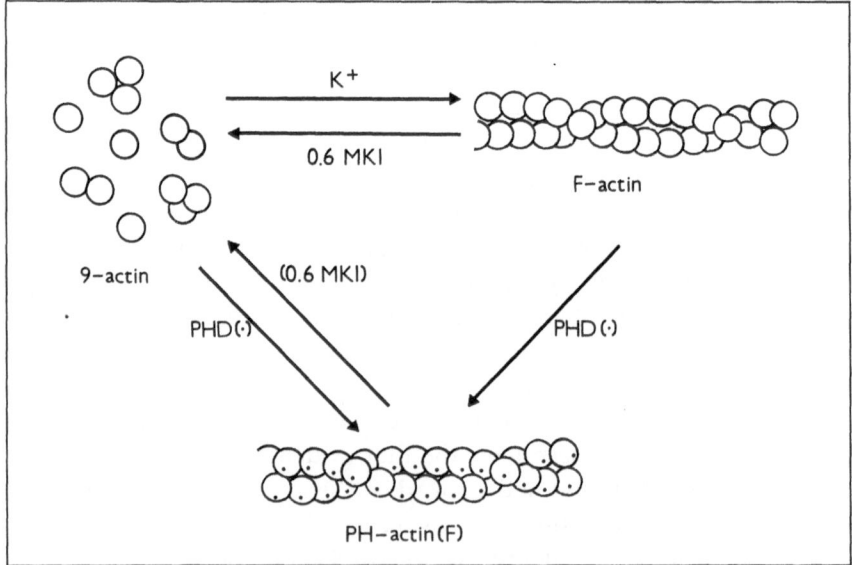

FIGURE 17.1   Proposed mechanism for the action of phalloidin on muscle actin

To summarise the mechanism, as we understand it today: phalloidin accelerates the polymerisation of monomeric or oligomeric units of G-actin to microfilaments (Figure 17.1); likewise phalloidin binds to natural microfilaments like F-actin, induced for example by interaction of K^+-ions and nucleotides. In both cases polymerisation is irreversible, at least to KI treatment. Whether it is that the equilibrium of monomeric and polymeric actin is essential for the liver cells, or that a thorough polymerisation to filaments makes a structural change in the membrane, which causes for example the loss of K^+-ions, it appears reasonable to believe that the polymerisation of actin is the first event in phallotoxin action, which consequently leads to the death of the liver cells in a way still unknown.

These findings open the field for phalloidin as an instrument in the molecular biology of membranes. I want to conclude with two experiments, performed recently in Heidelberg with phallotoxins attached to polymeric supports. Acidic phallotoxins were coupled to dextrane, mol. wt. 500 000, by an hexamethylendiamine spacer (Figure 17.2). The phallotoxin–dextrane derivative was non-toxic in the white mouse. When this compound was introduced into the viscosimetric study of Löw and Wieland, we got a polymerisation effect similar to that achieved when myosin was present in the incubation[5]. The time of outflow was increased to 145 sec and the solution almost became a gel. This effect, however, was reversible on addition of KI, which decreased the outflow time to 38 sec.

We cannot distinguish to date whether the non-toxicity of this compound is due to the reversibility of the polymerisation reaction, as in the

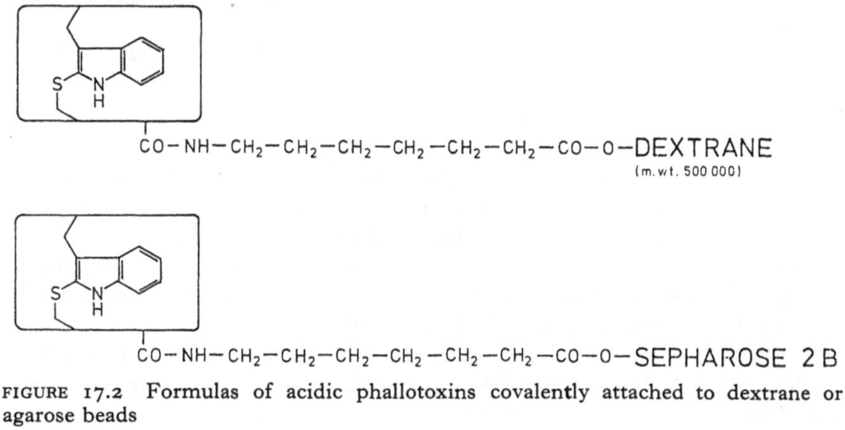

$\overset{|}{C}O-NH-CH_2-CH_2-CH_2-CH_2-CH_2-CH_2-CO-O-\text{DEXTRANE}$
(m.w.t. 500 000)

$\overset{|}{C}O-NH-CH_2-CH_2-CH_2-CH_2-CH_2-CH_2-CO-O-\text{SEPHAROSE 2 B}$

FIGURE 17.2 Formulas of acidic phallotoxins covalently attached to dextrane or agarose beads

case of the non-toxic sulphoxide, or, whether the dextrane coupled phallotoxin does not reach the actin molecules, situated, we assume, at the inner surface of the cell membrane. Nevertheless, the reversible binding of actin to phallotoxin–dextranes encouraged us to try an affinity chromatography on a Sepharose–phallotoxin column. Indeed, when a solution of G-actin was applied to a column of Sepharose-phallotoxins, part of the material was not bound to the column (Figure 17.3), and the main fraction was eluted by 0.6 M KI solution. Further studies must show whether this procedure is useful for the isolation of cell actin in different types of cells.

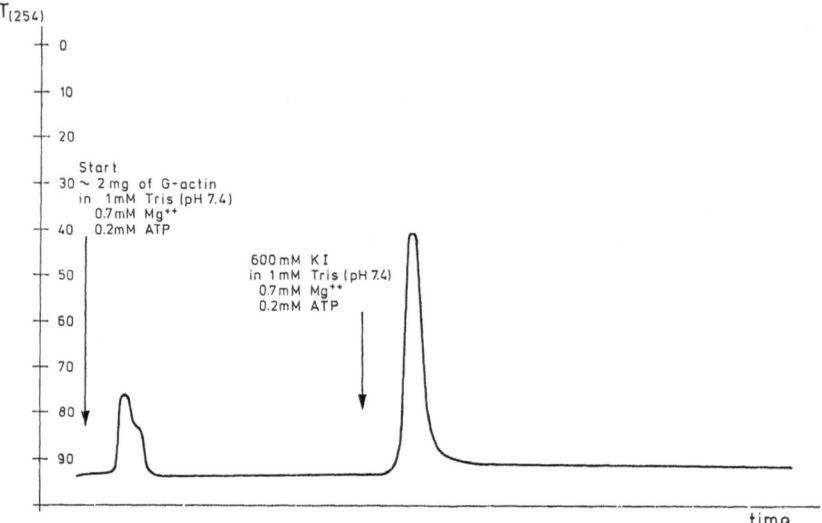

FIGURE 17.3   Elution diagram of muscle G-actin on a column of Sepharose-2B-phallotoxin

REFERENCES

1. Govindan, V. M., Faulstich, H., Wieland, Th., Agostini, B. and Hassel-bach, W. (1972). *In-vitro* effect of phalloidin on a plasma membrane preparation from rat liver. *Naturwissenschaften*, **59**, 521–522
2. Weiss, E., Sterz, I., Frimmer, M. and Kroker, R. (1973). Electron microscopy of isolated rat hepatocytes before and after treatment with phalloidin. *Beitr. Pathol. Anat. Allg. Pathol.*, **150**, 345–356
3. Faulstich, H., Wieland, Th., Walli, A. and Birkmann, K. (1974). Antamanide protects hepatocytes from phalloidin destruction. *Hoppe-Seyler's Z. Physiol. Chem.*, **355**, 1162–1163

4. Lengsfeld, A. M., Löw, J., Wieland, Th., Dancker, P. and Hasselbach, W. (1974). Interaction of phalloidin with actin. *Proc. Nat. Acad. Sci.* (*USA*), **71**, 2803–2807
5. Löw, I. and Wieland, Th. (1974). The interaction of phalloidin, some of its derivatives, and of other cyclic peptides with muscle actin as studied by viscosimetry. *FEBS Letters*, **44**, 340–343
6. Faulstich, H., Wieland, Th. and Jochum, C. (1960). Amanin und die Amanitine sind Sulfoxide. *Liebigs Ann. Chem.*, **713**, 186–195

Mechanism of necrosis induced by hepatotoxic bile acids

H. GREIM, L. SCHWARZ, P. CZYGAN AND H. POPPER

Cholestasis is accompanied by an increase in hepatic bile acid concentration. In the rat after bile duct ligation dihydroxylated chenodeoxycholic acid increases, but trihydroxylated cholic and β-muricholic acids become the major bile acids[1]. β-muricholic acid is formed from chenodeoxycholic acid by 6β-hydroxylation[2]. This reaction is mediated by the non-specific microsomal mixed function oxidase[3] and is thought to prevent accumulation of hepatotoxic chenodeoxycholic acid in the hepatocyte[1].

In human cholestasis no β-muricholic acid is formed and chenodeoxycholic acid as well as cholic acid become the major bile acids[4]. These differences in bile acid metabolism between rat and man result in differing consequences in extrahepatic and intrahepatic cholestasis. Whereas the rat removes chenodeoxycholic acid by 6β-hydroxylation, man tries to remove chenodeoxycholic acid by conjugating reactions such as sulphatation and glucuronidation. The consequences of these differing protective metabolic pathways as well as the mechanisms that result in rat and human cholestasis will now be discussed.

EXTRAHEPATIC BILIARY OBSTRUCTION

EXPERIMENTAL CHOLESTASIS

Hepatotoxicity of chenodeoxycholic acid has been demonstrated by different authors. Fisher and his co-workers showed hepatocellular necrosis after perfusion of isolated rat livers with chenodeoxycholic acid[5]. When we incubated isolated rat liver microsomes with 0.1 mM chenodeoxycholic acid, competitive inhibition of the microsomal drug metabolising enzyme system was observed[6]. Concentration of approximately 0.1 mM of chenodeoxycholic acid was found in rat liver after bile duct ligation[1], explaining observations of prolonged hexobarbital narcosis in rodents after bile duct ligation[7,8]. Furthermore, chenodeoxycholic acid concentrations exceeding 0.3 mM are detergent to microsomal suspensions[6,9]. At this concentration chenodeoxycholic acid inactivates cytochrome P_{450}, the terminal oxidase of the microsomal enzyme system, forming inactive cytochrome P_{420}. Additionally, other microsomal membrane components are solubilised such as cytochrome b-5 and NADPH cytochrome P_{450} reductase, that is required for NADPH-mediated cytochrome P_{450} reduction[10].

However, in cholestatic rat livers chenodeoxycholic acid levels do not exceed 0.1 mM (Figure 18.1) because of a sufficiently active 6β-hydroxylase forming non-toxic β-muricholic acid[1]. That is why hepatocellular necrosis is hardly ever seen in the rat after bile duct ligation[11].

EXTRAHEPATIC CHOLESTASIS IN MAN

Human liver however does not hydroxylate chenodeoxycholic acid at the 6β-position. Consequently this bile acid accumulates in cholestatic

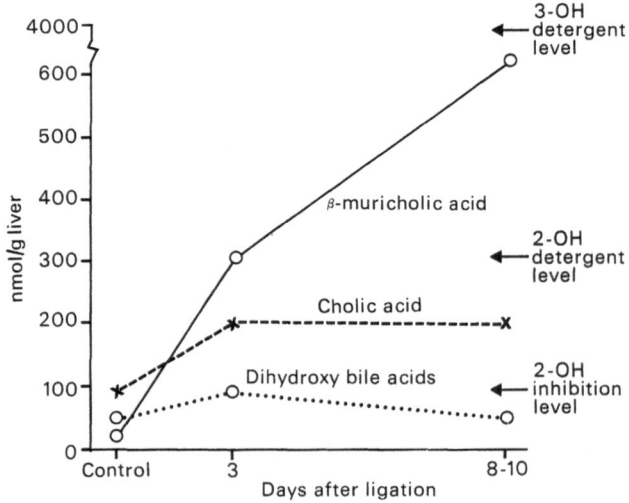

FIGURE 18.1   Alterations in hepatic bile acid concentrations after bile duct ligation in 200 g male Sprague–Dawley rats

diseases[4] (Table 18.1). In short-term cholestasis, sulphatation[12,13] and glucuronidation[14] may prevent accumulation of this bile acid. Both conjugating reactions form highly water soluble derivatives that can be excreted in the urine. Furthermore, sulphate esters seem to be less detergent than the original glycine or taurine conjugate of the bile acids and consequently are less hepatotoxic. Stiehl and Czygan recently showed no solubilising effect of lithocholic sulphates in microsomal preparations, whereas free lithocholic acid or its glycine or taurine conjugates affected drug metabolising enzymes[15]. These data support the observations of Fisher and his co-workers who demonstrated reduced cholestatic effect of lithocholic acid sulphates in the isolated

Table 18.1 CONCENTRATION OF BILE SALTS IN HUMAN LIVER (NMOL/G TISSUE MEAN ± SD)

Diagnosis	Weeks of jaundice	Serum bilirubin mg%	Deoxy-cholic acid	Cheno-deoxycholic acid	Cholic acid
			nmol/g ± SD		
Normal (7)	0	< 1.0	13 ± 7	20 ± 6	38 ± 14
Sclerosing cholangitis	7	27	10	28	218
Pancreas Ca	4	20	22	68	515
Sclerosing cholangitis	10	12	Trace*	190	280
Bile duct Ca	10	35	Trace*	162	580
Bile duct Ca	13	20	Trace*	380	660
Bile duct Ca	36	22	Trace*	380	315

* Present in less than 5 nmol/g liver

perfused rat liver[16]. Glucuronidation of the bile acids may also reduce hepatotoxicity but no data are available at the present time.

In prolonged cholestasis however protective formation of sulphate or glucuronide derivatives seem to be surpassed by an increased formation of chenodeoxycholic acid. Consequently high levels of this bile acid can be found in the livers of such patients[4] (Table 18.1). Concentrations exceed levels of 0.1 mM where competitive inhibition of drug metabolising enzymes can be seen *in vitro*[6]. In some cases even detergent levels exceeding 0.3 mM could be observed.

Correlation between such high levels of dihydroxylated bile acids— mainly chenodeoxycholic acid—and liver cell necrosis as indicated by feathery degeneration (Figure 18.2) strongly suggest detergent capability of elevated concentrations of dihydroxylated bile acids in cholestatic livers.

These observations still support the concept that increased levels of hepatic bile acids are responsible for most of the functional and morphological changes in the cholestatic liver[17]: inhibition of microsomal mixed function oxidase-mediated enzyme reactions at levels of 0.1 mM and destruction of structural components and enzyme activities at concentrations exceeding this level.

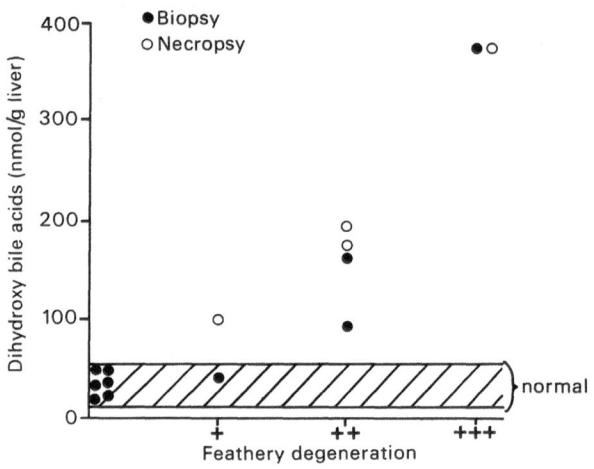

FIGURE 18.2   Correlation between the extent of feathery degeneration and concentration of dihydroxylated bile acids in human liver during cholestasis

INTRAHEPATIC CHOLESTASIS

In livers of patients with intrahepatic cholestasis similar patterns of bile acids are found[18]. Accordingly, similar consequences due to the increased bile acid concentrations can be expected in intrahepatic as in extrahepatic cholestasis. However, different preconditions result in these consequences: impaired bile flow in extrahepatic biliary obstruction and interaction of an hepatotoxic drug with cellular function in the case of intrahepatic cholestasis.

The initiating mechanism finally resulting in elevated bile acid levels in intrahepatic cholestasis is still not known. A few observations however may provide some arguments in favour of factors possibly involved in the initiation of intrahepatic cholestasis.

INTERFERENCE OF DRUGS WITH BILE ACID METABOLISM

Because of the close relationship between drug metabolism and bile acid hydroxylation reactions, one initiating step to intrahepatic cholestasis may be an interference of cholestatic drugs with bile acid metabolism. Most of the bile acid hydroxylation reactions are mediated by the non-specific microsomal P_{450} dependent drug metabolising enzyme system[19]. Since many drugs being metabolised by these enzymes interfere with each others metabolism[20], similar interference should occur between cholestatic drugs and bile acid hydroxylation, possibly resulting in increased hepatic bile acid levels by impaired metabolism.

To test whether cholestatic drugs interact with the non-specific enzyme system, the capacity of several of these compounds to inhibit aminopyrine demethylation—a typical substrate of the mixed function oxidase—was tested.

Rat or mouse liver microsomes were incubated at different concentrations of aminopyrine ranging from 0.1 to 10 mM to obtain kinetic data without the presence of an inhibitor. Turnover of the reactions was plotted against substrate concentrations according to Lineweaver-Burk. K_M of the aminopyrine demethylation is about 1 mM, V_{max} approximately 5 nmol/min × mg protein. Addition of cholestatic agents such as ANIT* in concentrations of 0.2 mM competitively inhibit aminopyrine demethylation[21] as well as addition of 1 mM norethandrolone. Similar effects were seen with 0.1 mM each of methyltestosterone or ethyltestosterone (Figure 18.3), and less markedly with chlorpromazine or tetracycline. When kinetics of a bile acid hydroxylation was determined in the presence of 0.05 mM methyltestosterone, a similar competition of the metabolism of taurodeoxycholate was observed (Figure 18.4). Ethyltestosterone had the same effect on the kinetics of this bile acid. This strongly suggests impairment of bile acid metabolism by cholestatic drugs possibly initiating elevation of hepatotoxic bile acids. To finally prove this assumption, other hydroxylation reactions have to be studied, especially that of the 12α-hydroxylation of the 7α-hydroxylated 3-keto derivative of cholesterol[22]. 12α-hydroxylation of this bile acid precursor determines whether chenodeoxycholic acid or cholic acid is

* α-naphthylisothiocyanate.

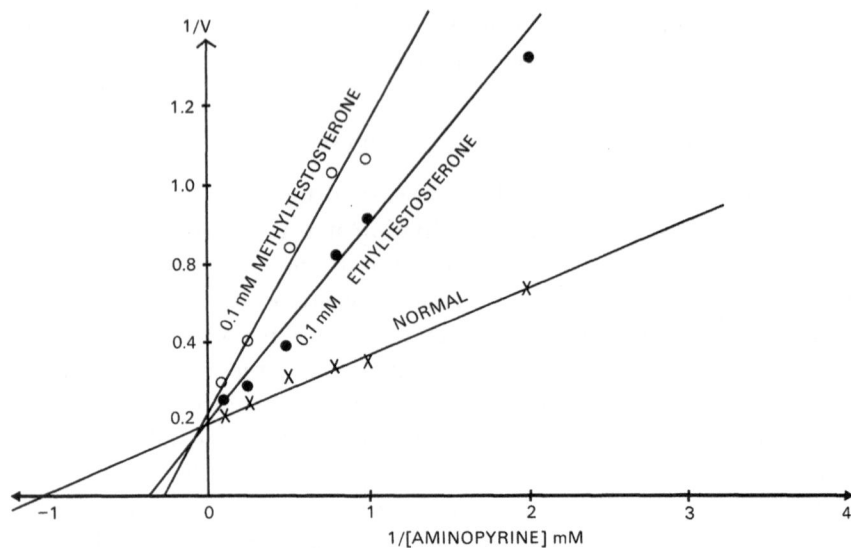

FIGURE 18.3   *In vitro* inhibition of microsomal aminopyrine demethylation by ethyl-testosterone and methyltestosterone. The incubation mixture contained in a final volume of 2 ml, 6 mg microsomal protein, isolated from the livers of non-treated rats, 5 mM $MgSO_4$, 0.66 mM $NADP^+$-Na_2, 16 mM DL-isocitrate-Na_3 and 400 mU isocitrate-dehydrogenase in 0.1 M phosphate buffer (pH 7.4) and was incubated for 6 min at 37 °C

formed[23]. Inhibition of this reaction would increase formation of cheno-deoxycholic acid. Unfortunately this reaction is difficult to measure and no kinetic data are available at the present time. However, Danielsson has some evidence that a 12α-hydroxylation is reduced in experimental rat cholestasis after bile duct ligation[24].

INTERFERENCE OF DRUGS WITH MEMBRANE FUNCTION

Another drug-induced mechanism that initiates intrahepatic cholestasis may be a direct interaction of the drugs with hepatocellular membrane function. Presently we try to evaluate this possible mechanism with isolated rat liver cells, separated by hyaluronidase and collagenase perfusion of the liver. The resulting cells are normal in regard of oxygen consumption, sodium–potassium distribution, lactate dehydrogenase permeability and trypan blue permeability of the cell membranes.

Incubation of the cells with ANIT or the sulphonylureas chlorpropamide and tolbutamide, affected membrane function at high concentra-

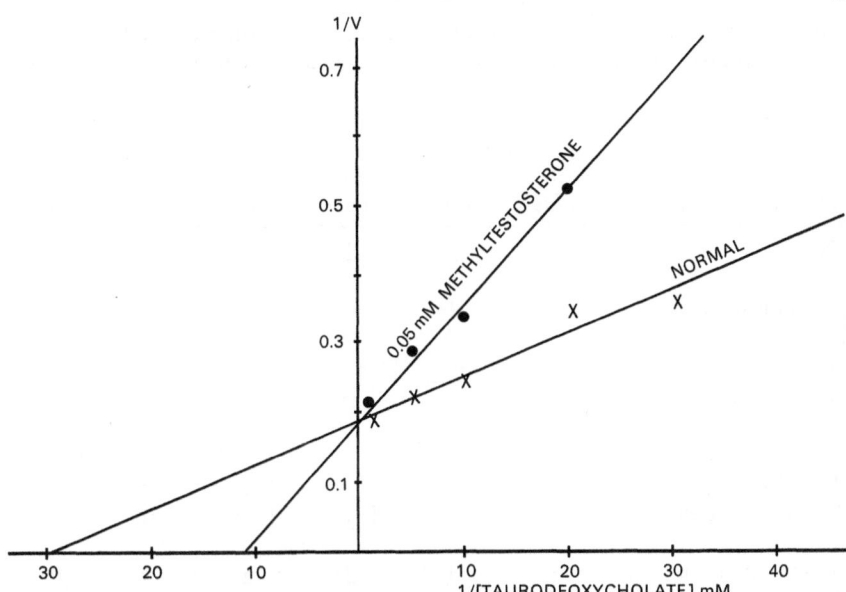

FIGURE 18.4 *In vitro* inhibition of microsomal 7α-hydroxylation of taurodeoxycholic acid. In a final volume of 1 ml the incubate contained 3.3 mg microsomal protein, isolated from rats pretreated with 0.1% phenobarbital in the drinking water for 7 days, and an NADPH-generating system as described in the legend of Figure 18.1. The reaction was terminated after 20 min incubation at 37 °C and the bile acids were extracted with methanol and quantitatively determined by gas-liquid chromatography as trifluoroacetylated derivatives

tions only (Table 18.2). The four antibiotics, being hepatotoxic by inhibition of protein synthesis, had no effect. By contrast, exposure to steroids at concentrations as low as 0.5 mM induced trypan blue staining as well as marked protrusions. These cells have one to four bulges surrounded by a thin membrane. The cell volume is increased almost twofold.

Trypan blue staining is a generally accepted criterion for impaired membrane function. Formation of bulges may be due to an interaction of the drug with the outer layer of the cell surface resulting in a protrusion of the inner membrane. Increased permeability of the latter to inorganic and organic ions and water may aggravate this process. These preliminary results have to be substantiated, determining uptake and release of bile acids by the cells exposed to cholestatic drugs. However, they strongly indicate direct interaction of such drugs with membrane function of the hepatocyte.

Table 18.2 ABILITY OF CHOLESTATIC DRUGS TO INDUCE TRYPAN BLUE
STAINING (BLUE) AND MEMBRANE PROTRUSIONS (PROT) IN ISOLATED RAT LIVER
CELLS

Drug concentration	2 mM		1 mM		0.5 mM	
	blue	*prot*	*blue*	*prot*	*blue*	*prot*
ANIT	+	+++	±	−	−	−
Chloramphenicol	−	±	−	−	−	−
Erythromycin	−	−	−	−	−	−
Griseofulvin	−	−	−	−	−	−
Tetracycline	−	−	−	−	−	−
Ethyltestosterone			++	+++	+	+++
Methyltestosterone			++	+++	±	±
Norethandrolone			+++	+++	+	+
Chlorpropamide	+	+++	±	±	−	−
Tolbutamide	±	±	−	−	−	−

The cause of intracellular accumulation of bile acids due to impaired
membrane function is not known at the present time. Non-limited
regurgitation as well as impaired secretion may account for this consequence of drug-induced intrahepatic cholestasis.

CONCLUSION

There is no doubt that increased bile acid levels are the consequences of
extrahepatic as well as of intrahepatic cholestasis. They affect liver
function by competitive inhibition of microsomal enzymes and by
detergent effects resulting in the hypoactive endoplasmic reticulum.
This impairs metabolism of exogenous compounds such as drugs and
of endogenous substrates such as steroids including bile acids, finally
resulting in hepatocellular necrosis. Protective mechanisms such as
sulphatation and glucuronidation do not seem to be sufficient in removing hepatotoxic bile acids during severe cholestasis. In extrahepatic
obstruction, impaired bile flow induces cholestasis by an elevation of
intrahepatic bile acid levels. In intrahepatic cholestasis either impaired
bile acid metabolism due to competitive inhibition of bile acid hydroxy-

lation reactions may be the initiating step or a direct interaction of such drugs with hepatocellular membrane function. Both factors may be capable of inducing changes in the patterns and distribution of intra-hepatic bile acid levels.

REFERENCES

1. Greim, H., Trülzsch, D., Roboz, J., Dressler, K., Czygan, P., Hutterer, F., Schaffner, F. and Popper, H. (1972). Mechanism of cholestasis. 5. Bile acids in normal rat livers and in those after bile duct ligation. *Gastroenterology*, **63**, 837–845
2. Samuelsson, B. (1959). On the metabolism of chenodeoxycholic acid in the rat. Bile acids and steroids 85. *Acta Chem. Scand.*, **13**, 976–983
3. Voigt, W., Hsia, S. L., Cooper, D. Y. and Rosenthal, O. (1968). Photo-reactivation spectrum of the CO-inhibited taurochenodeoxycholate 6β-hydroxylase system. *FEBS Letters*, **2**, 124–126
4. Greim, H., Trülzsch, D., Czygan, P., Rudick, J., Hutterer, F., Schaffner, F. and Popper, H. (1972). Mechanism of cholestasis. 6. Bile acids in human livers with or without biliary obstruction. *Gastroenterology*, **63**, 846–850
5. Fisher, M. M. and Yousef, I. M. (1971). Sex dependent differences in the bile acids of rats. *Fed. Proc.*, **30**, 582 (Abstr.)
6. Hutterer, F., Denk, H., Bacchin, P. G., Schenkman, J. B., Schaffner, F. and Popper, H. (1970). Mechanism of cholestasis. 1. Effect of bile acids on microsomal cytochrome P-450 dependent biotransformation system *in vitro*. *Life Sci.*, **9**, 877–887
7. McLuen, E. F. and Fouts, J. R. (1961). The effect of obstructive jaundice on drug metabolism in rabbits. *J. Pharmacol. Exp. Ther.*, **131**, 7–11
8. Becker, B. A. and Plaa, G. L. (1965). The nature of α-naphthylisothio-cyanate-induced cholestasis. *Toxicol. Appl. Pharmacol.*, **7**, 680–685
9. Hutterer, F., Bacchin, P. G., Denk, H., Schenkman, J. B., Schaffner, F. and Popper, H. (1970). Mechanism of cholestasis. 2. Effect of bile acids on the microsomal electron transfer system *in vitro*. *Life Sci.*, **9**, 1159–1166
10. Hutterer, F., Greim, H., Trülzsch, D., Czygan, P. and Schenkman, J. B. (1972). Microsomal biotransformation system in cholestasis. In: *Progress in Liver Diseases*, **Vol. IV** (H. Popper and F. Schaffner, editors) (New York: Grune and Stratton)
11. Popper, H. and Schaffner, F. (1970). Pathophysiology of cholestasis. *Human Pathol.*, **1**, 1–24
12. Palmer, R. H. (1967). The formation of bile acid sulfates: A new pathway of bile acid metabolism in humans. *Proc. Nat. Acad. Sci. (USA)*, **58**, 1047–1052
13. Stiehl, A. (1974). Bile salt sulphates in cholestasis. *Eur. J. Clin. Invest.*, **4**, 59–64

14. Fröhling, W. and Stiehl, A. (1974). Bile salt glucuronides in man. Identification and quantitative analysis. *Digestion*, **10**, 318
15. Czygan, P. and Stiehl, A. (1975). Untersuchungen zur Toxizität sulfatierter und nicht sulfatierter Lithocholsäure. *Zschr. Gastroenterologie* (in press)
16. Fisher, M. M., Magnussen, R. and Miyai, K. (1971). Bile acid metabolism in mammals. I. Bile acid-induced intrahepatic cholestasis. *Lab. Invest.*, **21**, 88–91
17. Schaffner, F. and Popper, H. (1969). Hypothesis: Cholestasis is the result of hypoactive hypertrophic endoplasmic reticulum in the hepatocyte. *Lancet*, **ii**, 355–359
18. Greim, H. and Czygan, P. (1974). Gallensäuren in der Leber und im Serum bei verschiedenen Lebererkrankungen. *Verh. Dtsch. Ges. Inn. Med.* (in press)
19. Greim, H., Trülzsch, D., Czygan, P., Hutterer, F., Schaffner, F., Popper, H., Cooper, D. Y. and Rosenthal, O. (1973). Bile acid formation by liver microsomal enzymes. *Ann. N.Y. Acad. Sci.*, **212**, 139–147
20. Rubin, A., Tephly, T. R. and Mannering, G. J. (1964). Kinetics of drug metabolism by hepatic microsomes. *Biochem. Pharmacol.*, **13**, 1007–1016
21. Czygan, P., Greim, H., Hutterer, F., Schaffner, F. and Popper, H. (1974). Comparison of two types of intrahepatic jaundice in rats with bile duct ligation. *Acta Hepato-Gastroenterol.*, **681**, 339–345
22. Berséus, O., Danielsson, H. and Einarsson, K. (1967). Synthesis and metabolism of cholest-5-ene-3 beta, 7 alpha, 12 alpha-triol. *J. Biol. Chem.*, **242**, 1211–1215
23. Mitropoulos, K. A. and Myant, N. B. (1967). The formation of lithocholic acid, chenodeoxycholic acid and α- and β-muricholic acids from cholesterol incubated with rat-liver mitochondria. *Biochem. J.*, **103**, 472–479
24. Danielsson, H., personal communication

CHAPTER 19

The role of lipid peroxidation in liver injury

T. F. SLATER

INTRODUCTION

The peroxidative degradation of polyunsaturated fatty acids (I) involves (a) an initiating reaction leading to the formation of polyunsaturated fatty acid free radical (II); (b) subsequent reaction of II with oxygen to yield a peroxy radical (III); (c) reaction of III with another molecule of I to produce a hydroperoxide (IV) and a further molecule of II that can repeat the reaction with O_2 as already described; (d) a variety of other reactions leading to the breakdown of the polyunsaturated fatty acid molecules, and chain terminations that inhibit the overall process of lipid peroxidation (for review see Tappel[1]). A simplified scheme showing initiation and propagation reactions is given in Figure 19.1.

The peroxidative degradation of polyunsaturated fatty acids (PUFA) outlined above may result in severe disruption of the normal, highly organised structure of lipid-rich biomembranes with associated disturbances to many important metabolic processes. Lipid peroxidation of biomembranes may also involve peroxidative changes in membrane components other than PUFA, in cholesterol for example.

An increased rate of lipid peroxidation has been implicated[2-5] (with varying amounts of experimental evidence to support such contentions) in many types of cellular injury: for example in the liver disturbances following exposure to CCl_4, ethyl alcohol, hydrazine, white phosphorus, orotic acid, iron overload; and in other types of tissue damage produced by exposure to ozone, nitrogen dioxide, high oxygen pressures, irradiation and so on. It is of some considerable importance therefore to understand more about the underlying mechanisms that are involved in lipid peroxidation, and to assess critically the significance of lipid peroxidation

Initiation

(i) $PUFA(H) + R \cdot \longrightarrow PUFA \cdot + RH$

Propagation

(ii) $PUFA \cdot + O_2 \longrightarrow PUFAO_2 \cdot$

(iii) $PUFAO_2 \cdot + PUFA(H) \longrightarrow PUFAO_2H + PUFA \cdot$

Chain termination

(iv) $2PUFA \cdot$

(v) $2R \cdot$

(vi) $PUFA \cdot + PUFAO_2 \cdot$

(vii) $2PUFAO_2 \cdot$ $\longrightarrow$ non-initiating or

(viii) $PUFA \cdot + S$ non-propagating products

(ix) $PUFAO_2 \cdot + S$

(x) $R \cdot + S$

FIGURE 19.1   A simplified scheme indicating the main events in lipid peroxidation of polyunsaturated fatty acids [PUFA(H)]. In (i) the initiating event results in the forma-tion of the PUFA· radical that can interact with oxygen as in (ii); reaction with a second PUFA(H) in (iii) results in the formation of a new PUFA· radical thereby propagating the chain reaction. The chain reaction may be terminated in a variety of ways as indicated in (iv)–(x). S is a free radical scavenger molecule

in relationship to cell injury. In discussing the role of lipid peroxidation in tissue injury I shall restrict my remarks to peroxidative damage to liver endoplasmic reticulum but, in fact, much of my discussion will have more general applicability. There are four fundamental questions that I wish to consider:

(i) Can the rate of lipid peroxidation be stimulated in liver endo-plasmic reticulum under conditions *in vivo* in various types of liver intoxication?

(ii) If so, what types of initiation mechanisms are involved?

(iii) Is the resultant lipid peroxidation damaging to cell components?

(iv) Is the stimulation of lipid peroxidation of major significance to the onset and development of the various types of liver injury that I shall discuss?

If much of what is discussed here appears to have little *direct* relation-ship to the end results of cell injury as observed by the pathologist—fatty liver, necrosis, cirrhosis etc.—this does not mean that the reactions to be outlined are irrelevant to our general aims. I believe it important that we should try to deduce the chemical mechanisms underlying tissue injury, to take the numerous question marks out of our speculative schemes that are designed to show how tissue injuries develop from primary metabolic disturbances, and this has led me over the last few years to the study of the chemical behaviour of transient metabolic intermediates. What I hope to demonstrate in this article is that by using the techniques of fast reaction kinetics we may be able to make rational decisions as to the significance of key metabolic disturbances as opposed simply to a demonstration that they may or may not occur. The four questions listed above will now be discussed in turn.

(i) $\underline{PUFA(H)} + R\cdot \longrightarrow PUFA\cdot + RH$
(ii) $\overline{PUFA\cdot + O_2} \longrightarrow PUFAO_2\cdot$
(iii) $PUFAO_2\cdot + PUFA(H) \longrightarrow \underline{PUFAO_2H} + PUFA\cdot$
(iv) $PUFAO_2\cdot \longrightarrow \underline{diene\ conjugation}$
(v) $PUFAO_2\cdot \longrightarrow \underline{aldehydes,\ hydroxy\text{-}alkenals,\ ethane}$

FIGURE 19.2   The main reactions involved in the initiation and propagation of lipid peroxidation are shown to indicate the components of the complex series of reactions that have been used to follow the course of the reactions involved. Components that have been so measured are shown underlined: (i) destruction of PUFA(H); (ii) utilisation of O_2; (iii) production of hydroperoxide; (iv) appearance of a conjugated diene bond; (v) formation of aldehyde products (generally malonaldehyde is measured), and the formation of ethane [29]

CAN THE RATE OF LIPID PEROXIDATION BE INCREASED *IN VIVO?*

The short answer here is an unequivocal yes! A variety of experimental techniques may be used to follow the course of lipid peroxidation under conditions *in vitro* and *in vivo*; these techniques are outlined in Figure 19.2. The major parameters used to show changes in lipid peroxidation under conditions *in vivo* have been the decreased content of PUFA[6], the increased level of hydroperoxide[7], the increase in diene conjugation[8], and the production of malonaldehyde and malonaldehyde-like materials[9].

Early attempts to demonstrate increased malonaldehyde production *in vivo* were largely defeated by the rapid metabolism of malonaldehyde by mitochondria. However, by rapidly extracting liver samples with acid, the changes in liver malonaldehyde content following exposure to CCl_4 can be demonstrated. The time course of such changes and the relative stimulations caused by CCl_4, $CHCl_5$ and $CBrCl_3$, are very similar to those found using the diene conjugation technique. Some data for malonaldehyde changes are shown in Figure 19.3 to illustrate the above points.

WHAT SITES OF INITIATION ARE INVOLVED FOR LIPID PEROXIDATION IN LIVER ENDOPLASMIC RETICULUM?

In attempting to answer this apparently simple question we run into major experimental difficulties in that the initiation process in liver microsomes appears generally to involve the interaction of PUFA with a free radical moiety of high chemical reactivity. As a result of this

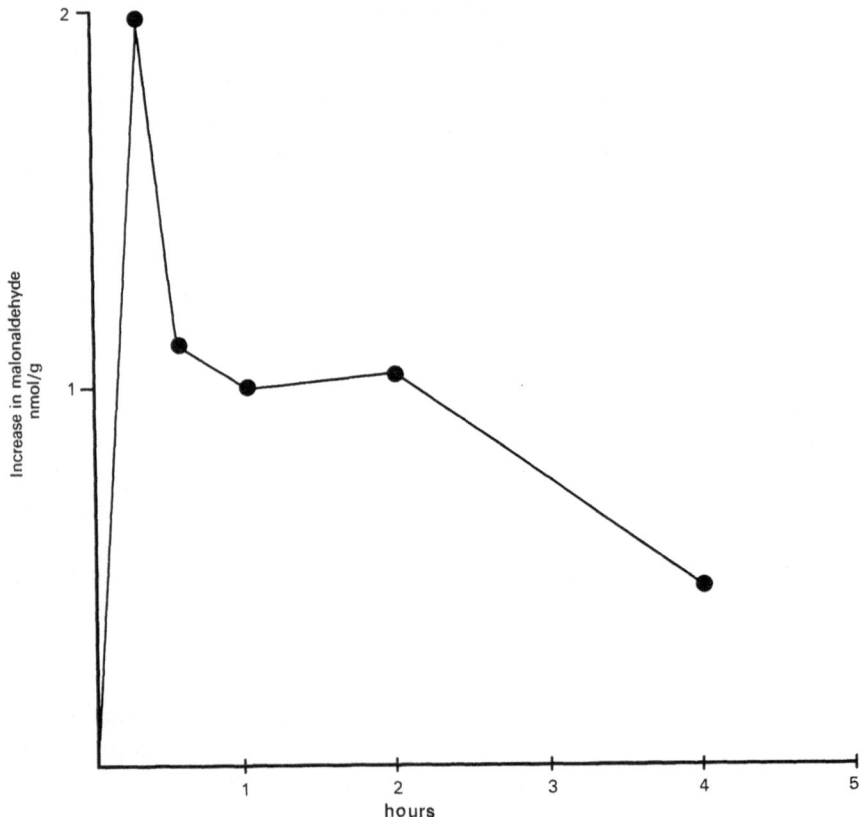

FIGURE 19.3   The concentration of malonaldehyde in female rat liver at various times after dosing with 2.5 ml CCl_4/kg body wt. The method used is that described by Jose and Slater[10] and the data shown are unpublished data of the author and P. J. Jose.

intrinsically high reactivity, the initiating species has only a transient existence often in the range 10^{-3}–10^{-6} sec. Moreover, the most probable types of initiating species in liver endoplasmic reticulum may undergo rapid interconversions and interactions so that any meaningful discussion of the mechanism of lipid peroxidation, that is other than in a chemically trivial and naive way, has to deal with events that occur in very short time periods. Such studies, of course, appear to be far detached from the changes seen by the pathologist in his tissue sections, but nonetheless they are of key importance when we come to consider the primary reactions involved in tissue injury.

The types of experimental approach that we are using in analysing such fast reactions include stopped flow spectrophotometry in the millisecond range, and pulse radiolysis in the microsecond range. I can illustrate our studies by briefly describing the reaction between the trichloromethyl radical $CCl_3^{\cdot}$ and the reducing free radical scavenger Promethazine (or Phenergan). It has been known for a long time that Promethazine can attenuate some of the damaging reactions of CCl_4 on the liver, particularly those reactions that are related to the stimulatory action of CCl_4 on lipid peroxidation[11]. It appeared probable that Promethazine exerted this protective action by scavenging $CCl_3^{\cdot}$; a direct analysis of this reaction using pulse radiolysis was therefore of some interest.

A diagrammatic representation of the principle of pulse radiolysis is shown in Figure 19.4. The short pulse of high energy electrons generates free radicals in the sample cuvette (the radical species that predominate such as the hydrated electron e_{aq}^{-} depend on the experimental conditions used in the cuvette). Provided that there is a measurable change in the light absorption spectrum during the course of the reaction then the interaction of the generated radicals with the molecular species under study can be followed as a function of time at a selected wavelength of incident light (or, if necessary, by the change in some other parameter such as conductivity). By repeating the experiment at different wavelengths of incident light the absorption spectrum of the reaction products may be obtained under suitable circumstances. In collaboration with Dr R. L. Willson the following reactions were studied:

(a) $e_{aq}^{-} + CCl_4 \longrightarrow CCl_3^{\cdot} + Cl^{-}$

(b) $CCl_3^{\cdot} + \text{Promethazine} \rightarrow CCl_3^{-} + \text{Promethazine}^{+\cdot}$

(c) $2 \text{ Promethazine} + S_2O_8{}^{2-} \longrightarrow 2 \text{ Promethazine}^{+\cdot} + 2SO_4{}^{3-}$

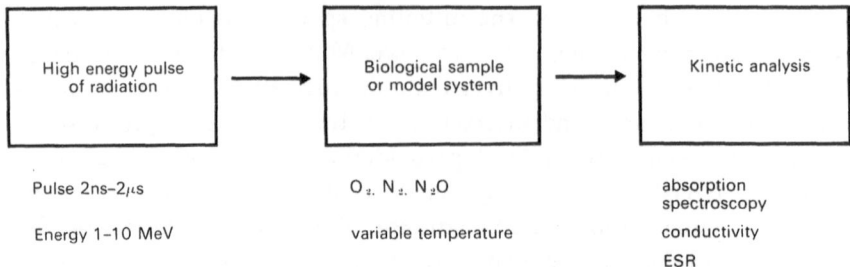

Pulse 2ns–2μs	O_2, N_2, N_2O	absorption spectroscopy
Energy 1–10 MeV	variable temperature	conductivity
		ESR

FIGURE 19.4   A much simplified and diagrammatic representation of the technique of pulse radiolysis using a linear accelerator. A short pulse (generally of duration 2 ns–2 μs) of high energy (1–10 MeV) is delivered to the sample, which in biological studies in generally in aqueous solution. The radical species so generated may be modified by including or excluding in the sample mixture components such as O_2, N_2, nitrous oxide, isopropanol etc. The reactions of the primary radical products with the biolmolecules under study can be followed using techniques such as absorption spectroscopy, conductivity, polarography or electron spin resonance. For details of the procedures used see Ref. 30

Reaction (b) was found to be very fast, with a rate constant of 10^9 M^{-1} s^{-1}. The absorption spectra of the Promethazine$^{+\cdot}$ species formed in (b) and (c) were identical[12]. It was thereby demonstrated by direct kinetic spectroscopy that Promethazine efficiently scavenges CCl_3^- by reaction (b) above.

In considering what initiation mechanisms for lipid peroxidation operate in liver microsomes we are faced with an apparent paradox at the outset. The primary reaction in PUFA initiation is one of oxidation:

$$PUFA\ (H) + R^\cdot \rightarrow PUFA^\cdot + RH$$

By contrast the microsomal NADPH-P_{450} chain is primarily a reductive pathway concerned with electron flow. It may be concluded that the PUFA initiation stage must involve a component R that becomes further reduced:

$$(NADPH - P_{450}) + e^- \longrightarrow R_{reduced} \xrightarrow{PUFA(H)} R_{reduced}^{-\cdot} + PUFA^\cdot + H^+$$

There is of course no objection to R being a *component* of the NADPH-P_{450} chain rather than a side-product as long as it is re-oxidisable to allow repetition of the initiating event. However, if R is indeed a component of the chain, and thereby largely immobilised within the membrane plane, the initiation process would be diffusion controlled through the migration to R of the PUFA molecules. From such considerations I feel it more probable for R to be side-product formed from the $NADPH\text{-}P_{450}$ sequence, which is itself readily diffusible away from its site of formation.

Reductive electron flow from the $NADPH\text{-}P_{450}$ chain can be considered to occur at several loci; possible exit points being the flavine enzyme, thiol and non-haem iron groups, as well as P_{450}. Such reductive electron flow from the $NADPH\text{-}P_{450}$ chain can interact with neighbouring molecules such as oxygen which can then diffuse away before entering into other reactions. The trapping of the electron flow by oxygen is only one way in which the reductive flow can be directed and Figure 19.5 illustrates the overall complexity that may result at just one exit site of the $NADPH\text{-}P_{450}$ chain, that is the flavoprotein region. The

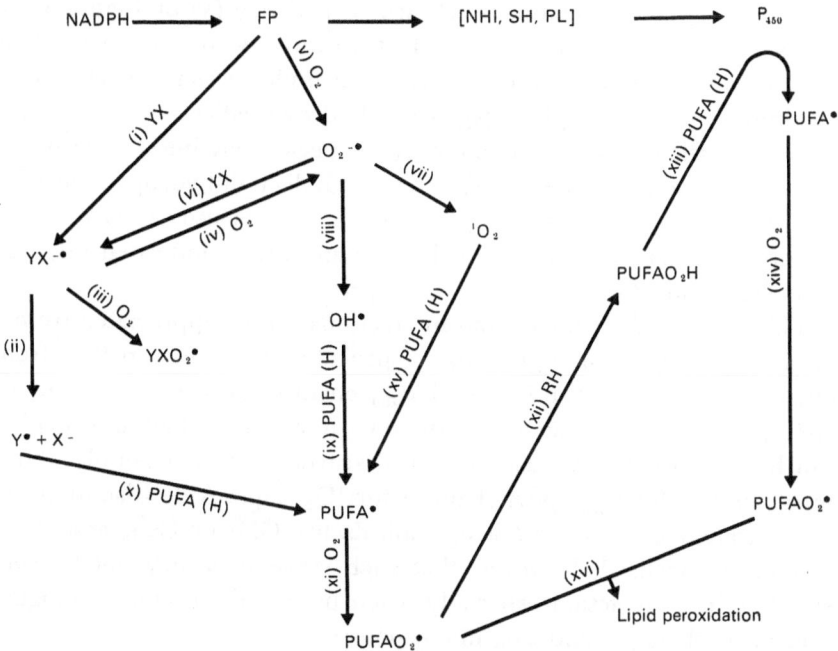

FIGURE 19.5 A diagrammatic scheme to indicate the complexity of possible electron flow from one component of the $NADPH\text{-}P_{450}$ electron transport chain. Only flow from the NADPH-flavoprotein is indicated but similar outflows can be expected from other and more distal sites along the chain. In (i) component YX accepts an electron to form the anion radical $YX^{-\cdot}$; this may undergo bond scission as in (ii) or react with oxygen to give a peroxy radical (iii) or superoxide (iv). Oxygen itself may be reduced to superoxide (v) and this may reduce YX as in (vi) or form singlet O_2 (vii)[14] or $OH^{\cdot}$ (viii)[15]. The hydroxyl radical or $Y^{\cdot}$ may initiate lipid peroxidation as in (ix) and (x) which can go to the hydroperoxide (xi) and (xii); the hydroperoxide itself may initiate further lipid peroxidation processes through reaction with P_{450} acting as a peroxidase (xiii) and (xiv)[16]

discussion that follows for this site could equally well be applied in general terms to other exit sites from the microsomal electron transport chain. The flavoprotein may feed electrons directly to some acceptor (i)YX which for example could be cytochrome c, or a nitroimidazole, or CCl_4. The end results in these three examples would be:

(a) $e^- + $ ferri-cytochrome $\longrightarrow$ ferrocytochrome c
(b) $e^- + $ nitroimidazole $\longrightarrow$ nitroimidazole$^{-\cdot}$
(c) $e^- + CCl_4 \longrightarrow CCl_3^{\cdot} + Cl^-$

Compounds formed as in (b) may then react quickly with O_2 thereby regaining their original oxidised state and forming the superoxide anion radical, $O_2^-\cdot$ Free radicals formed as in (c) may be sufficiently reactive to initiate lipid peroxidation as shown in pathway (x) of Figure 19.5. The superoxide radical $O_2^-\cdot$ may be formed directly from a flavoprotein interaction[13] and this may be transformed under certain experimental conditions either to singlet oxygen[14] or hydroxy radicals, a particularly strong oxidising species[15]. These oxygen species may initiate peroxidation as indicated in pathway (ix). The metabolism of hydroperoxides by a peroxidatic reaction involving cytochrome P_{450} is also associated with initiating events and lipid peroxidation[16] and this is indicated in pathways (viii) and (xiv).

The complexity of the overall interactions can be appreciated from a brief consideration of Figure 19.5 especially when electron flow from other components of the NADPH-P_{450} chain is taken into account. In attempting to analyse such interactions, much important information can be obtained by the use of radical scavengers: for example, tetranitromethane for e^-_{aq} diphenyl furan for $^1O_2$, superoxide dismutase for $O_2^-\cdot$, Promethazine for oxidising radicals like $OH\cdot$ or $CCl_3^{\cdot}$ and so on It must be realised, however, that such scavengers may not be very selective in their action especially when used with complex biological systems such as peroxidising microsomes.

Because there are various electron flow possibilities in a system as complex as liver microsomes it can be realised that if we dam up one route we can force the reductive flow into new and often unusual directions. As a consequence it is necessary to be very careful, when distorting the experimental conditions, that one is not consequently studying a quite abnormal pathway. Obvious causes for concern here are where the oxygen tension is changed in anaerobic experiments, or where electron flow *along* rather than *away* from the chain is blocked. The effect of oxygen tension on the major routes for chain termination in olefin oxidation are discussed by Bateman[17] and illustrate the overall point being made about the influence of experimental conditions on the types of reaction being considered here. The use of metabolic inhibitors to decide whether a competition for electron flow exists between drug metabolism at P_{450} and lipid peroxidation also requires careful interpretation. Some substrates for P_{450} metabolism, and also a variety of products of such metabolism, are quite strong free radical scavengers and can interfere with lipid peroxidation directly thereby making suspect any simple interpretation as to the mechanism of these inhibitory effects.

So far in this section I have outlined various pathways that may be involved in initiation without saying much about relative rates of reaction. It is worth stressing how reactive are some of the intermediate species so far mentioned; Table 19.1 gives some rate constants relevant

Table 19.1 RATE CONSTANTS FOR REACTIONS INVOLVING CCl_4 AND $O_2^{-\cdot}$

	$k(M^{-1} s^{-1})$	*Reference*
$e_{aq}^- + CCl_4 \longrightarrow CCl_3^{\cdot} + Cl^-$	3×10^{10}	25
$CCl_3^{\cdot} + Prom \longrightarrow CCl_3^- + Prom^{+\cdot}$	1.1×10^9	12
$CCl_4 + isoProp \longrightarrow CCl_3^{\cdot} + Cl^- + H^+ +$ acetone	0.7×10^9	12
$CHCl_3 + isoProp \longrightarrow CHCl_2^{\cdot} + Cl^- + H^+ +$ acetone	$< 10^7$	12
$2O_2^{-\cdot} + 2H^+ \text{ (spontaneous)} \longrightarrow H_2O_2 + O_2$	$< 10^5$	26
$2O_2^{-\cdot} + 2H^+ \text{ (SDM)} \longrightarrow H_2O_2 + O_2$	2×10^9	27
$OH^{\cdot} + d\, GMP \longrightarrow d\, GMP^{+\cdot}$	5×10^9	28
$OH^{\cdot} + Prom \longrightarrow Prom\, (OH)^{\cdot}$	10^{10}	28

to this discussion. Such rates are so fast that we must seriously consider the effect that diffusion processes have on the overall course of events. Factors that require consideration in this context include the diffusion in of oxygen, diffusion away of excited species like $O_2^{-\cdot}$, the penetration of free radical scavengers and the diffusions of the PUFA and initiating sites such as P_{450} within the membrane that are closely related to membrane fluidity generally. The spin label studies particularly of Stier and co-workers[18] have demonstrated that regions of differential fluidity may occur within microsomal membranes. As a consequence we may expect marked differences to occur in the rate of lipid peroxidation from one region of the endoplasmic reticulum to another, at any particular instant in time, depending on such features as relative diffusion rates and membrane fluidity. To this variability must be added the different reductive flow patterns that are available under various experimental conditions as described in Figure 19.5.

It is possible therefore to introduce the concept that lipid peroxidation in liver endoplasmic reticulum occurs through a dynamic set of interactions that may change substantially to affect both the rate and the mechanisms of lipid peroxidation according to the micro-environment of the membrane and the surrounding medium.

The concept outlined above can be represented diagrammatically (Figure 19.6) in terms of the intractions between sets; the areas of overlap of the individual component with one another representing the effective molecular interactions. The extent of the various types of overlap will then be affected by the fluidity of the interaction species within the membrane as discussed by Stier and Sackmann[18] for the interaction of the $NADPH^-$-flavoprotein and P_{450}. Thus by modifying the membrane fluidity or by changing the local concentration of an interacting species (in Figure 19.6 this is equivalent to the area of the component in question) we may expect large differences in set–set

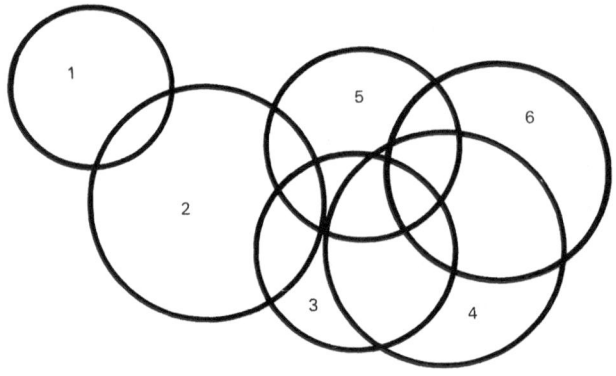

1 NADPH
2 FP
3 NHI, SH, PL
4 P_{450}
5 O_2
6 BS

FIGURE 19.6   Each circle represents a component (s) of the NADPH-cytochrome P_{450} electron transport chain; the overlap between circles indicates the interactions between the relevant components. If the components are allowed a certain amount of translational motion within the plane of the membrane of the endoplasmic reticulum (see Ref. 18), then the areas of overlap (i.e. potential interactions) will change and different pathways of electron flow may be relatively more favoured. The numbers in the figure refer to (1) NADPH   (2) the NADPH-flavoprotein   (3) a composite set of components including non-haem iron, sulphydryl-groups and phospholipid   (4) cytochrome P_{450} (5) oxygen   (6) a drug binding site having hydrophobic character

interactions which will determine the electron flows through the system as a whole.

IS LIPID PEROXIDATION DAMAGING?

This question is far easier to answer than the question posed at the start of the last section. Lipid peroxidation is indeed a damaging process that can cause cellular disturbances through a number of separate mechanisms.

Firstly, the peroxidative degradation of PUFA may cause substantial damage to the structure and metabolic functions of biomembranes. In particular this may adversely affect metabolic integrations which are dependent on intracellular compartmentation.

Secondly, the peroxy radicals and hydroperoxides formed during lipid peroxidation can affect susceptible enzymes and proteins by oxidising thiol groups and by degrading haem groups[19]. The latter reaction may be of relevance to the loss of cytochrome P_{450} during microsomal lipid peroxidation[20].

Thirdly, lipid peroxidation results in the production of a variety of water soluble materials some of which have considerable biological reactivity[21]. One generally appreciated product is malondialdehyde which can produce cross-linking reactions in proteins[22]. In addition among the peroxidation products there are hydroxy unsaturated aldehydes such as 4-hydroxy-oct-2-en-1-al. These compounds react rapidly with thiol groups[22] and may thereby strongly inhibit enzyme activities. In addition the hydroxy-alkenals react with primary amines including spermine and spermidine (G. W. White and T. F. Slater, unpublished data). These reactions of the aldehyde products of peroxidation may be of direct relevance to the known action of lipid peroxidation on nucleotide and protein synthesis. Figure 19.7 illustrates the above remarks in a diagrammatic manner.

IS LIPID PEROXIDATION OF MAJOR
SIGNIFICANCE IN TISSUE INJURY?

In certain types of tissue injury this question is also easy to answer in the affirmative, for example in photosensitised damage to lysosomes in

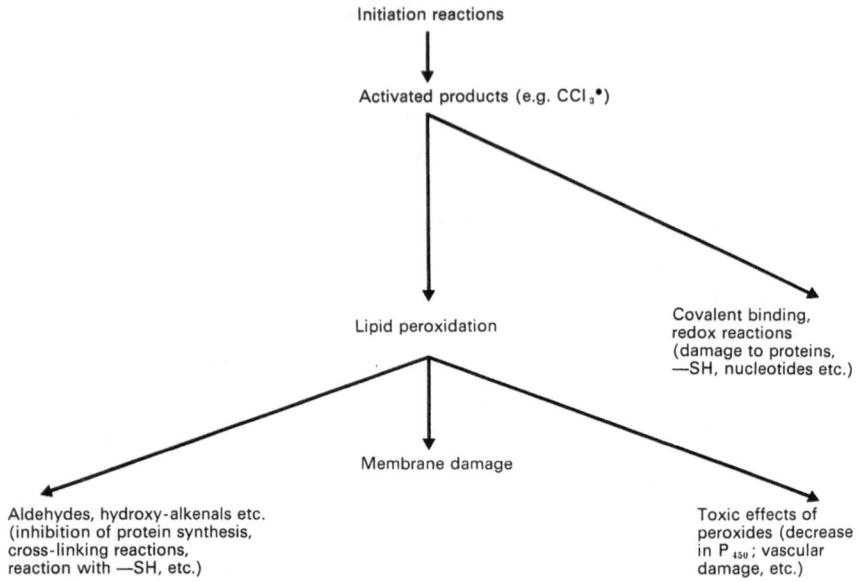

FIGURE 19.7   A simplified scheme indicating some major routes by which an activated intermediate (e.g. $CCl_3^.$ from CCl_4) formed in the endoplasmic reticulum may produce metabolic disturbances within the endoplasmic reticulum and, through the agency of comparatively long-lived secondary products (alkenals) to relatively distant sites

skin epithelium[23]. In that case the excited photosensitiser initiates lipid peroxidation of the lysosomal membrane with subsequent release of damaging acid hydrolases into the cytoplasm. As may be imagined the process is markedly attenuated by decreasing oxygen tension, and by including suitable scavengers in the system. This particular example clearly illustrates how peroxidative attack on the membrane of one class of intracellular organelle can result in severe injury to the cell as a whole.

The situation described above for photosensitisation is unusual in being fairly clear cut and relatively easy to interpret. With many other examples of tissue injury, however, for example following exposure to CCl_4, to ethanol, to orotic acid etc., the data are not so easy to interpret.

With CCl_4 intoxication there seems no doubt that lipid peroxidation is stimulated in liver endoplasmic reticulum very early on after exposure of the animal to the toxic agent[2]. This peroxidative damage is probably a major contribution to the morphological changes seen in liver endoplasmic reticulum, to the decreased glucose-6-phosphatase and P_{450} activities, and to an inhibition of drug metabolising activity generally[24]. The primary reaction appears to be the production of $CCl_3^.$ but this free radical species is chemically so reactive that many other damaging reactions occur in addition to initiating lipid peroxidation: covalent binding of $CCl_3^{\cdot}$, reaction with neighbouring nucleotides and thiol groups etc. In my opinion, in this type of injury, lipid peroxidation is only one factor, albeit an important one, in the overall sequence of early damaging events. The occurrence and significance of lipid peroxidation in CCl_4 induced liver injury have been discussed extensively by Recknagel[2] and the author[4].

With other types of liver injury, as in ethanol-reduced fatty liver or during orotic acid intoxication the overall mechanisms linking an increased lipid peroxidation with the tissue injury seem even more blurred than discussed above for CCl_4. Above all we have to remember that when we measure increased *content* of lipid peroxides, or diene conjugates, or malonaldehyde rather than the *rate* of production, we are measuring the result of a competition between the rate of production *v.* the rate of degradation. Some small stimulations in lipid peroxidation reported in certain types of tissue injury may thus result from inhibitions of rates of catabolism of the component in question rather than small increases in rates of formation.

In this article I have outlined my views on the complex area of lipid peroxidation in biomembranes. In attempting to explain in reasonably detailed terms the mechanisms involved, and the significance of such disturbances to various types of liver injury, we have much to learn and a long hard road to travel.

REFERENCES

1. Tappel, A. L. (1973). Lipid peroxidation damage to cell compartments. *Fed. Proc.*, **32**, 1870–1874
2. Recknagel, R. O. and Glende, E. A. (1973). Carbon tetrachloride hepatotoxicity: an example of lethal cleavage. *C.R.C. Critical Reviews in Toxicology*, **2**, 263–297
3. Di Luzio, N. R. (1973). Antioxidants, lipid peroxidation and chemical induced liver injury. *Fed. Proc.*, **32**, 1875–1881
4. Slater, T. F. (1972). In: *Free Radical Mechanisms in Tissue Injury* (London: Pion Ltd.)
5. Dianzani, M. U. (1973). Biochemical aspects of fatty liver. *Trans. Biochem. Soc.*, **1**, 903–908
   Dianzani, M. U. and Ugazio, G. (1973). Lipoperoxidation after CCl_4 poisoning in rats previously treated with anti-oxidants. *Chem. Biol. Interactions*, **6**, 67–79

Torrielli, M. V., Ugazio, G., Gabriel, L. and Burdino, E. (1974). Effect of drug pre-treatment on $CBrCl_3$-induced liver injury. *Toxicology*, **2**, 321–326

6. Horning, M. G., Earle, M. J. and Maling, H. M. (1962).
7. Patterson, D. S. P., Allen, W. M., Berrett, S., Sweasey, D. and Dore, J. T. (1971). The toxicity of parenteral iron preparations in the rabbit and the pig with a comparison of the clinical and biochemical responses to iron-dextran in 2-day old and 8-day old piglets. 261 *Vet. Med. A.*, **18**, 453–464
8. Srinivasan, S. and Recknagel, R. O. (1971). A note on the stability of conjugated diene absorption of rat liver microsomal lipids after CCl_4 poisoning. *J. Lipid Res.*, **12**, 766–767
9. May, H. E. and Reed, D. J. (1973). A kinetic assay of TPNH-dependent microsomal lipid peroxidation by changes in difference spectra. *Anal. Biochem.*, **55**, 331–337
10. Jose, P. J. and Slater, T. F. (1972). Increased concentrations of malon-aldehyde in the livers of rats treated with CCl_4. *Biochem. J.*, **128**, 141P
11. Slater, T. F. (1969). The effects of CCl_4 on rat liver microsomes during the first hour of poisoning *in vivo* and the modifying actions of pro-methazine. *Biochem. J.*, **111**, 317–324
Slater, T. F. and Sawyer, B. C. (1971). The stimulatory effects of carbon tetrachloride on peroxidative reactions in rat liver fractions *in vitro*. *Biochem. J.*, **123**, 823–828
12. Slater, T. F. and Willson, R. L. (1974). Carbon tetrachloride and bio-logical damage: pulse radiolysis studies of associated free radical reactions.
13. Massey, V., Strickland, S., Mayhew, S. G., Howell, L. G., Engel, P. C., Mathews, R. G., Schuman, M. and Sullivan, P. A. (1969). The produc-tion of superoxide anion radicals in the reaction of reduced flavins and flavoproteins with molecular O_2. *Biochem. Biophys. Res. Commun.*, **36**, 891–897
14. Khan, A. U. (1970). Singlet molecular oxygen from superoxide anion and sensitized fluorescence of organic molecules. *Science*, **168**, 476–477
15. Fong, K.-L., McCay, P. B., Poyer, J. L., Keele, B. B. and Misra, H. (1973). Evidence that peroxidation of lysosomal membranes is initiated by hydroxyl free radicals produced during flavin enzyme activity. *J. Biol. Chem.*, **248**, 7792–7797
16. Hrycay, E. G. and O'Brien, P. J. (1973). Microsomal electron transport: reduced NADP-cytochrome c reductase and cytochrome P-450 as electron carriers in microsomal NADPH-peroxidase activity. *Arch. Biochem. Biophys.*, **157**, 7–22
17. Bateman, L. (1954). Olefin oxidation. *Q. Revs. Chem. Soc. (London)*, **8**, 147–167
18. Stier, A. and Sackmann, E. (1973). Spin labels as enzyme substrates. *Biochim. Biophys. Acta.*, **311**, 400–408
19. Kokatnur, M. G., Bergan, J. G. and Draper, H. H. (1966). *Proc. Soc. Exp. Biol. Med.*, **123**, 314–317

20. De Matteis, F. and Sparks, R. G. (1973). Iron-dependent loss of liver cytochrome P-450 haem *in vivo* and *in vitro*. *FEBS Letters*, **29**, 141–144
21. Schauenstein, E. (1967). Autoxidation of polyunsaturated esters in water: chemical structure and biological activity of the products. *J. Lipid Res.*, **8**, 417–428
22. Esterbauer, H. (1970). Kinetik der Reaktion von Sulfydrylverbindungen mit α, β-ungesättigten Aldehyden im wässrigem System. *Monat. Chemie*, **101**, 782–810
23. Slater, T. F. and Riley, P. A. (1966). Photosensitisation and lysosomal damage. *Nature (London)*, **209**, 151–154
24. Sesame, H. A., Castro, J. A. and Gillette, J. R. (1968). Studies on the destruction of liver microsomal cytochrome-P-450 by carbon tetrachloride administration. *Biochem. Pharmacol.*, **17**, 1759–1768
25. Lesigne, B., Gilles, L. and Woods, R. J. (1974). Spectra and decay of trichloromethyl radicals in aqueous solutions. *Can. J. Chem.*, **52**, 1135–1139
26. Rabani, J. and Nielson, S. O. (1969). Absorption spectra and decay kinetic of O_2^- and HO_2^- in aqueous solutions by pulse radiolysis. *J. Phys. Chem.*, **73**, 3736–3744
27. Rotilio, G., Bray, R. C. and Fielden, E. M. (1972). A pulse radiolysis study of superoxide dismutase. *Biochim. Biophys. Acta*, **268**, 605–609
28. Willson, R. L., Wardman, P. and Asmus, K.-D. (1974). Interaction of d GMP radical with cysteamine and promethazine as possible model of DNA repair. *Nature (London)*, **252**, 323–324
29. Riely, C. A., Cohen, G. and Lieberman, M. (1974). Ethane evolution: a new index of lipid peroxidation. *Science*, **183**, 208–210
30. Swallow, A. J. (1973). *Radiation Chemistry: An Introduction* (London: Longmans)

CHAPTER 20

Inhibition of protein synthesis in carbon tetrachloride-induced liver injury

M. U. Dianzani and E. Gravela

One of the most intriguing aspects of CCl_4 toxicity is the problem of the relationships between the metabolism of this substance, the development of the block in protein synthesis and the onset of fatty infiltration. It is well known that CCl_4 is homolytically cleaved in the smooth endoplasmic reticulum of hepatocytes and that lipid peroxidation develops as a consequence of this attack[1-4]. As a morphological and biochemical consequence of lipid peroxidation, the membranes of the smooth endoplasmic reticulum become damaged and their function is compromised. As a chemical consequence, several unstable and reactive substances, such as lipoperoxides, lipohydroxyperoxides and aldehydes, are produced. These substances may initiate secondary damages to other cell structures.

The onset of lipid peroxidation in microsomal membranes was the very first sign of cell damage ever to be detected in the liver of CCl_4-poisoned animals. According to Rao and Recknagel[5], the diene conjugation band, which represents the chemical evidence for the presence of lipid peroxidation, is detectable in microsomal phospholipids as early as five minutes after giving the poison by stomach tube. Radioactive metabolites of labelled CCl_4 have also been detected in microsomal phospholipids five minutes after poisoning[6]. Impairment of protein synthesis is seen at 15–30 min after poisoning[7,8]. The onset in triglyceride accumulation is chemically evident, however, only at one hour after poisoning[9,10]. The chronology in the development of these damages suggests the possibility of sequential relationships. The fact that the impairment in protein synthesis, as well as the onset in triglyceride accumulation, are to be considered as consequences of the development of lipid peroxidation, is suggested also by the fact that pretreatment with

antioxidants, such as reduced glutathione (GSH), propylgallate (PG) and
N,N'-diphenyl-p-phenylenediamine (DPPD), exerts different actions
on the different types of damages[8,11]. GSH and PG, which are water
soluble, do protect against the loss in protein synthesis, as well as
against the development of fatty infiltration, but are unable to prevent
the appearance of the diene conjugation band in microsomal lipids. Also
the fixation of $^{14}CCl_4$ labelled metabolites into microsomal phospholipids
is not significantly modified by previous administration of PG and of
GSH. DPPD, a lipid-soluble substance, can protect, however, not only
against the loss of protein synthesis and fat accumulation, but also
against the appearance of the diene conjugation band. This last protection is neither constant nor complete, but it could reflect a different
distribution of DPPD in cell structures. In fact, DPPD, which is lipid-
soluble, might possibly arrive at cell sites (microsomal phospholipids)
where lipid peroxidation takes place. This seems to be less easy in the
case of water-soluble PG and GSH. While PG and DPPD probably
also act by interfering with the metabolism of CCl_4 in the smooth
endoplasmic reticulum, this is not the case with GSH. The dissociation
in protection against different types of damages suggests: (i) that the
impairment in protein synthesis and the onset of triglyceride accumulation are the consequence of the metabolism of CCl_4 leading to lipid
peroxidation and (ii) that these changes are mediated through some
events occurring outside the membranes, in the water-soluble phase of
the cell. These conclusions are substantiated by the fact that CCl_4 is
only able to block protein synthesis *in vivo*. Smuckler and Benditt[7] have
shown that ribosomal changes never occur when CCl_4 is added directly
to the polysomal preparations *in vitro*. The dissociation of polyribosomes does not occur even when CCl_4 is added to the whole homogenate, conditions in which its metabolism stimulates lipid peroxidation,
as is shown by accumulation of malonyldialdehyde[8].

The mechanism by which CCl_4 acts in producing the block in protein
synthesis may be considered from two angles: (i) the major site of its
inhibiting action and (ii) the nature of the substance(s) directly responsible for the inhibition.

Data reported in Table 20.1 suggest that the inhibiting action of
CCl_4 is not primarily concerned with the phases of protein synthesis
preceding the fixation of aminoacyl-tRNA to ribosomes. In fact, the
in vitro phenylalanine incorporation into liver microsomes is not modified when microsomes from normal liver are challenged by the so-called

Table 20.1   *In vitro* INCORPORATING ACTIVITY OF LIVER MICROSOMES OBTAINED FROM CONTROL OR CCl_4-POISONED RATS. Male rats, Wistar strain, weighing 150–200 g, were starved 16–18 hours before being given 0.25 ml CCl_4/100 g body wt. by stomach tube. CCl_4 was diluted 1:1 (v:v) with mineral oil. Control animals received mineral oil alone. The rats were killed 30 min after poisoning. Liver microsomes and pH 5 fraction were isolated as previously described[12,13]. The incubation medium for amino acid incorporation contained 20 mM tris-HCl buffer pH 7.6, 100 mM KCl, 5 mM $MgCl_2$, 2 mM ATP, 10 mM phosphocreatine, 0.25 mM GTP, 25 μg creatine phosphokinase, 20 mg equiv microsomes, 20 mg equiv pH 5 fraction. Final volume was 0.5 ml. 0.1μCi of [14][C]phenylalanine (Radiochemical Centre, Amersham), diluted with unlabelled phenylalanine in order to get a final concentration of 5 μM, were added to the zero time. Incubation was done at 37 °C for 15 min; the reaction was stopped by addition of 5% trichloroacetic acid. The protein-bound radioactivity was measured with a liquid scintillation system (L.S. spectrometer, Mark-I, Nuclear Chicago Corp.) as previously described[12]

Source of microsomes	Source of pH 5 fraction	Number of experiments	cpm/mg microsome protein mean + SD
Control	Control	5	976 ± 95
CCl_4	CCl_4	5	420 ± 62
Control	CCl_4	3	949 ± 84
CCl_4	Control	3	395 ± 78

'pH 5 fraction' from CCl_4-treated rats; on the contrary, a heavy inhibition is seen when microsomes from CCl_4-treated rats are challenged by the 'pH 5 fraction' from normal rats, as well as by that from the same CCl_4-damaged liver. This experiment clearly shows that the CCl_4-induced damage is sited in the microsomal fraction.

A heavy polyribosomal dissociation is seen as early as 15 min after giving 250 μl CCl_4/100 g body wt. by stomach tube[8]. This damage is prevented not only by the previous administration of antioxidants, but also by a cycloheximide pretreatment. Cycloheximide is known to be a translation inhibitor. Other substances acting on translation in a similar way, such as emetine[14,15] and tenuazoic acid[16], are also able to prevent the CCl_4-induced polyribosomal dissociation. These results show that the ribosomes-mRNA complex is not directly affected by CCl_4 treatment. A direct ribonuclease-like action can therefore be excluded. CCl_4-induced polysomal dissociation therefore seems to be the consequence of something happening when ribosomes and mRNA are still free in the cytoplasm. So, CCl_4 may be considered as a poison of recycling. In other words, the initiation reaction seems to be one among the main sites for the action of CCl_4 on protein synthesis. Ribosomes from CCl_4-treated rats behave *in vitro* like ribosomes devoid of mRNA activity. In fact, they work at normal rate in incorporating phenylalanine into proteins when poly(U) is used as a messenger[12,17]. As the initiation reaction for polyphenylalanine synthesis directed by poly(U) does not seem to be identical to that involving endogenous mRNA, these results do not exclude that the initiation reaction is primarily affected. If this is true, a potentiation in the action would be expected by giving CCl_4 and well-established inhibitors of initiation simultaneously. Among such substances, we used, in a few experiments, aurintricarboxylic acid (ATA) and pyrocathecol violet (PV). ATA was injected intraperitoneally into rats in the amount of 4 mg/100 g body wt., while PV was injected in the amount of 20 mg/100 g body wt. No potentiation was seen either in the extent of the block in protein synthesis or in triglyceride accumulation within the liver. It was found, however, that these substances, which are very active *in vitro*, are unable to cross the normal liver cell membranes[18].

The initiation reaction involves the collaboration of different substances. The most important are ribosomes, mRNA and the initiation factors. The mechanism of the initiation reaction is not completely understood, but it seems evident that enzymatic systems are involved in catalysing the single steps. It has been established that free SH groups are needed for the reaction[19,20]. This fact could explain the protective action of GSH in CCl_4-treated animals.

We are now attempting to discover which step of the initiation reaction is primarily damaged by CCl_4 poisoning. In 1973 Gravela[21] published the results of some experiments indicating the informosomal protein as a possible target for the primary damage. Gravela injected labelled orotate, 30 min before killing, into rats poisoned with CCl_4 (1–6 hours before killing). In these conditions, in which practically only mRNA becomes labelled in the cytoplasm, he found an increase in the extent of labelling of polyribosomes and a decrease in the labelling of the subribosomal particles. This result shows that ribosomes of CCl_4-treated rats bind well with newly synthesised mRNA. In another experiment, Gravela injected the [3H]orotate 30 min before giving actinomycin D in order to stop the further synthesis of RNA; one minute after actinomycin he administered CCl_4. In these rats treated Gravela found a shift of radioactivity from the polysomes to the 40 S region of the gradient. This fraction is usually referred to as 'informosomal fraction'. By combining the results of these experiments, Gravela concluded that ribosomes of CCl_4-treated rats bind preferentially with the recently synthesised ('new') mRNA. The 'old' mRNA remains mainly unbound in the informosomal fraction. These experiments seem to indicate that one of the main effects of CCl_4 is a decrease in the recycling time of informosomes.

Notwithstanding the heavy polyribosomal dissociation found in the liver of CCl_4-treated animals, the ribosomes did not appear to be detached from the endoplasmic membranes more than in untreated animals. In fact, the ratio of free to membrane-bound ribosomes remains unmodified[21,22]. This fact suggests that the attack of polysomes on the endoplasmic membranes is not a primary target for the CCl_4-induced damage.

At present, we have no knowledge of the behaviour of the initiation factors or of the combining enzymatic system. The fact that the damage to the protein synthesis system as provoked by CCl_4 can be prevented by the pretreatment with GSH might imply that its nature is oxidative. A few experiments were done in order to study the behaviour of SH groups in different fractions of the system. For this purpose, we used labelled N-ethyl-maleimide, a well-known sulphydryl reagent. This was added *in vitro* to ribosomes obtained, either from normal or from CCl_4-treated rats, by incubation with puromycin according to Metlas *et al*[23]. Then ribosomes were dissociated into 40 S and 60 S subunits. It is clear from Table 20.2 that there was no difference in the uptake of N-ethyl-maleimide by both 40 S and 60 S subunits isolated either from control or from poisoned rats. Neither was any difference found with regard to the N-ethyl-maleimide uptake by the 40 S fraction of the postmitochondrial supernatant (informosomal fraction). These negative results, however, cannot be considered as definite proof that the CCl_4-induced damage is other than oxidative. In fact, denaturation of proteins may have complicated the intramolecular distribution of SH groups available to N-ethyl-maleimide. In addition, the damage might involve only very few specific SH groups sited in key positions of the molecules.

The problem of the substances responsible for the impairment in protein synthesis also remains unresolved. As the impairment seems to be a consequence of CCl_4 metabolism, leading to the production of free radicals, as well as to lipid peroxidation, the following hypotheses may be advanced: (i) the impairment is due to free radicals produced by the

Table 20.2   *In vitro* UPTAKE OF N-ETHYL-MALEIMIDE BY RIBOSOMAL SUBUNITS OBTAINED FROM CONTROL OR CCl_4-POISONED RATS. Animals and treatments were as in Table 20.1. The liver postmitochondrial supernatant (PMS), prepared as described elsewhere[21], was incubated for one hour at 37 °C in a medium similar to that described in Table 20.1, except that 0.25 mg/ml puromycin were added to the zero time (in order to release ribosomes from mRNA according to Metlas *et al.*[23]). The mixture was then treated with 1 % Triton × 100 and 1 % Na-deoxycholate, and ribosomes were isolated as described else-where.[21] Ribosomes were then suspended into a 20 mM tris-HCl buffer pH 7.6, containing 0.2 M KCl and 1mM $MgCl_2$, in order to obtain the separation of the subunits. These were incubated in a final volume of 1 ml (about 1 mg ribosomes) with 1 μCi of [14][C]N-ethylmaleimide (Radiochemical Centre, Amersham) diluted with unlabelled N-ethylmaleimide in order to get a specific activity of 1 Ci/M. Incubation was carried out for one hour at 0 °C with continuous stirring. The subunits were then separated on a linear sucrose gradient (0.5–1.5 M sucrose, containing buffer, KCl and $MgCl_2$ as in the above described incubation medium) by centrifuging at 95 000 g for 20 hours. Gradients were fractionated as described elsewhere[21]. The fractions corresponding to 40 S and 60 S particles were collected, treated with excess unlabelled N-ethyl-maleimide, and then purified with 5 % trichloroacetic acid before counting radioactivity as in Table 20.1. Results are given as nmol N-ethyl-maleimide/mg of subunits

	Mineral oil		CCl_4	
	40 S	*60 S*	*40 S*	*60 S*
1° experiment	17.4	29.1	18.3	30.2
2° experiment	22.5	28.7	21.4	29.6

homolytic cleavage of CCl_4 (ii) it is due to substances produced by the peroxidative disintegration of lipids or (iii) it is due to some other substances secondarily involved.

In order to check the first possibility, we injected labelled CCl_4 into rats and checked the eventual presence of radioactivity in the subcellular fractions involved in protein synthesis. While a consistent binding of the label to the phospholipid fraction of microsome was evident, no binding at all was detected as regards ribosomes or informosomal fractions. In addition, the hypothesis that the damage to the protein synthesis system is provoked by CCl_4 free radicals themselves seems improbable if one considers the very high reactivity of these substances, which are produced in cell sites (the smooth endoplasmic reticulum metabolic system) relatively far from those involved in protein synthesis.

The possibility that the damages are provoked by products of the disintegration of lipids has also been tested. Table 20.3 shows the results of an experiment in which labelled acetate was injected into rats 13 hours before giving CCl_4. It was seen that the degree of labelling of ribosomal subunits and of informosomal fractions was not different in poisoned and control animals. This experiment is, however, not conclusive, as acetate may have been incorporated into molecules other than fatty acids. The relatively high degree of labelling seen in fractions from both poisoned and control rats indicates, for instance, the incorporation of acetate into messenger and ribosomal RNAs and/or proteins. So, a small amount of lipid-derivative radioactivity bound to the

Table 20.3 RADIOACTIVITY IN LIVER RIBOSOMAL SUBUNITS OBTAINED FROM FASTED RATS INJECTED WITH LABELLED ACETATE 14 HOURS BEFORE KILLING. Wistar male rats, weighing 100–120 g, were fasted for eight hours and then treated intraperitoneally with $^{14}[C]$acetate (sodium salt), in the amount of 50 μCi, corresponding to 8.3 μmol. After 13 hours further fasting, 0.25 ml CCl_4, diluted 1:1 (v:v) with mineral oil, were given by stomach tube. Control animals received mineral oil alone. Liver lipids labelling corresponds, in these conditions, to about 3000 cpm/mg total lipids. Ribosomes and subunits were isolated as described in Table 20.2. Results are given as cpm/mg subunits

	Mineral oil		CCl_4	
	40 S	*60 S*	*40 S*	*60 S*
1° experiment	3940	2100	3140	1580
2° experiment	2880	2080	3130	1990

subribosomal particles cannot be detected. In addition, a limiting factor may have been represented by the low extent of incorporation of acetate into polyunsaturated fatty acids, which are the main precursors of lipoperoxides.

Under a general point of view, the hypothesis that the damaging factors are lipoperoxides themselves seems improbable, due to their rather high molecular mass and to their high reactivity. These are not good conditions for easy diffusibility of these substances. The hypothesis which seems the most probable one is that the damaging substances are not the lipoperoxides themselves, but some easily diffusible product of their disintegration. Among such substances, we first considered aldehydes. These substances are known to react with free SH groups, so producing cyclic inactive compounds[24,25]. A lot of different aldehydes have been shown to be able to inhibit protein synthesis *in vitro*[26-29]. It is also known that aldehydes are present in rather high amount among the products of peroxidative degradation of lipids[30,31]. The production of malonyldialdehyde is used, for this reason, as a measure of the extent of peroxidation. Among the aldehydes derived from the peroxidative disintegration of unsaturated lipids, we first tested malonyldialdehyde (MDA). Table 20.4 shows that MDA is able to consistently inhibit the incorporation of labelled amino acids into proteins of the postmitochondrial supernatant *in vitro*, only at concentration ranges exceeding 5 mM. Lower concentrations are ineffective. MDA, is however, not very reactive. Professor Slater suggested testing two unsaturated aldehydes, which, according to Schauenstein[30], are derived from the peroxidative

Table 20.4 EFFECT OF MALONYLDIALDEHYDE *in vitro* ON AMINO ACID INCOR-
PORATION INTO RAT LIVER POSTMITOCHONDRIAL SUPERNATANT. The rat liver
postmitochondrial supernatant was prepared according to Richardson *et al.*[32].
Incubation was carried out for 15 min at 37 °C in a medium containing in a
final volume of 0.4 ml: 2 mM ATP, 10 mM phosphocreatine, 0.25 mM GTP,
20 μg creatine phosphokinase, 2 mM magnesium acetate, 100 mM KCl,
20 mM tris-HCl buffer pH 7.4, 33 mg equiv postmitochondrial supernatant.
Amino acids source was a protein hydrolysate of *Chlorella* (Radiochemical
Centre, Amersham. Specific activity 52 mCi C14/mAtom carbon). It was
added to the zero time, in the amount of 0.2 μCi, diluted with a mixture of
16 unlabelled L-amino acids in order to reach a final concentration of 10 μM.
Radioactivity was determined on hot trichloroacetic acid precipitates, collected and purified on Millipore filters[21]. Results are given as cpm/mg equiv
postmitochondrial supernatant. Malonyldialdehyde was prepared from
tetraethoxypropane (with Dowex WX 2); double experiments with malonyldialdehyde and with the corresponding amount of tetraethoxypropane were
done in each case

Concentration	Malonyldialdehyde	Tetraethoxypropane
0.0	236	236
0.08 mM	251	249
0.15 mM	242	252
0.30 mM	240	253
0.50 mM	247	244
1.25 mM	232	244
2.50 mM	227	245
5.00 mM	226	236
12.50 mM	102	233
25.00 mM	24	228

disintegration of unsaturated natural lipids. These two aldehydes, i.e. 4-hydroxy-2,3-trans-penten-1-al (HPE) and but-2-en-1,4-dial or maleylaldehyde (MA) are much more reactive than MDA and were very effective in reacting with thiol groups, and in inhibiting the incorporation of labelled precursors into DNA, RNA and protein in suspensions of tumour cells[29]. Professor Slater generously provided samples of these substances. The results of preliminary experiments show a marked inhibition of *in vitro* amino acid incorporation into liver proteins by both substances at very low concentrations (0.05–0.2 mM). It is interesting that the inhibition site is not related to the steps of the protein synthesis scheme preceding the fixation to ribosomes of aminoacyl-RNA. In fact, the two tested aldehydes are ineffective in the *in vitro* synthesis of ^{14}[C]aminoacyl-tRNA, whereas they inhibit the incorporation of preformed ^{14}[C]aminoacyl-tRNA into microsomal proteins. In this respect, the two aldehydes behave in a way similar to CCl_4. Notwithstanding the fact that we cannot say at present to what extent our results on protein synthesis *in vitro* is due to a block in the initiation reaction, these preliminary experiments suggest that continuation of our work in this direction would be worthwhile.

Another aspect of the problem of the block in protein synthesis by CCl_4 is that of its real participation in producing the onset of triglyceride accumulation. Fat accumulation represents the result of a balance between the income and the outcome of triglyceride from the liver cell pool. An increased income may be the consequence of an increased arrival of non-esterified fatty acids from the blood plasma, or of an increased synthesis of these substances within the liver cell itself, or also of a decreased oxidation in mitochondria. All these situations can increase the free fatty acid concentration within the liver, so producing the conditions for an increased local synthesis of triglycerides. A decreased outcome of triglycerides can be related to a block in the release of lipoproteins from the liver cell into the blood plasma. Both increased income and decreased outcome may provoke the same result, that is to say an increase in the actual concentration of triglycerides within the liver. Many among the described factors may be present in the same pathological condition. CCl_4 mainly acts by blocking lipoprotein secretion, but it is also able to increase the arrival of non-esterified fatty acids from the blood stream[33,15]. Cycloheximide, a powerful inhibitor of protein synthesis, is a poor steatogenic agent, notwithstanding the fact it is a good inhibitor of lipoprotein secretion[33], probably because it depresses the blood concentration of non-esterified fatty acids[33], and slowly inhibits the synthesis of triglycerides within the liver[34]. Cycloheximide has a strong extrahepatic action[15,35], that might be important in decreasing the release of non-esterified fatty acids from the adipocytes. Emetine, another inhibitor of protein synthesis, is, on the contrary, a powerful steatogenic agent, notwithstanding the fact it is an even stronger depressor of the blood level of non-esterified fatty acids[14,15,35]. Possibly, the strong steatogenic power of emetine is due to the fact that it inhibits the lipoprotein release more than the fatty acids supply to the liver cell. Moreover, emetine and cycloheximide could exert a different effect on the triglyceride synthesis within the liver.

In any case, a block in protein synthesis may act in provoking triglyceride accumulation mainly by decreasing in the liver the pool of available apolipoprotein molecules, which are necessary for the formation of very low density lipoproteins (VLDL). We don't know at present at which time the block in the synthesis of new apolipoprotein molecules becomes relevant in provoking triglyceride accumulation. In fact, it seems clear that each of these molecules can act several times in extracting triglycerides from the liver and in vehiculating them throughout the plasma to the extrahepatic utilisation tissues. The problem of deciding if the block in apolipoprotein synthesis is important in explaining the onset of triglyceride accumulation and is therefore strictly dependent upon the knowledge of the life-span of pre-existing molecules. Unfortunately, the state of our knowledge about this problem is still inconclusive. According to recent data by Eisenberg and Rachmilewitz[36], who studied the distribution and the half-lives of several apolipoprotein subfractions from VLDL previously labelled and injected into recipient animals, these subfractions undergo rapid redistribution among the other lipoprotein fractions. Their half-lives are somehow different. Generally, after an initial period in which a dilution of the subfractions in the organism and a distribution among the various lipoprotein fractions occurs, a period of less rapid decay takes place. It is, however, difficult to decide if the half-lives of the apolipoprotein subfractions are consistent with the view that the onset in triglyceride accumulation is only dependent on the block of their synthesis.

If we compare the onset times for triglyceride accumulation as shown by other steatogenic substances, being also inhibitors of protein synthesis (see Table 20.5), we never found onset times as early as those seen in the case of CCl_4 or of $CBrCl_4$, another very active haloalkane. Most

Table 20.5 RELATIONSHIP BETWEEN DOSE SIZE AND THE LAG PERIOD BEFORE THE ONSET OF FATTY LIVER AS DETERMINED BY SEVERAL STEATOGENIC TREATMENTS. Data of our laboratory. Data with puromycin have been reported by Robinson and Seakins[37]

Treatments	Dose (per 100 g body wt.)	Onset of fatty liver (hours after poisoning)
CCl_4	2.58 mmol	1
$CBrCl_3$	0.26 mmol	1
CS_2 (males)	2.58 mmol	12
CS_2 (females)	2.58 mmol	6
White phosphorus	1 mg	6
Ethionine (females)	100 mg	7
Puromycin°	7.5–20 mg	5–16
N-dimethylnitrosamine	20 mg	6
cycloheximide	0.1 mg	6
emetine	2 mg	3
aflatoxin B_1	0.1 mg	6
ethanol	800 mg	6
-amanitine	0.5 mg	24
choline deficiency		12

inhibitors of protein synthesis provoke the onset of fatty liver between five and six hours after poisoning. Only emetine, among the substances used in our laboratory, provoked fatty liver at three hours. The delayed onset, with respect to haloalkanes poisoning, might be explained by different impacts on the various factors of the balance discussed above. It might also imply, however, an action of CCl_4 on lipoprotein secretion other than the impairment in the synthesis of new apolipoprotein molecules. In experiments published a few years ago[11] we were able to show that isolated lipoperoxides or CCl_4 metabolites inhibit the *in vitro* recombination between delipidated lipoprotein and lipids. This fact might be related to the denaturating action of lipoperoxides or of CCl_4 metabolites on apolipoproteins. It is impossible to say at present if this mechanism has a real value *in vivo*. As lipoperoxides are produced at the level of the membranes of the endoplasmic reticulum, that are thought to be also the sites for lipoprotein assembly, the hypothesis may be tenable. Other possibilities do, however, exist. For instance, damage in plasma membranes might also be considered as responsible for the accumulation within the liver of well-formed lipoprotein micelles. Another possibility might also be a decreased mobility of these micelles throughout the cytoplasm, due to the impairment of some intracellular system necessary for their transport. In other words, the early accumulation of fat might also be a problem of intracellular traffic. Some experiments to test this possibility are now being processed in our laboratory.

ACKNOWLEDGMENT

The experiments described in this paper were aided by a grant from Consiglio Nazionale delle Ricerche, Roma.

REFERENCES

1. Comporti E., Saccocci, C. and Dianzani, M. U. (1965). Effect of CCl₄ *in vitro* and *in vivo* on lipid peroxidation of rat liver homogenates and subcellular fractions. *Enzymologia*, **29**, 185–204
2. Ghoshal, A. K. and Recknagel, R. O. (1965). Positive evidence of acceleration of lipoperoxidation in rat liver by carbon tetrachloride: *in vitro* experiments. *Life Sci.*, **4**, 1521–1530
3. Slater, T. F. (1966). *In vitro* effects of carbon tetrachloride on rat liver microsomes. *Biochem. J.*, **101**, 16P
4. Slater, T. F. (1972). *Free Radical Mechanisms in Tissue Injury*, 1–283 (London: Pion Ltd.)
5. Rao, K. S. and Recknagel, R. O. (1968). Early onset of lipoperoxidation in rat liver after carbon tetrachloride administration. *Exp. Molec. Pathol.*, **9**, 271–278
6. Rao, K. S. and Recknagel, R. O. (1969). Early incorporation of carbon-labelled carbon tetrachloride into rat liver particulate lipids and proteins. *Exp. Molec. Pathol*, **10**, 219–228
7. Smuckler, E. A. and Benditt, E. P. (1965). Studies on carbon tetrachloride intoxication. III. A subcellular defect in protein synthesis. *Biochemistry*, **4**, 671–679
8. Gravela, E. and Dianzani, M. U. (1970). Studies on the mechanism of CCl₄-induced polyribosomal damage. *FEBS Letters*, **9**, 93–96
9. Artizzu, M. and Dianzani, M. U. (1962). The changes in the mitochondria and lysosomes in the fatty livers of rats fed with carbon tetrachloride and their independence of ribonuclease activation. *Biochim. Biophys. Acta*, **63**, 453–464
10. Lombardi, B. and Ugazio, G. (1965). Serum lipoproteins in rats with carbon tetrachloride-induced fatty liver. *J. Lipid. Res.*, **6**, 498–505
11. Dianzani, M. U. and Ugazio, G. (1973). Lipoperoxidation after carbon tetrachloride poisoning in rats previously treated with antioxidants. *Chem. Biol. Inter.*, **6**, 67–79
12. Gravela, E., Gabriel, L. and Ugazio, G. (1971). Protection by glutathione and propylgallate on the impaired *in vitro* aminoacid incorporation into

liver microsomal protein of CCl₄-poisoned rats. *Biochem. Pharmacol.*, **20**, 2065–2070

13. Gravela, E. (1968). Azione della tossina difterica sulla sintesi di poli-fenilalanina diretta da poli(U) in ribosomi di embrione di pollo. *Lo Sperimentale*, **118**, 43–56

14. Gravela, E. and Poli, G. (1974). Modifications of carbon tetrachloride-induced liver steatosis and necrosis by cycloheximide and emetine. *IRCS*, **2**, 1534

15. Dianzani, M. U. (1974). Il punto attuale sul problema della steatosi epatica. *Atti Giornate Mediche di Montecatini*, **17**, 2–25

16. Farber, E., Liang, H. and Shinozuka, H. (1971). Dissociation of effects on protein synthesis and ribosomes from membrane changes induced by carbon tetrachloride. *Amer. J. Pathol.*, **64**, 601–622

17. Weksler, M. E. and Gelboin, H. V. (1967). Carbon tetrachloride-induced loss of microsomal messenger-ribonucleic acid activity. *Biochim. Biophys. Acta*, **145**, 184–187

18. Grollman, A. P. and Huang, H. T. (1973). Inhibitors of protein synthesis in eukariotes: tools in cell research. *Fed. Proc.*, **32**, 1673–1678

19. Bermek, E., Mönkemeyer, H. and Berg, R. (1971). The role of SH-groups of human ribosomal subunits in polypeptide synthesis. *Biochem. Biophys. Res. Comm.*, **45**, 1294–1299

20. Kosower, N. S., Vanderhoff, G. A. and Kosower, E. M. (1972). Gluta-thione. VIII. The effects of glutathione disulphide on initiation of protein synthesis. *Biochim. Biophys. Acta*, **272**, 623–637

21. Gravela, E. (1973). Evidence for a reduced active life-span of messenger-RNA in liver of rats poisoned with carbon tetrachloride. *Exp. Molec. Pathol.*, **19**, 79–93

22. Sarma, D. S. R., Reid, I. M., Verney, E. and Sidransky, H. (1972). Studies on the nature of attachment of ribosomes to membranes in liver. I. Influence of ethionine, sparsomycin, CCl₄ and puromycin on mem-brane-bound polyribosomal disaggregation and on detachment of membrane-bound ribosomes from membranes *Lab. Invest.*, **27**, 39–47

23. Metlas, R., Popic, S. and Kanazir, D. (1973). Preparation of ribosomal subunits from rat liver postmitochondrial supernatant. *Anal. Biochem.*, **55**, 539–543

24. Loreti, L., Ferioli, E. M., Gazzola, G. C. and Guidotti, G. G. (1971). Studies on the anti-tumour activity of aliphatic aldehydes. III. Formation of thiazoidine-4-carboxylic acid in tissues. *Eur. J. Cancer*, **7**, 281–284

25. Buttkus, H. (1972). The reaction of malonaldehyde or oxided linolenic acid with sulphydryl compounds. *J. Amer. Oil Chem. Soc.*, **49**, 613–614

26. Guidotti, G. G., Fonnesu, A. and Ciaranfi, E. (1964). Inhibition of aminoacid incorporation into protein of Yoshida ascites hepatoma cells by glyceraldehyde. *Cancer Res.*, **24**, 900–905

27. Moulè, Y. and Frayssinet, C. (1971). Effects of acrolein on transcription *in vitro*. *FEBS Letters*, **16**, 216–218

28. Comi, P., Ottolenghi, S., Gianni, A. M., Giglioni, B. and Guidotti, G. G.

238 *Pathogenesis and mechanisms of liver cell necrosis*

(1973). Inhibition of protein synthesis by aliphatic aldehydes. *Biochimie*, **55**, 507–508

29. Slater, T. F., Conroy, P , Fraval, H., Jose, P. J., McBrien, D., Nodes, J. T., Sawyer, B. and White, G. W. (1974). Biochemical and antitumour properties of hydroxy- and keto-aldehydes (in press)

30. Schauenstein, E. (1967). Autoxidation of polyunsaturated esters in water: chemical structure and biological activity of the products. *J. Lipid. Res.*, **8**, 417–428

31. Ellis, R., Gaddis, A. M., Currie, G. T. and Powell, S. L. (1968). Carbonyls in oxidizing fat. XIII. The isolation of free aldehydes from autoxidized triolein, trilinolein and trilinolenin *J. Amer. Oil Chem. Soc.*, **45**, 553–559

32. Richardson, A., McGown, E., Henderson, L. M. and Patricia, B. (1971). *In vitro* aminoacid incorporation by the postmitochondrial supernatant from rat liver. *Biochim. Biophys. Acta*, **254**, 468–477

33. Gravela, E., Pani, P., Ferrari, A. and Mazzarino, C. (1971). Effects of the CCl_4-cycloheximide interaction on protein synthesis and lipid metabolism in rat liver. *Biochem. Pharmacol.*, **20**, 3423–3430.

34. Bar-On, H., Stein, O. and Stein, Y. (1972). Multiple effects of cycloheximide on the metabolism of triglycerides in the liver of male and female rats. *Biochim. Biophys. Acta*, **270**, 444–452

35. Gravela, E., Bertone, G. and Poli, G. (1974). Inhibitori della sintesi proteica e steatosi epatica: differenze tra cicloesimide, emetina e N-dimetilnitrosamina. *Boll. Soc. Ital. Biol. Sper.*, **50**, 1674–1679

36. Eisenberg, S. and Rachimlewitz, D. (1973). Metabolism of rat plasma very low density lipoprotein. I. Fate in circulation of the whole lipoprotein. II. Fate in circulation of apoprotein subunits. *Biochim. Biophys. Acta*, **326**, 378–390 and 391–405

37. Robinson, D. S. and Seakins, A. (1962). Inhibition of plasma lipoprotein synthesis and the occurrence of fatty livers in the rats. *Biochem. J.*, **83**, 36P–37P

CHAPTER 21

Mechanism of hepatic necrosis induced by halogenated aromatic hydrocarbons

J. R. GILLETTE

Many drugs and other foreign compounds may be converted in the body to various metabolites, some of which may evoke pharmacological and toxicological effects in addition to those caused by the parent substances. When the metabolites are chemically inert, they exert their effects by combining reversibly with action sites and thus the magnitude of their effects may often be related to their concentration in blood plasma. However, several chemically inert foreign compounds are converted in the body to chemically reactive metabolites that combine covalently with various micromolecular and macromolecular substances in tissues and thereby cause changes which result in various toxicities including cancer, mutagenesis, cellular necrosis, immunological reactions, blood dyscrasias and foetal damage[1-3]. Because of the seriousness of these toxicities, our laboratory has been engaged in developing a general approach by which we can determine whether a given toxicity is mediated by chemically reactive metabolites.

Because chemically reactive metabolites presumably exert their toxic effects by combining irreversibly with target macromolecular substances, the severity and the incidence of the toxicity should be related to the number or concentration of target macromolecules that ultimately combine with the reactive metabolite. Thus, the severity and incidence of the toxic reaction should not necessarily be related to the concentration of the chemically reactive metabolite in blood plasma even if we were fortunate enough to devise analytical procedures for the assay of such highly chemically reactive substances in plasma and tissues.

In attempting to relate the formation of chemically reactive metabolites with their toxicities, my colleagues and I have found it useful to think of the incidence rate and the severity of the toxicity as the product of two mathematical functions: (1) the proportion of the dose of the parent compound that becomes covalently bound to the target macromolecule and (2) the probability that a given amount of chemically reactive metabolite that is covalently bound to the target macromolecules in a tissue will result in the toxicity in that tissue. The second of these mathematical functions, of course, is complex and depends on a number of factors. For example, with carcinogenic substances the value of the second function would depend on the presence of promoters (such as croton oil), on whether repair mechanisms of DNA introduce translational errors into DNA or prevent them, on the rate of cellular division, and the rate of repair of other cellular processes such as protein synthesis. Because of the complex interrelated factors that are represented by the second function, it seems likely that its value will vary not only with the compound but also from one tissue to another and from one animal species to another.

The first mathematical function is also complex but may be viewed as the mathematical product of a series of ratios. The length of the series depends on the number of reactions by which the foreign compound is converted to its chemically reactive metabolite. For example, 2-acetylaminofluorene (2-AAF) is converted first to N-hydroxy-2-acetylaminofluorene (NOH-2-AAF) which in turn is conjugated with sulphate to form N-O-sulphate-2-acetylaminofluorene (N-O-sulphate-2-AAF) which is thought to be the major chemically reactive metabolite that reacts with tissue macromolecules[4]. Thus, in this case, the equation for the incidence or severity of the toxicity may be viewed as:

$$(I) \text{ or } (S) = \text{Dose ABCMP}$$

In which A is the proportion of the dose of 2-AAF that is converted to NOH-2-AAF, B is the proportion of N-OH-2-AAF that is converted to N-O-sulphate-2-AAF, C the proportion of N-O-sulphate-2-AAF that becomes covalently bound to tissue macromolecules, M is the proportion of covalently bound metabolites that are attached to target macromolecule and P is the probability that a given amount of target macromolecule-metabolite conjugate results in the toxicity.

Very highly chemically reactive metabolites react with various tissue macromolecules including protein, the various RNAs, DNA, glycogen and lipids. Thus, it is difficult, if not impossible to determine which macromolecule is the target macromolecule for a given toxicity. Moreover, the target macromolecule may be present in some organs and not in others. For this reason, it is not possible to determine when a given amount of covalently bound metabolite will result in toxicity and when it won't. For example, if M or P is very low, large amounts of covalently bound metabolite may be found in a tissue even though the substance does not cause toxicity in that tissue. On the other hand, if both M and P are high, toxicity may occur even when very little covalently bound metabolite is found in that tissue. It is evident, therefore, that by itself the amount of covalent binding found in a tissue cannot be used to predict toxicity.

Nevertheless, it occurred to us that when a substance is known to cause a toxicity, we might be able to determine whether the toxicity was mediated by a chemically reactive metabolite, by a chemically stable metabolite or by the parent compound. It seemed likely that changes in the concentration of the reactive metabolite within a given tissue would alter not only the rate of covalent binding of the reactive metabolite to the target macromolecule, but also its rate of covalent binding to other macromolecules. Thus, treatments that alter the pattern of metabolism of the toxicant in animals should cause parallel *changes* in the amount of covalent binding to both the target macromolecules and other macromolecules. According to this view *changes* in the amount of covalent binding of the reactive metabolite to tissue proteins should parallel *changes* in the incidence or severity of the toxicity even though the target macromolecule might be a minor tissue protein or even when the target macromolecule is not a protein at all.

Changes in the amount of covalent binding of a chemically reactive metabolite to tissue macromolecules after a given dose of the toxicant can occur only by changing one or more of the ratios, A, B etc. However, each ratio depends on the relative rates at which the toxicant or metabolite is converted to the next compound along the pathway leading to the covalent binding and is eliminated from the body by innoxious pathways[5-7]. When one or more of the pathways are catalysed by enzymes or transport systems that become saturated by the toxicant or metabolite or when one or more of the pathways are catalysed by enzyme systems that require co-substrates which may become depleted in the tissues, the ratios may vary with time and thus are difficult to visualise. In order to gain an insight into the interrelationships among the various pathways, however, let us assume that all processes are first order, i.e. the rates are directly proportional to the concentration of the parent compound or the metabolite. Under these conditions each ratio equals the rate constant for the formation of the next metabolite along the pathway leading to the covalent binding of the drug to tissue macro-molecules divided by the sum of the rate constants for this reaction and the other pathways by which the toxicant or the metabolite is eliminated from the body (Table 21.1).

Inspection of the equation for these ratios leads to several principles that frequently have been misunderstood.

(1) Increases or decreases in the activity of the enzyme that catalyses a reaction along the pathway leading toward covalent binding of the chemically reactive metabolite will have their greatest effect when the reaction represents a relatively minor route of elimination of the toxicant or metabolite (that is the numerator of the ratio is markedly changed but the denominator is not). Thus, increases or decreases in the activity of the 'activating' enzyme may result in marked changes in the toxicity of the substance without markedly changing the half-life of the toxicant in the body. On the other hand, when the reaction leading to the forma-tion of covalently bound metabolite is the only mechanism by which the toxicant or metabolite is eliminated from the body, then increases or decreases in the activity of the enzyme would not alter the toxicity even though they would markedly change the half-life of the toxicant or the metabolite (that is the ratio would still be 1.0 because the numerator and the denominator would be increased or decreased to the same extent).

(2) Increases or decreases in the activity of an enzyme (or process) that leads to the formation of innoxious metabolites would have their greatest effect when the reaction represents the major pathway by which the toxicant or metabolite is eliminated from the body. Thus, the doubling of the activity of such an enzyme would have a greater effect on the toxicity when the product represents 90% of the total elimina-tion of the toxicant or metabolite than when it represents 10%.

(3) When the ultimate reactive metabolite is converted to only one innoxious metabolite, increases or decreases in the activity of the enzyme that catalyses the formation of the metabolite may markedly alter the toxicity without appreciably altering the pattern of urinary metabolites. Thus, a toxicity may appear in one animal species but not in another even when the pattern of urinary metabolites of the toxicant is indistinguishable in the two species.

With these general concepts in mind, it is also important to consider the effects of plasma levels of the toxicant or metabolite that saturate

Table 21.1 THEORETICAL ASPECTS OF THE RATIOS IN THE EQUATION:
INCIDENCE= DOSE ABC . . . MP

Each ratio equals the amount of foreign compound or metabolite that is converted to the next substance on the pathway leading to the formation of covalently bound metabolite divided by the amount of foreign compound administered or the amount of metabolite formed in the body.
For example,

$$A = \frac{\text{Amount of Metabolite } (M_a)}{\text{Dose of Foreign Compound } (D)}$$

In turn the ratios depend on the relative rates at which the next substance is formed and the foreign compound or metabolite is eliminated from the body.
For example,

$$A = \frac{\int F_{ai} D \, dt}{\int F_{ai} D \, dt + \int F_{aii} D \, dt + \ldots}$$

and

$$B = \frac{\int F_{bi} M_a \, dt}{\int F_{bi} M_a \, dt + \int F_{bii} M_a \, dt + \ldots}$$

in which

$$\int F_{ai} [D] \, dt = \int F_{bi} [M_a] \, dt + \int F_{bii} [M_a] \, dt + \ldots$$

The Functions, F_{ai}, F_{aii} . . ., F_{bi}, F_{bii} . . ., etc,
usually fit one of the following kinds of processes.

I is a first order process: $F_I = k$

II is a saturable process: $F_{II} = \dfrac{V_{max}}{K + [X]}$

in which $[X]$ is the concentration of the foreign compound or the metabolite.
III is a process that requires a depletable endogenous cosubstrate (S):

$$F_{III} = \frac{V_{max}(S)}{K_1 + K_2(X) + K_3(S) + K_4(X)(S)}$$

When all of the processes are first order and when the body may be viewed kinetically as a one-pool system* the ratios depend on the relative values of the first order rate constants:

For example,

$$A = \frac{k_{ai}}{k_{ai} + k_{aii} + k_{aiii} \ldots}$$

and

$$B = \frac{k_{bi}}{k_{bi} + k_{bii} + k_{biii} \ldots}$$

* For a two pool linear system see Ref. 7

various drug metabolising enzymes or deplete the body of the co-substrates required in the conjugation pathways.

(4) A large single dose of the toxicant may saturate the enzyme that catalyses the formation of a metabolite that leads to its covalent binding to tissue macromolecules. Under these conditions, the proportion of the dose of the toxicant that becomes covalently bound to tissue macro-molecules may decrease as the size of the dose is increased. Thus, the amount of covalently bound metabolites may be greater when the drug dosage is divided and given repetitively than when it is given as a large, single dose.

(5) A large single dose of a toxicant may result in plasma concentra-tions that saturate binding sites on plasma proteins, active transport systems in kidneys or enzymes that catalyse the conversion of the toxicant to an innoxious metabolite. In these situations, the proportion of the dose of the toxicant that becomes covalently bound to tissue macromolecules may increase as the size of the dose is increased. Indeed, there may be a dose threshold below which very little covalent binding occurs.

(6) A large single dose of a toxicant may deplete the body of a co-substrate (such as sulphate or phosphoadenosine phosphosulphate) required for the formation of the chemically reactive metabolite. Thus, the proportion of the dose of toxicant that becomes covalently bound to macromolecules may decrease as the size of the dose is increased. Administration of the dose in divided doses given repetitively may increase the proportion of the dose that becomes covalently bound because the concentration of the co-substrate should depend not only on the rate at which it is consumed in the reaction but also on the rate at which it is mobilised from body stores or resynthesised. Moreover, increases or decreases in the activity of the enzyme that catalyses the formation of the chemically reactive conjugate may or may not affect the proportion of the dose of the toxicant that becomes covalently bound depending on the relative rates at which the co-substrate is consumed in the reaction and resynthesised.

(7) A large single dose of the toxicant may deplete the body of a co-substrate (such as glutathione) required for the formation of an innox-ious metabolite. In this situation, the proportion of the dose of the parent compound or the proportion of the metabolite that becomes covalently bound to tissue macromolecules may increase as the size of the dose is increased. Indeed, there may be a dose threshold below

which very little covalent binding occurs. When a toxic dose is divided and given repetitively, the covalent binding and the toxicity may be decreased, depending on the rate at which the co-substrate is resynthesised or mobilised from body stores. Moreover, increasing the activity of the enzyme that catalyses the formation of the metabolite that combines with the co-substrate usually will increase the proportion of the dose that becomes covalently bound but the magnitude of the increase will depend upon the relative rates at which the co-substrate is consumed in the formation of the innoxious metabolite and is resynthesised. On the other hand, increases in the activity of the enzyme that catalyses the formation of the conjugate may or may not decrease the covalent binding, depending on the rate of synthesis of the co-substrate.

Thus, the values of the various ratios depend on a number of inter-related reactions. Moreover, the problem of evaluating the ratios is further complicated when a treatment alters the rates of more than one of the various metabolic reactions. Thus, a given treatment may cause an increase in one ratio and a decrease in another. Moreover, a treatment may increase a ratio with one dosage and decrease it with another.

Many of these principles have been illustrated with studies on the hepatic necrosis induced by halogenated aromatic hydrocarbons, such as bromobenzene. Although the urinary metabolites of bromobenzene were identified many years ago[8-10], recent studies have revealed that nearly all of the bromobenzene administered to animals is converted to its chemically reactive metabolite, bromobenzene-3,4-epoxide[11-13] by a cytochrome P_{450} enzyme system localised mainly in the endoplasmic reticulum of liver. Thus, ratio A for this reaction equals nearly 1.0.

Some of the epoxide rearranges non-enzymatically to form 4-bromophenol. Some is converted to a dihydrodiol by an epoxide hydrolase in liver endoplasmic reticulum; the dihydrodiol in turn is dehydrogenated to a 4-bromocatechol by an enzyme in the soluble fraction of liver. But about 70% of the epoxide formed in rats receiving a non-toxic dose of bromobenzene is converted to a glutathione conjugate by one or more glutathione transferases in the soluble fraction of liver; the conjugate is then hydrolysed to its cysteinyl derivative, which in turn is acetylated to form the mercapturic acid that is excreted into urine[11]. Thus, ratio B depends on the relative rates at which bromobenzene-3,4-epoxide becomes covalently bound to hepatic macromolecules and is converted to 4-bromophenol, 3,4-dihydro-3,4-dihydroxy-bromobenzene and 3,4-dihydro-3-hydroxy-4-glutathionyl-bromobenzene (Figure 21.1).

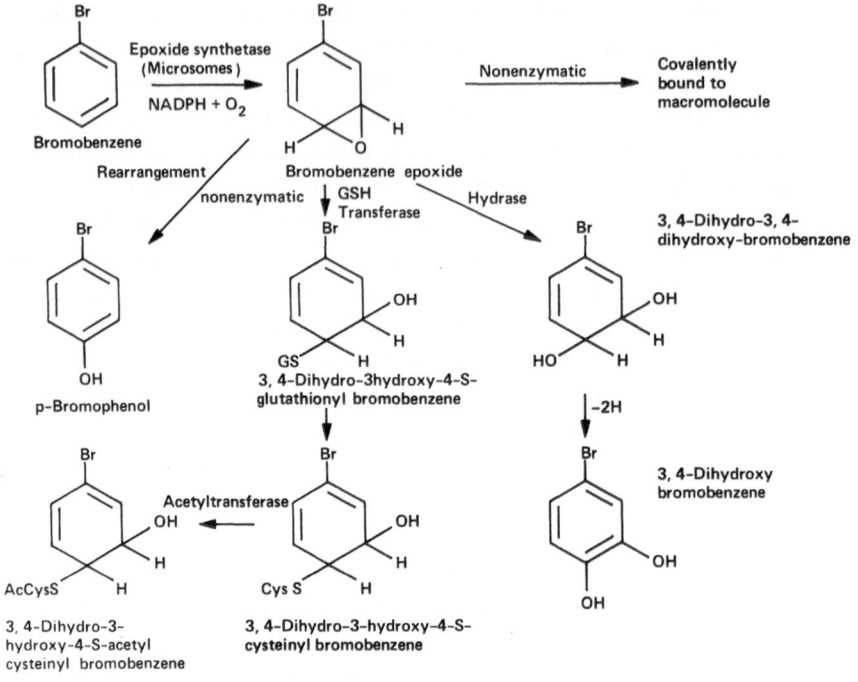

FIGURE 21.1   Pathways of bromobenzene metabolism

If all of the reactions by which bromobenzene is metabolised were first order, the proportion of the dose of bromobenzene that becomes covalently bound should be independent of the dose. However, Reid and Krishna[14] found that the proportion of the dose that became covalently bound to liver proteins in rats remained relatively constant only until a dose of 1.2 mmol/kg of bromobenzene was administered and was markedly increased when doses greater than 1.2 mmol/kg were administered. They also found that centrilobular necrosis in liver did not occur unless doses greater than the threshold dose of 1.2 mmol/kg were given. These findings thus suggested that the metabolic reactions of bromobenzene were first order with the low, non-toxic doses of bromobenzene but that at least one of the reactions was not first order at the higher, toxic doses.

Since ratio A for the covalent binding of bromobenzene in rat liver is nearly 1.0 when non-toxic doses are used, increasing the dose cannot cause a further increase in A. Thus the increase in the proportion of the dose that became covalently bound must be due to an increase in ratio

B. Since the major urinary metabolite of bromobenzene after non-toxic doses is the mercapturic acid, it seemed likely that the increase in ratio B was due to a decrease in the rate of formation of the glutathione conjugate of bromobenzene epoxide. In accord with this view, the proportion of the dose of bromobenzene excreted as the mercapturic acid decreased from about 70% to about 50% as the dose was increased from a non-toxic to a toxic dose[11]. However, the decrease in the rate of formation of the glutathione conjugate was not due to the saturation of the glutathione transferases by bromobenzene-3,4-epoxide. Instead, the decrease was caused by a decrease in the concentration of glutathione in liver[12]. After the administration of a toxic dose of bromobenzene, the glutathione concentration in liver is markedly decreased to about 15% of normal. Moreover, pulse-labelling experiments have shown that the rate of covalent binding of radiolabelled bromobenzene is greater when the glutathione concentrations are low than when they are high. Furthermore, *in vitro* experiments have shown that the rate of covalent binding is decreased by the addition of glutathione[12].

Pretreatment of rats with phenobarbital, which hastens the metabolism of bromobenzene, increases the severity of the centrilobular necrosis and the amount of covalently bound metabolite after the administration of threshold toxic doses of bromobenzene[11-14]. Although these results indicate that the increase in covalent binding of the radiolabelled metabolite is caused by an increase in the rate of formation of bromobenzene-3,4-epoxide, the reason for the increase in covalent binding is rather subtle. Since an increase in the rate of bromobenzene metabolism cannot increase ratio A, it must cause an increase in ratio B, presumably by decreasing the rate of formation of the glutathione conjugate. However, a decrease in the amount of the glutathione conjugate would be expected only when the rate of synthesis of glutathione was appreciable in comparison with the rate of formation of the bromobenzene-3,4-epoxide. Thus, the steady-state concentration of the epoxide depends on the relative rates at which the epoxide is formed and the glutathione is synthesised.

Since the pretreatment of rats with phenobarbital increases the activity of microsomal epoxide hydrolase[15], the ratio of B would be expected to decrease under conditions in which the concentration of glutathione does not limit the rate of formation of the glutathione conjugate. In accord with this view, the pretreatment of rats with phenobarbital decreases the covalent binding of radiolabelled bromobenzene when low, non-toxic doses of bromobenzene are administered, has little affect on the covalent binding when intermediate doses are given and increases the covalent binding when high doses of the toxicant are injected[14].

These studies on the covalent binding and toxicity of bromobenzene have thus illustrated several of the principles enumerated above. Other studies by my colleagues have illustrated how the saturation of the enzyme that catalyses the acetylation of isoniazid limits the liver toxicity caused by isoniazed[16], how saturation of the reversible binding sites on plasma proteins increases the toxicity furosemide[17] and how pretreatment with phenobarbital can increase the toxicity and covalent binding of acetaminophen in mice and decrease them in hamsters[18,19]. Elucidation of these mechanisms would have been considerably more difficult without the concept of the ratios which determine the proportion of the dose of toxicant that becomes covalently bound to proteins and other macromolecules in liver.

Our attempts to elucidate the mechanisms by which chemically reactive metabolites cause cellular necrosis (that is those processes represented by M and P) have been less successful. It is commonly believed that the chemically reactive metabolite of carbon tetrachloride causes centrilobular necrosis by promoting peroxidation of lipids particularly in the endoplasmic reticulum of liver. However, this mechanism of cellular necrosis cannot be the only mechanism by which chemically reactive metabolites cause liver necrosis because lipid peroxidation as measured by increases in diene conjugation does not occur in liver after the administration of toxic doses of bromobenzene, dimethylnitrosamine, acetaminophen or furosemide (Table 21.2). More-

Table 21.2 DIENE CONJUGATION OF HEPATIC MICROSOMAL LIPIDS (Data of H. M. Maling and J. R. Mitchell, unpublished results)

| Toxicant | $A_{240/mmol}PL*$ | | Dose | Hours after toxicant |
	control	toxicant		
CCl$_4$ (rats)	196	342†	2.0 ml/kg	0.5
CBr Cl$_3$ (rats)	187	303†	0.1 ml/kg	0.5
Dimethyl nitrosamine (rats)	207	211	300 mg/kg	2.0
Bromobenzene (rats)	200	195	1.0 ml/kg	2.0
Acetaminophen (mice)	193	196	400 mg/kg	2.0
Furosemide (mice)	194	208	400 mg/kg	2.0

* Absorbance/mmol phospholipid. Mean of 3–9 animals
† Significantly different from control values. P < 0.05

over, carbon tetrachloride in rats pretreated with phenobarbital causes a selective destruction of cytochrome P_{450} in liver endoplasmic reticulum, whereas other substances that cause centrilobular hepatic necrosis, including bromobenzene, do not (Table 21.3). Thus, there are probably several different mechanisms by which chemically reactive metabolites cause hepatic necrosis.

When the covalent binding of the bromobenzene metabolite to liver proteins was measured at various times after the administration of a toxic dose of bromobenzene to mice, the amount of covalent binding increased with time until a maximum was reached at about 12–16 hours, at which time the histopathological changes first began to become apparent in the centrilobular regions of the liver[14]. After that time, however, the amount of covalent binding decreased until only

Table 21.3 EFFECT OF VARIOUS TOXICANTS ON CYTOCHROME P_{450} IN LIVER
(Data of B. Stripp and R. H. Menard, unpublished results

Substance	Time	Cytochrome P_{450}
		%
None	—	100
CCl_4	3	60
Bromobenzene	3	100
Bromobenzene	12	93
Allyl alcohol	3	95
Allyl alcohol	12	64

small amounts of covalently bound bromobenzene remained at 96 hours after the administration of the toxicant. At first it seemed possible that the decrease in the covalent binding might be associated with the loss of protein from necrotic cells but autoradiographic studies indicated that this interpretation was unlikely. At five hours after the administration of toxic doses of radiolabelled bromobenzene, the amount of covalent binding was only slightly greater in the centrilobular regions of liver than in the periportal regions. The amounts of covalently bound bromobenzene gradually increased in both regions of the liver as the radiolabelled bromobenzene was metabolised until a maximum was reached at about 12–16 hours. After that time, however, the covalently bound radiolabelled bromobenzene metabolites decreased preferentially in the periportal regions until almost all of the remaining covalently bound radiolabel was localised in the necrotic centrilobular regions by

24–96 hours[14]. Thus, the decrease in radiolabel appeared to be due mainly to the selective replacement of damaged protein in those cells that were destined to survive.

In accord with this view autoradiograms after the intravenous injection of [14][C]L-leucine at various times after the administration of a toxic dose of unlabelled bromobenzene revealed a striking decrease in the [14][C]L-leucine labelled proteins in the centrilobular regions as early as six hours after the administration of bromobenzene when no cellular damage was apparent[14]. This preferential decrease in the relative rates of protein synthesis in the centrilobular regions probably accounts for the inability of the hepatocytes in these regions to replace the damaged proteins and suggests that impairment of protein systhesis may be a necessary though not sufficient cause of cellular necrosis.

Studies on the synthesis and release of proteins during perfusion of livers from rats treated with bromobenzene have revealed another aspect of the interrelationships between the covalent binding of bromobenzene-3,4-epoxide to liver proteins and protein repair mechanisms in hepatocytes[20]. The incorporation of radiolabelled amino acids into hepatic proteins and serum albumin in living animals depends not only on the rates of their uptake and incorporation into protein by the liver but also on their uptake and incorporation into proteins of other tissues in the body. Thus, the finding that hepatotoxicants decrease the amount of radiolabelled amino acid incorporated into hepatic protein and serum albumin may be due to a decrease in the rate of protein synthesis in the liver provided that the hepatotoxicants do not appreciably affect protein synthesis in other tissues. By contrast, the uptake and incorporation of radiolabelled amino acids into proteins during the perfusion of isolated liver depends solely on their rates of uptake and incorporation into liver protein and serum albumin. Ultimately nearly all of the radiolabel is incorporated into protein regardless of the rate of protein synthesis provided that the radiolabelled amino ācids are not appreciably converted to other metabolic products.

Davis *et al.*[20] found that the uptake of [14][C]L-leucine added to the perfusion medium by liver from untreated rats was initially very rapid and then slowed to negligible rates after about 30–40 min (Figure 21.2). Ultimately about 75–80% of the total radiolabel was taken up by the liver (Table 21.4). During the initial phases, the incorporation of the radiolabelled leucine into protein was also very rapid; approximately 70% of the total amount of [14][C]L-leucine was incorporated during the

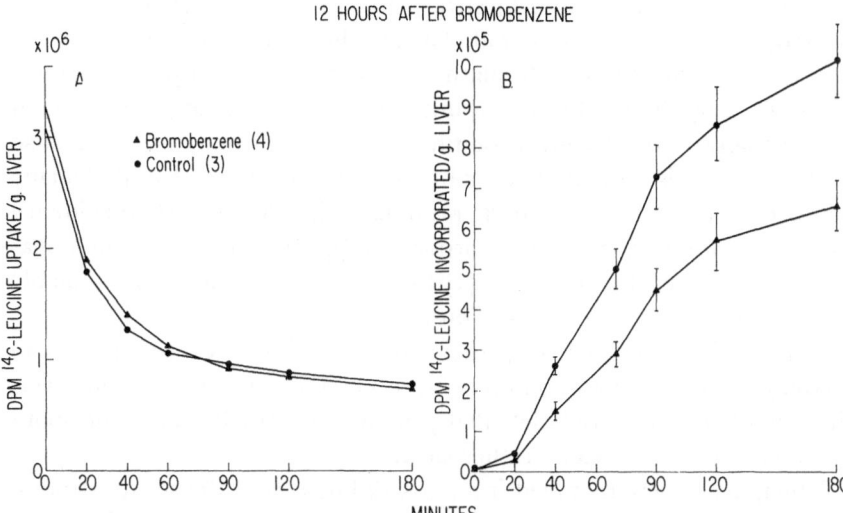

FIGURE 21.2 Effect of bromobenzene treatment on the formation and release of ^{14}[C]L-leucine labelled protein in perfused rat liver

Table 21.4 EFFECT OF BROMOBENZENE TOXICITY ON THE INCORPORATION OF ^{14}[C]L-LEUCINE INTO HEPATIC AND SERUM PROTEINS OF RAT LIVER DURING LIVER PERFUSION (From Davis, *et al.*[20], by courtesy of *Biochem. Pharmacol.*)

	Control (3)	*Bromobenzene** (4)
^{14}[C]L-leucine uptake		
k (10^3/g liver) (min^{-1} g^{-1})	3.89 ± 0.64	4.20 ± 0.33
Total (%)	74 ± 3	77 ± 2
^{14}[C]L-leucine incorporated (3 hours)		
Liver (DPM/g liver × 10^{-5})	12.1 ± 0.8	16.4 ± 1.9†
Serum (DPM/g liver × 10^{-5})	10.2 ± 1.7	6.6 ± 1.2†
(Serum/total) × 100 (3 hours)	45.6 ± 4.0	28.9 ± 6.1†

Time of perfusion (*min*)	$\dfrac{(Serum/total)\ Experimental}{(Serum/total)\ control}$
60	0.68
90	0.63
120	0.66
180	0.63

* Livers were removed from rats 12 hours after the administration of bromobenzene (1.0 ml/kg, i.p.)
† Significantly different from control values. P < 0.05
Numbers in parentheses are the number of animals used

first 30 min of perfusion. Moreover, 30 min after the perfusion was started, only 15% of the total radiolabel in the liver was not incorporated into protein, and the liver to plasma ratio of the unincorporated radiolabel was 1.67. Thus, the incorporation of ^{14}[C]L-leucine into protein had virtually stopped within the first hour of perfusion, either because protein synthesis had stopped or because the remaining ^{14}[C]L-leucine had been converted to metabolic products. Since there was no evidence for the accumulation of unincorporated ^{14}[C]L-leucine within hepatocytes, the rate of uptake of ^{14}[C]L-leucine was used as a reasonable estimate of its rate of incorporation into protein.

Very little radiolabelled protein was released into the perfusion medium during the first 20 min (Figure 21.2). After the delay, however, the rate of release of radiolabelled protein was initially rapid for about one hour and then became rather slow.

When livers were removed from rats 12 hours after the administration of a dose of bromobenzene (1.0 ml/kg) that causes minimal hepatic damage[11,12] and perfused with ^{14}[C]L-leucine, there was little or no change in the rate constant of uptake or total uptake of the radiolabelled amino acid or in the total amount of radiolabelled protein synthesised (Table 21.4). But the release of ^{14}[C]labelled protein into the perfusion medium was decreased (Figure 21.2). Indeed after the livers were perfused for 3 hours, the amount of radiolabelled protein in the medium was about 35% lower with livers from the bromobenzene-treated rats than with those from untreated rats (Table 21.4). However, the decrease in the release of the radiolabelled proteins did not appear to be caused by a decrease in either the rate of synthesis of the radiolabelled protein or to an impairment of its release into the medium, because the percentage decrease in the rate of release did not change with time (Table 21.4). It, therefore, seems likely that the decrease in the release of radiolabelled protein is caused by a change in the relative rates of synthesis of serum and hepatic proteins.

It seems unlikely that the alteration in the pattern of protein synthesis in these minimally damaged livers is due to the formation of new hepatocytes. Indeed, if the time-course for the development of liver necrosis in rats is similar to that in mice, these changes in the pattern of protein synthesis occur before the first signs of liver necrosis appear histologically. The apparent alteration in the pattern of protein synthesis thus raises the possibility that the liver possesses mechanisms by which it can switch from the serum protein synthesis to hepatic protein synthesis and thereby accelerate the replacement of proteins damaged by chemically reactive metabolites. If this is the case, then liver necrosis caused by chemically reactive metabolites may not occur when either the intracellular proteins are damaged or protein synthesis is impaired, but may occur only when the intracellular proteins are damaged and the cells are incapable of replacing them.

REFERENCES

1. Miller, E. C. and Miller, J. A. (1966). Mechanisms of chemical carcinogenesis: Nature of proximate carcinogens and interactions with macromolecules. *Pharmacol. Rev.*, **18**, 805–838
2. Gillette, J. R., Mitchell, J. R. and Brodie, B. B. (1974). Biochemical basis for drug toxicity. *Ann. Rev. Pharmacol.*, **14**, 271–288
3. Mitchell, J. R., Potter, W. Z., Hinson, J. A., Snodgrass, W. R., Timbrell, J. A. and Gillette, J. R. (1975). Toxic drug reactions. In: *Handbuch der experimentellen Pharmacologie XXVIII. Concepts in Biochemical Pharmacology Part 3*, 383–419 (J. R. Gillette and J. R. Mitchell, editors) (Berlin, Heidelberg, New York: Springer-Verlag)
4. Miller, J. A. (1970). Carcinogenesis by chemicals: An overview. G. H. A. Clowes Memorial Lecture. *Cancer Res.*, **30**, 559–576
5. Gillette, J. R. (1973). Factors that affect the covalent binding and toxicity of drugs. In: *Pharmacology and the Future of Man*, Proc. Fifth Intl. Cong. on Pharmacol., San Francisco 1972, **Vol. 2**, 187–202 (T. A. Loomis, editor) (Basel: S. Karger)
6. Gillette, J. R. (1974). A perspective on the role of chemically reactive metabolites of foreign compounds in toxicity. I. Correlation of changes in covalent binding of reactive metabolites with changes in the incidence and severity of toxicity. *Biochem. Pharmacol.*, **23**, 2785–2794
7. Gillette, J. R. (1974). A perspective on the role of chemically reactive metabolites of foreign compounds in toxicity. II. Alterations in the kinetics of covalent binding. *Biochem. Pharmacol.*, **23**, 2927–2938
8. Baumann, E. and Preusse, C. (1879). Über Bromphenylmercaptursäure. *Ber. Dtsch. Chem. Ges.*, **12**, 806–810
9. Azouz, W. M., Parke, D. V. and Williams, R. T. (1953). Studies in detoxification. 51. The determination of catechols in urine and the formation of catechols in rabbits receiving halogenobenzene and other compounds. Dihydroxylation *in vivo*. *Biochem. J.*, **55**, 146–151
10. Knight, R. H. and Young, L. (1958). Biochemical studies of toxic agents. 11. The occurrence of premercapturic acids. *Biochem. J.*, **70**, 111–119
11. Zampaglione, N., Jollow, D. J., Mitchell, J. R., Stripp, B., Hamrick, M. and Gillette, J. R. (1973). Role of detoxifying enzymes in bromobenzene-induced liver necrosis. *J. Pharmacol. Exp. Ther.*, **187**, 218–227
12. Jollow, D. J., Mitchell, J. R., Zampaglione, N. and Gillette, J. R. (1974).

Bromobenzene-induced liver necrosis. Protective role of glutathione and evidence for 3,4-bromobenzene oxide as the hepatotoxic metabolite. *Pharmacology*, **11**, 151–169

13. Brodie, B. B., Reid, W. D., Cho, A. K., Sipes, G., Krishna, G. and Gillette, J. R. (1971). Possible mechanism of liver necrosis caused by aromatic organic compounds. *Proc. Nat. Acad. Sci.* (*Wash.*), **68**, 160–164

14. Reid, W. D. and Krishna, G. (1973). Centrolobular hepatic necrosis related to covalent binding of metabolites of halogenated aromatic compounds. *Exp. Molec. Pathol.*, **18**, 80–99

15. Daly, J. W., Jerina, D. M. and Witkop, B. (1972). Arene oxides and the NIH shift: The metabolism toxicity and carcinogenicity of aromatic compounds. *Experientia* (*Basel*), **28**, 1129–1149

16. Mitchell, J. R. and Jollow, D. J. (1975). Metabolic activation of drugs to toxic substances. *Gastroenterology*, **68**, 390–410

17. Mitchell, J. R., Potter, W. Z., Hinson, J. A. and Jollow, D. J. (1974). Massive hepatic necrosis caused by furosemide, a furan-containing diuretic. *Nature* (*London*), **251**, 508–511

18. Potter, W. Z., Thorgeirsson, S. S., Jollow, D. J. and Mitchell, J. R. (1974). Acetaminophen-induced hepatic necrosis. V. Correlation of hepatic necrosis, covalent binding and glutathione depletion in hamsters. *Pharmacology*, **12**, 129–143

19. Jollow, D. J., Thorgeirsson, S. S., Potter, W. Z., Hashimoto, M. and Mitchell, J. R. (1974). Acetaminophen-induced hepatic necrosis. *Pharmacology*, **12**, 251–271

20. Davis, D. C., Hashimoto, M. and Gillette, J. R. (1973). Effects of bromobenzene and carbon tetrachloride on the synthesis and release of proteins by perfused rat liver. *Biochem. Pharmacol.*, **22**, 1989–2001

Index